CLASSICS FROM JONA

Readings in Nursing Administration

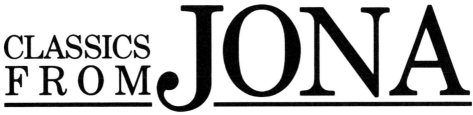

CLASSICS FROM JONA

Readings in Nursing Administration

Edited by

SUZANNE SMITH BLANCETT, R.N., Ed.D.

Editor-in-Chief
Journal of Nursing Administration

J. B. LIPPINCOTT COMPANY   Philadelphia

London   Mexico City   New York   St. Louis   São Paulo   Sydney

Sponsoring Editor: Nancy Mullins
Manuscript Editor: Marjory I. Fraser
Indexer: Norman Duren, Jr.
Design Coordinator: Anita Curry
Production Manager: Kathleen P. Dunn
Production Coordinator: Ken Neimeister
Compositor: Digitype
Printer/Binder: RR Donnelley & Sons Company

1 3 5 6 4 2

Library of Congress Cataloging-in-Publication Data

Classics from JONA.

    Collection of articles previously published in the Journal of nursing
administration.
    Includes index.
    1. Nursing services—Administration. 2. Nursing services—
Economic aspects. I. Blancett, Suzanne Smith. II. Journal of
nursing administration. [DNLM: 1. Nursing—collected
works. 2. Nursing, Supervisory—collected works. WY 5 C614]
RT89.C57   1988   362.1′73′068   87-2684
ISBN 0-397-54665-3

CONTRIBUTORS

Darlene I. Anderson, R.N.
Director of Quality
Assurance Services
United Hospitals
St. Paul, MN

John E. Baird, Jr., Ph.D.
Baird Consulting Group
Gutnee, IL

Joy D. Calkin, R.N., Ph.D.
Associate Professor of Nursing and
Health Services Administration
University of Wisconsin
Madison, WI

Catherine R. Carpenter, R.N., M.S.
Army Nurse Corps
Tripler Army Medical Center
Honolulu, HI

Linda J. Corey, R.N.
Formerly Head Nurse
Veterans Administration
Medical Center
San Diego, CA

Lu Ann W. Darling, Ed.D.
Consultant in Leadership and
Organizational Development
Los Angeles, CA

Ronald L. DeWald, M.D.
Professor, Department of
Orthopedic Surgery
Rush Medical College
Chicago, IL

Erica L. Drazen
Manager, Health Care
Technology Unit
Arthur D. Little, Inc.
Cambridge, MA

Linda Edmunds, R.N., M.S.
Travenol Laboratories, Inc.
Hauppauge, NY

Sandra R. Edwardson, R.N., Ph.D.
Associate Professor
University of Minnesota
School of Nursing
Minneapolis, MN

Ellen H. Elpern, R.N., M.S.N
Assistant Professor
Department of Medical Nursing
Rush University College of Nursing
Chicago, IL

Nancy Ertl, R.N.
Director, Patient Care
Mercy Health Center
St. Joseph's Unit
Dubuque, IA

Jane A. Fanning, R.N., M.S., C.N.A.A.
Vice President
Formerly Patient Care
Bayfront Medical Center, Inc.
St. Petersburg, FL

Barbara Feltman, R.N., M.S.N
Quality Assurance Coordinator
Nursing Department
Foster G. McGaw Hospital
Loyola University Medical Center
Maywood, IL

Frances Fisher, R.N., M.S.
Clinical Director, Surgical Nursing
St. Elizabeth's Hospital
Boston, MA

Dorothy H. Fox, R.N., Ph.D.
Nursing Management Consultant
St. Louis, MO

Richard T. Fox, Ph.D.
Professor, Department of Hospital
and Health Care Administration
Saint Louis University
St. Louis, MO

Cynthia M. Freund, R.N., Ph.D.
Associate Professor
School of Nursing
University of North Carolina
Chapel Hill, NC

George Glusko, B.S.
Vice President of Finance
Polyclinic Medical Center
Harrisburg, PA

Kathryn Hegedus, R.N., D.N.S.
Director of Staff Development
and Research,
Children's Hospital Medical Center
Boston, MA

Nancy J. Higgerson, R.N., M.A.
Vice President for Nursing
Abbot–Northwestern Hospital
Minneapolis, MN

Frances Hoffman, M.A.T., M.H.A.
Administrator, Division of
Developmental Disabilities
University of Iowa Hospitals
and Clinics
Iowa City, IA

Valerie Hunt, R.N., M.S.
Director, Nursing Education
St. Elizabeth's Hospital
Boston, MA

JoAnn Johnson, R.N., D.P.A.
Professor of Nursing
California State University
Los Angeles, CA

Phillippa Ferguson Johnston, R.N., M.S.
Assistant Administrator
Capital Hill Hospital
Washington, DC

Loretta Joy, R.N., M.S.N.
Nursing Quality Assurance/
Special Projects Coordinator
New England Baptist Hospital
Boston, MA

Diane K. Kjervik, R.N., M.S., J.D.
Director, Governmental Affairs
American Association of
Colleges of Nursing
Washington, DC

Elaine Larson, R.N., Ph.D., F.A.A.N
Nutting Chair in Clinical Nursing
The Johns Hopkins University
School of Nursing
Baltimore, MD

Kathy Luciano, R.N., M.S.N., C.N.A.A.
Vice President, Patient Services
Presbyterian Intercommunity
Hospital
Whittier, CA

Loraine G. McGrath, R.N., M.S.
Senior Consultant in Human
Relations and Personal Effectiveness
Management Consultants
San Diego, CA

Joan Quinn McClelland, R.N., B.S.N.
Public Health Nurse
Washtenaw County Health
Department and the Huron Valley
Visiting Nurses Association, MI

Barbara Hazard Munro, R.N., Ph.D.
Associate Professor
Center For Nursing Research
University of Pennsylvania
Philadelphia, PA

Sallie M. Olsen, R.N., Ph.D.
Nursing Consultant and
Senior Associate
McManis Associates
San Francisco, CA

Anita Werner O'Toole, R.N., Ph.D.
Professor of Nursing
Kent State University
Kent, OH

Richard O'Toole, Ph.D.
Professor of Sociology
Kent State University
Kent, OH

Karen Rajki, R.N., M.S.
Nursing Staff Development Instructor
Foster G. McGaw Hospital
Loyola University Medical Center
Maywood, IL

Mary Riley, Ph.D.
President, Morgan Method, Inc.
Sebastopol, CA

Mary F. Rodts, R.N., M.S.
Assistant Professor
Department of Surgical Nursing
Rush University College of Nursing
Chicago, IL

Julie Wine Schaffner, R.N., M.S.N.
Assistant Administrator
Lutheran General Hospital
Park Ridge, IL

Susan G. Sheedy, R.N., M.P.H.
Vice President, Nursing
Baptist Medical Center
Birmingham, AL

Donna Richards Sheridan, R.N., M.S.
Management Development
Coordinator
Stanford University Hospital
Palo Alto, CA

Carol H. Smeltzer, R.N., Ed.D., F.A.A.N.
Senior Associate Hospital Director
University of Arizona
Health Sciences Center
Tucson, AZ

Margaret D. Sovie, R.N., Ph.D., F.A.A.N.
Associate Dean for Nursing Practice
University of Rochester
Rochester, NY

Carol D. Spengler, R.N., Ph.D.
Associate Hospital Administrator
University of Michigan
Medical Center
Ann Arbor, MI

June L. Stark, R.N., B.S.N.
Critical Care Instructor
New England Medical Center
Boston, MA

Ann Van Slyck, R.N., M.S.N.
Formerly Assistant Administrator for
Nursing Services
St. Luke's Hospital Medical Center
Phoenix, AZ

Hollie Vanderzee, R.N., M.S.N.
Private Consultant in
Nursing Administration
Formerly Vice President of Nursing
Glens Falls Hospital
Glens Falls, NY

Katherine W. Vestal, R.N., Ph.D.
Vice President, Nursing
Northwestern Memorial Hospital
Chicago, IL

**Duane D. Walker, R.N., M.S.,
F.A.A.N.**
Vice President, Patient Services
Queen's Medical Center
Honolulu, HI

Mary A. Wallace, R.N., M.S., C.S.
Psychiatric Nursing Supervisor
Veterans Administration
Medical Center
San Diego, CA

Judith J. Warren, R.N., M.S.
Assistant Professor of Nursing
University of Hawaii
Honolulu, HI

Lin Carney Weeks, R.N., M.S.
Director, Nursing Staff Development
Hermann Hospital
Houston, TX

James W. West, M.D.
Assistant Professor
Department of Medicine
Rush Medical College
Chicago, IL

Harold C. White, Ph.D.
Professor, Department
of Management
Arizona State University
Tempe, AZ

Karyl Woldum, R.N., M.S.
Vice Chairman of Nursing
New England Medical Center
Boston, MA

Michael N. Wolfe, Ph.D.
Assistant Professor
Department of Management
Arizona State University, AZ

Rita D. Zielstorff, R.N., M.S.
Assistant Director
Laboratory of Computer Science
Massachusetts General Hospital
Boston, MA

PREFACE

Since its start over 15 years ago, *The Journal of Nursing Administration* (JONA) has published some of the most innovative and creative, as well as classic, literature in nursing administration. With a focus on quality, JONA has consistently delivered useful, relevant, and timely information to top-level, as well as aspiring, nurse executives. JONA is nursing administration's journal—contemporary, visionary, and dynamic.

Like most journals, each article in an issue of JONA addresses a different topic. This increases the probability that all readers of any particular issue will find some content of personal or professional interest. However, this formatting approach does have a drawback—the diversity and development of thought on any particular issue is often lost over time. For example, the JONA article on characteristics of young graduate nurses will not be indexed in the health care literature under a recruitment or retention heading. The content of this article has the potential then of not being seen or used within the broader context of recruitment and retention. The idea of an anthology emerged from the realization of the value that nursing administration practitioners, teachers, and students could gain from having the best of JONA articles categorized according to general theme areas.

The themes in this book—Recruitment and Retention, Managing Others, Quality Assurance, The Cost of Nursing Services, Nurse–Physician Relations, Computers, and Trends and Issues—were chosen to reflect recurring areas of concern in nursing administration service and education, as well as some of the more cutting edge and rapidly changing areas. The classification is not inclusive but rather presents some important components of the whole domain of nursing administration. Likewise, the articles chosen reflect a range of opinions on the theme.

To give readers an overview of each theme area, I invited leaders in nursing administration practice and education to write a state-of-the-art opinion paper on the theme. These leaders were asked to place the diversity of ideas expressed in the articles within the context of the broader theme. Each section introduction has thus become another unique view on the theme.

It is with pleasure that I present the writings of so many creative and innovative leaders in nursing administration.

Suzanne Smith Blancett, R.N., Ed.D.
Editor-in-Chief

CONTENTS

INTRODUCTION

DUANE D. WALKER

This is an exciting time for nursing. It is a time of disorder and discomfort and a time of difficult changes. It offers unusual opportunities for both individual professional development and development of the profession. It demands creativity, courage, and innovation. It is a time for change.

Directly in the middle of the turbulence and undoubtedly the key participant in efforts that will bring about change is the nurse who is in an administrative position. In this era of disquiet, these nurses are the people who must confront the challenges and find creative ways to turn them into gains.

From the top nursing administrator to the assistant nursing manager, these nurses are important people within a health care agency. They set the tone and pace of the nursing department, and they have the potential for strongly influencing the goals of the organization and its movement toward those goals. Moreover, they have both the potential and the responsibility for fostering and contributing greatly to the growth of individuals with whom they work and to the continuing evolution and maturation of the profession.

The fine collection of articles in this anthology accurately reflects nursing's current state of flux and the key role of nurses who are in administrative positions. These selections correctly represent the genuine concerns and interest of nursing leaders in service settings today, and they accurately describe the future directions that nursing may take. In addition, because not all nursing leaders agree on the most useful ways to proceed, the articles highlight some of the unresolved issues and accompanying controversy.

This collection thus presents a clear, comprehensive view of the intricacies of the "real world" of nursing management. Anyone who is interested in or involved in the nursing profession in any capacity would benefit from reading these selections.

The articles are grouped in categories whose titles, in themselves, give a clear overview of the complex realm of nursing as part of the health care industry. In addition, these categories are presented in a thoughtful sequence that begins with the most fundamental, long-standing concerns; builds to the more advanced and more recent concerns; and ends with a view of assorted trends that have widespread implications.

For example, the first topic area deals with recruitment and retention, which are long-time, ongoing, basic matters of concern to all nurses in management positions. Managers have long recognized that excessive turnover among nurses is costly, both in dollars and cents and in quality of care. Moreover, in the absence of highly competent, motivated nurses to provide patient care, the remainder of the topics described in this anthology would become somewhat academic; the development of the profession and its future as a profession depend heavily on the quality and dedication of its practicing membership.

In recent years, nursing administrators have increasingly recognized that an adequate salary and decent working conditions are simply not enough to attract and assure retention of first-class nurses. Many leaders, therefore, began to develop and implement programs designed to recognize the needs and professional characteristics of practicing nurses and to provide career development opportunities within the profession. The works presented here discuss some of these efforts.

The next topic, Managing Others, is closely related to recruitment and retention issues, because the degree of skill and wisdom with which nursing management is practiced has a strong effect on nurses' job satisfaction and desire to remain in the organization and the profession. Of particular interest in this section are Darling's and McGrath's articles concerning the trauma of promotion, together with Ertl's article on the selection of managers. Although most people view promotion to a management position as desirable, it can also be traumatic in that it requires giving up or letting go of things that have been important. According to these authors, a participatory process of selecting managers and specific supportive actions during the transition to the new role will help assure the new manager's success. Other works under this topic relate to the important process of managing others and requirements for successful management.

Quality assurance, which is another increasingly important concern for nursing, is the subject of the next section. Since 1982, when the Joint Commission for Accreditation of Hospitals left the type of quality assurance activity up to the discretion of the institution, the door has been open to new approaches to meeting the requirement for assuring quality in nursing care. Articles in this section contain descriptions of nurses' traditional views of their quality assurance activities, as well as details of some of the newer ways to meet this requirement.

Quality of care and the next topic, cost of care, go hand-in-hand; they have become virtually inseparable in nursing administrators' daily challenges. With the advent of prospective pricing, the pressure is on nursing managers at all levels to contain costs, while — at the same time — maintaining or improving quality. In response, several innovators in nursing are devising methods for billing for nursing care on the basis of a patient's classification. They are focusing on development of facts and figures that will demonstrate the financial and health care value of nursing and show its cost-effectiveness. Articles in this section describe these efforts in relation to cost-containment.

Prospective pricing, the topic of the next group of articles, is also likely to have a significant effect on the relationship between nurses and physicians. In hospitals, particularly, both physicians' and nurses' roles will probably change, with each becoming more interdependent. Although a result may be conflict, a greater degree of sharing and cooperation is equally possible and, as noted in these selections, nursing managers can help to foster such collaboration.

The use of computers, the next topic area, is intimately related to the concepts in all of the preceding articles, because computers are the tools that are essential to facilitate the envisioned changes and to help resolve the concerns. As Carpenter points out, information is a vital resource in any enterprise, and computerization is necessary to organize and communicate information quickly and accurately. The articles presented here propose integrated, agency-wide, computerized systems that will aid nurses in clinical, as well as administrative, decision making, and the authors stress the importance of intimate involvement of nursing managers in planning and implementing such systems.

The final group of articles concerns various trends and issues that have significant implications for nursing management. These range from national economic trends and their impact on the health care industry to issues concerning the unionization of nurses and collective bargaining. Other articles deal with cooperation between health care agencies in the provision of care and in the development of nursing research. And finally, nursing authors stress the need for a taxonomy of nursing diagnoses and for systematic, formal planning for the achievement of administrative nursing goals.

As a nursing administrator, I find this compilation impressive. Without doubt, it dramatizes the infinite complexity of the world of nursing management today, and those who read these selections will surely gain in understanding of this world.

Appreciation is due to the editor for choosing and presenting this collection with obvious care and good judgment. Special gratitude should also be given to the many excellent authors, each of whom has written clearly, thoughtfully, and imaginatively about complicated subjects.

CLASSICS FROM JONA
Readings in Nursing Administration

UNIT ONE

KATHY LUCIANO

Recruitment and Retention

The achievement of nursing department objectives depends on the competence and availability of human resources. Nurse staffing for clinical, educational, research, and administrative programs is the foundation for departmental activities. Nursing administrators should recognize recruitment and retention of nurses as the most essential components of an organizational plan — if objectives are to be accomplished.

The nature of nursing department objectives, organizational hierarchies, clientele served, financial reimbursement, and educational networks are many and varied among health care agencies. The nurses who staff these agencies represent different backgrounds of education, career goals, and life-styles. A challenge of contemporary nursing managers is the integration of departmental (and agency) objectives with the employment expectations of diverse nursing staff. The ability to achieve this integration rests with strategies used for recruitment and retention of the nurses who will effect the objectives.

Recruitment and retention are discussed frequently as a *single* entity. Recruitment of staff, however, is usually a distinct activity to fill vacant positions; in other words, a nurse was not retained and must be replaced. Turnover among staff is inevitable and is sometimes welcomed; but an annual turnover that exceeds 15% to 20% can create havoc for those managers with objectives for quality patient care by stable, competent care givers.

The nursing shortages of the past three decades caused many hospitals to scramble for strong nurse recruitment programs. The competitive, aggressive, and costly advertising often overshadowed the real issue of the need for strong nurse retention practices. Fortunately, within the past few years, nursing administrators have shifted their attention and budgets to programs for increased job satisfaction and subsequent nurse retention.

1

The *retention* of staff is the objective for the 1980s. A large part of this movement is due to the findings and recommendations from hundreds of nurse surveys about job satisfiers and dissatisfiers. Topics and questions for surveys vary among nursing groups and across the country, but some central themes are evident. Nurses at all organizational levels want administrative support, job security, challenging work environments, continuing education, and career mobility.

The most laudable retention programs in hospitals during the past decade are for career development. Nurses, by their own choices and with managerial coaching, can progress through their organizations laterally to other specialties, vertically to promotions, or downward to other positions. The key component of these career programs is recognition of nurses' needs with the concurrent commitment to retain competent staff. The nurse who chooses to remain in a direct care-giving role is given the same attention and support as the nurse who wants to progress up a career ladder to administrative or educational roles.

The effectiveness of career development programs depends primarily on the needs assessment of the nurses. New graduate nurses will demonstrate professional goals that are different from those of the more experienced nurses. Experienced nurses will require individualized programs, too, based on their past work and educational histories. The advanced clinicians, the managers, and the educators will present additional requirements in career planning. In many agencies, high nurse retention is a direct result of what the agencies have done to ensure the retention of individual nurses and the nursing department staff as a whole.

Nurses seeking employment are looking for agencies with programs that are congruent with the nurses' professional values and career goals. The reputation of an institution for advancing its nursing practice and for assuring recognition of the nurses can be the drawing power for both recruitment and retention of staff.

A measure used for nurse (RN) retention effectiveness is the average length of employment. If the average "length of RN stay" in a hospital is 4.0 years, then the nursing administrator has a starting point for establishing a retention standard. This standard needs to be a key component of departmental objectives, especially for quality assurance and fiscal control. A stable staff should provide patient care that is predictable for high quality. A stable staff should reduce recruitment/orientation expenses, and this expense reduction should exceed or match that required for staff development programs of existing employees.

The future of nursing manpower expertise in health care agencies will be a reflection of the administrative direction to promote retention programs while cutting back on recruitment gimmicks.

CHAPTER 1

Young Graduate Nurses: Who Are They and What Do They Want?

by Barbara Hazard Munro

Who are our young registered nurses? What are their attitudes and opinions, and what do they want from their jobs? A randomly drawn national sample was used to answer these questions. This group was dedicated to nursing, wanted to further their education, and desired important, challenging jobs in which they could continue to grow and develop professionally.

Turnover among nurses has been recognized as a very serious problem in relation to the cost of delivery of care and in relation to its quality. The rates of turnover that have been reported vary. The National Commission on Nursing and Nursing Education estimated a yearly resignation rate among hospital staff nurses of 70 percent[1]. The turnover is especially prevalent among the younger nurses—the 25 to 34 age range[2]. Hospital nurses have more than three times the turnover rate of teachers and one and one-half times the turnover rate of social workers[3]. What can hospital administrators do to alleviate this problem? A study by C. Emory Burton and Dorothy T. Burton focused on the factors that influenced job selection among new AD and BSN graduates[4]. They were able to offer suggestions for administrators about attracting and retaining these new graduates. The five schools they studied were in one geographic area.

This study builds on the Burton and Burton study by studying the characteristics and attitudes of nurses who have been in the work force from three to five years. It uses a randomly selected national sample and compares diploma, associate degree (AD), and baccalaureate (BS) graduates. It focuses on the group with the highest turnover rate.

Barbara Hazard Munro, R.N., Ph.D., is Associate Professor and Chairperson, Program in Nursing Research, Yale University School of Nursing, New Haven, Connecticut.

Employee turnover

Employee turnover has been extensively studied and has been found to be largely dependent upon job satisfaction[5–11]. Opportunities for professional growth, advancement, achievement, and recognition have all been shown to be related to satisfaction among nurses[12–18]. Job dissatisfaction has been found to be related to inadequate salaries, poor supervision, inadequate staffing, poor inservice programs, poor administrative support, and lack of opportunities for further education[19–25].

Some studies have found that graduates of diploma, associate degree, and baccalaureate nursing programs differ in the factors that would induce them to change jobs[26,27], whereas other investigators have found few differences among these groups[28–30].

Employee turnover is responsible for the greatest amount of fiscal loss in personnel management[31]. Because nurses outnumber all other health care workers, their turnover rate has a great impact on the cost of health care. Although some of this turnover is due to factors outside the control of hospital administrators, it has been reported that 64 to 75 percent of turnover among nurses is voluntary and therefore could be reduced[32]. It is extremely important for nursing administrators to know what nurses want, what will attract them to a particular job, and what will affect their decision to remain at the job.

Methodology

This ex post facto study uses data collected in the National Longitudinal Study of the High School Class of 1972 (NLS). The NLS was designed to discover what happens to young people after they leave high school and to relate this information to their personal and biographical characteristics and their educational experiences. Over 20,000 high school seniors of the class of 1972 were included in the sample. The sample design for the NLS was a stratified, two-stage probability sample of all schools, public and private, in the 50 states and the District of Columbia that contained twelfth graders during the 1971-72 school year. The design called for over 21,000 seniors in 1200 schools. Follow-up data have been collected so far in four waves over a period of seven years. The response rates ranged from 94 percent for the first follow-up to 89 percent for the fourth follow-up. The fourth follow-up resulted in a sample of 18,630[33]. The study reported here contained all those who had attained the status of registered nurse (RN) by the fourth follow-up, which took place from October 1979 to the spring of 1980. Included were 62 diploma, 180 associate degree, and 137 baccalaureate graduates for a total sample of 379. In general, the AD graduates had been out of school for five years; the Diploma graduates, four; and the BS graduates, three years.

The NLS questionnaires contain over 150 questions arranged in seven sections—General, Education and Training, Work, Family, Military, Activities and Opinions, and Background Information. The base-year and follow-up questionnaires have been similar in form and have been mailed to the respondents. Personal contact was made with those who did not return them.

Data analysis

Description of the sample

Ninety-six percent of the sample were female and 89 percent were white. Blacks comprised 5.5 percent; subjects of Spanish origin, 1.6 percent; Asian-Americans, .4 percent; and the rest were unspecified. Because all subjects were drawn from the same high school class, they were homogeneous in terms of age. Eighty-one percent were 25 years of age (range was 24–28). About half (51 percent) were married to their first spouse; 39 percent were unmarried; 7 percent divorced, widowed, or separated; and 3 percent remarried. Twenty-six percent had children. Of those, 74 percent had one child, 21 percent had two, and 5 percent had three. When asked how many children they planned to have, half the sample said two, another 24 percent said three, and 8.6 percent said none. In October 1979, 73 percent were working full-time, 17 percent part-time, and 10 percent were unemployed.

Women's issues

The subjects were asked to give their opinions on issues related to women. A four point Likert Scale ranging from disagree strongly to agree strongly was used to measure

---

EXHIBIT 1.
WOMEN'S ISSUES

It is usually better if man is achiever outside the home and woman takes of home and family.

	Diploma		AD		BS	
	n	%	n	%	n	%
Agree strongly	2	3	3	2	4	3
Agree	17	29	33	19	24	19
Disagree	30	50	111	66	60	47
Disagree strongly	11	18	22	13	40	31
Totals	60	100	169	100	128	100

$X^2 = 19.83$, 6 df, $p = .0030$

It is more important for a wife to help her husband than to have a career herself.

	Diploma		AD		BS	
	n	%	n	%	n	%
Agree strongly	1	2	7	4	1	1
Agree	17	28	24	14	16	12
Disagree	29	48	114	68	79	63
Disagree strongly	13	22	23	14	30	24
Totals	60	100	168	100	126	100

$X^2 = 17.26$, 6df, $p = .0084$

Most women are happiest when they are making a home and caring for children.

	Diploma		AD		BS	
	n	%	n	%	n	%
Agree strongly	4	7	2	1	2	2
Agree	16	27	26	16	19	15
Disagree	33	56	116	70	90	71
Disagree strongly	6	10	22	13	15	12
Totals	59	100	166	100	126	100

$X^2 = 12.16$, 6 df, $p = .0586$

Men should be given first chance at most jobs because they have the primary responsibility for providing for a family.

	Diploma		AD		BS	
	n	%	n	%	n	%
Agree strongly	2	3	3	2	1	1
Agree	13	22	19	11	10	8
Disagree	26	43	110	66	72	56
Disagree strongly	19	32	36	21	45	35
Totals	60	100	168	100	128	100

$X^2 = 17.383$, 6 df, $p = .0080$

these opinions. The responses of the three groups of subjects, diploma, AD, and BS, to these items were compared to see if their opinions differed. The diploma graduates differed significantly from AD and BS graduates on three of the items and on a fourth; the difference approached significance. Throughout this study, chi-square was used to test for differences among the groups and the .05 level was considered significant. Where significant differences existed, the results are presented for each group. Where the three groups did not differ, the results are given for the entire sample. See Exhibit 1 for the items on which the three educational groups differed.

Although the majority in all groups disagreed with the statement that said it is usually better if the man is the achiever outside the home and the woman takes care of the home and family, fewer diploma graduates (68 percent) disagreed than did AD (79 percent) or BS (78 percent) graduates. Similarly, fewer diploma graduates (70 percent) than ADs (82 percent) or BSs (87 percent) did not agree that it is more important for a wife to help her husband than to have a career herself. More diploma graduates (34 percent) than ADs (17 percent) or BSs (17 percent) agreed that most women are happiest when they are making a home and caring for children. This item approached significance (p = .0586). Also, more diploma graduates (25 percent) than ADs (13 percent) or BSs (9 percent) agreed that men should be given first chance at most jobs because they have the primary responsibility for providing for a family.

Eighty-two percent of all the subjects agreed that a working mother of preschool children can be just as good a mother as the woman who doesn't work. Fifty-four percent agreed that young men should be encouraged to take jobs that are usually filled by women, such as nursing. Eighty-five percent disagreed with the statement that most women are just not interested in having big and important jobs. Seventy-two percent believed that men with the same skills have less trouble getting jobs than women.

Although, in general, the respondents took a liberal view of women's issues, the diploma graduates were somewhat more conservative in their thinking.

Changes they would make

The subjects were asked if they had a chance to do things over again, what changes they would make. Although the majority of all groups said they would *not* take more academic and fewer technical courses, a greater percentage of diploma graduates (18 percent) and ADs (11 percent) said they would take more academic and fewer technical courses than did BSs (1.5 percent) (X^2 = 16.73, 2 df, p = .0002).

Only 18 percent of the entire group said they would not study nursing again, 26 percent said they would attend a different school, and 57 percent said they would get more education. Only 4 percent said they would start work sooner, and just 17 percent said they would choose a different type of work. More than 80 percent of the respondents

are happy with their choice of a career in nursing. Unfortunately, this is not reflected in the turnover rate for nurses.

Further education

Ninety percent of all the nurses said they were interested in further education. However, about half (53 percent) said financial considerations would interfere, and 46 percent felt their present job prospects were good enough. Only 23 percent were not sure what they wanted to study and even less (13 percent) were unsure about what career they wanted to pursue. Twenty-eight percent were tired of school. Only 3 percent said their academic background wasn't good enough, and just 1.4 percent said they didn't think they had the ability to succeed. The rest, an overwhelming 98.6 percent felt they could succeed at further education. Thus, you have a group of nurses who are interested in further education and have confidence in their own ability.

They were also asked what factors were important to them in their decisions about more schooling. They rated these items as follows: the determining factor, important, not important, or wouldn't even consider. There was general agreement among the three groups. They differed only on how important the quality of a particular department was to them. More BS graduates (51 percent) said that it would be a determining factor in their choice of school than did ADs (26 percent) or diploma (28 percent) graduates (X^2 = 23.91, 6 df, p = .0003).

Cost was a determining or important factor to 93 percent of the respondents. Financial aid was important for 51 percent and the determining factor for another 23 percent. The recommendation of an undergraduate professor was considered unimportant by 52 percent and another 13 percent said they wouldn't even consider it. The presence of a particular professor at an institution was either unimportant or not considered by 87 percent of the respondents. On the other hand, the reputation of the institution was important or the determining factor for 97 percent of the subjects. Location was almost equally important, with 96 percent rating it as important or the determining factor. Library facilities were considered important by 78 percent of the group. The group was divided in its assessment of the importance of proximity of the school to the spouse's school or work. Fifty-nine percent rated it as important or determining factor, and 41 percent rated it as unimportant or not considered. Cost, the availability of financial aid, and the institution's location and reputation were of most importance in deciding about furthering their education.

Factors relating to type of work they plan to do

They were asked the importance of various factors in determining the kind of work they plan to be doing. The three groups disagreed on three of these factors. It was less important to ADs and BSs that their work matched their hobby, and a good income was less important to BS graduates. Not one subject said that interesting and important work was unimportant to them, but fewer ADs rated this factor as very important. The great majority of all three groups, however, rated this as very important. See Exhibit 2. Previous work experience was rated as somewhat to very important by 99 percent of the subjects, but having a relative or friend in the same line of work was considered unimportant (80 percent). Having job openings available, job security and permanence, the freedom to make their own decisions, opportunities for promotion and advancement, and working with sociable people were considered somewhat or very important by 96 to 99.7 percent of the respondents.

Reasons for choosing current job

The 329 subjects who were working during the fourth data collection period responded to questions about their current job. When asked to give the reasons for choosing their job, 97 percent said it was what they were trained for, 94 percent said it was what they were looking for, and 83 percent said it was what they wanted to do. Very few indicated difficulties in securing a desired job. Only 3 percent said it was the only job they could find, 3 percent said they didn't have enough training to get what they wanted, and just 1 percent said they couldn't get the job for which they were trained. Two individuals stated that racial discrimination was encountered, and one female claimed discrimination because of sex. About one-third said it was the best paying job they could find. Job security was given as a reason by about half the sample.

Relationship of schooling to job

The respondents were asked how their schooling related to their job. Significantly more BS graduates (35 percent) than diploma (21 percent) or AD (20 percent) graduates said some of their courses weren't helpful ($X^2 = 7.15$, 2 df, $p = .0280$). Significantly less BS (70 percent) than diploma (81 percent) or AD (83 percent) graduates agreed that most of what they did on the job they learned at school ($X^2 = 6.81$, 2 df, $p = .0331$). Ninety-four percent of the sample said they were able to apply most of what they learned at school. Thirty-five percent said they would have liked more job related training. Twenty-five percent found the job was done differently from the way they were trained. An overwhelming number (96 percent) said they did as well as others with similar training.

Finding a job

When trying to attract applicants, it is important to know the way in which they seek opportunities for employment. Sixty-five percent found their jobs by direct application to employers, 23 percent used information from friends, and 13 percent used advertisements. See Exhibit 3 for a complete breakdown of these results.

Job satisfaction

The working RNs were asked to rate their satisfaction with various aspects of their jobs. They rated them on a scale of one to four, with one being very dissatisfied and four being very satisfied. The rank order of the items is given in Exhibit

EXHIBIT 2. FACTORS RELATING TO TYPE OF WORK NURSES PLAN TO DO							
		Diploma		AD		BS	
		n	%	n	%	n	%
Work matches hobby	Very important	11	19	15	9	10	8
	Somewhat important	19	32	35	21	31	24
	Not important	29	49	117	70	88	68
	Totals	59	100	167	100	129	100
	Note: $X^2 = 10.51$, 4 df, $p = .0326$						
Good income	Very important	34	57	94	56	56	43
	Somewhat important	25	42	71	43	64	50
	Not important	1	1	2	1	9	7
	Totals	60	100	167	100	129	100
	Note: $X^2 = 11.50$, 4 df, $p = .0215$						
Work important & interesting	Very important	58	97	145	86	122	95
	Somewhat important	2	3	23	14	7	5
	Totals	60	100	168	100	129	100
	Note: $X^2 = 8.91$, 2 df, $p = .0116$						

EXHIBIT 3.
HOW RESPONDENTS FOUND THEIR JOBS

	Yes		No	
	n	%	n	%
Direct application to employers	215	65	114	35
Friends	77	23	252	77
Newspaper, TV, or radio	44	13	285	87
School placement service	35	11	294	89
Professional periodicals or organizations	26	8	303	92
Relatives	25	8	304	92
Private employment service	4	1	325	99
Public employment service	3	1	326	99
Civil Service application	3	1	326	99

4. They were most satisfied with the pride and respect they received from their families, the opportunities to use past training and education, and the importance and challenge of the job. As a group, they were also satisfied with the progress they had made, job security, opportunities to develop new skills, and the overall job. They were less satisfied with working conditions, pay, opportunities for promotion and advancement, fringe benefits, and their supervisors. Nevertheless, these items were still rated closer to satisfaction (three) than to dissatisfaction (two). The three groups of nurses did not differ in their rating of job satisfaction.

Implications

Almost half (48 percent) of these young graduate nurses graduated from associate degree programs. Thirty-six percent are baccalaureate graduates, and 16 percent are diploma school graduates. Although their educational preparation varies, they do not differ very much in their attitudes and opinions.

They are mostly white, about half are married, and about one-fourth have children. The great majority of all these nurses believe that women should have equal opportunities for a rewarding career and that women are interested in important jobs. They do not agree that the husband's work should take precedence over the wife's. Although the majority of diploma nurses agreed with these views, more of them took the opposing stance than did nurses from the other two groups. These young nurses, then, are a group to whom opportunity and advancement are very important. They will not be satisfied with mediocre jobs.

Only 10 percent are unemployed. They are pleased with their choice of nursing as a career, feel well prepared for the jobs they hold, and have little difficulty in finding a job they want. They tend to apply directly to the institutions in which they seek employment. Because they have little difficulty in finding jobs, they can change jobs if not satisfied. It is thus incumbent upon administrators to find ways to make the job and its benefits attractive to them.

One area that has much attraction for this group is education. Further education is of interest to 90 percent of this sample, and they believe they have the background and intelligence to succeed at it. The opportunity to continue to grow professionally and to do important and challenging work was of paramount importance to them. Administrators are faced with a highly motivated group of individuals. To recruit and retain them, their needs for further education and professional growth must be met. Administrators need to look for ways to assist their nurses to become enrolled in educational institutions. The nurses need financial assistance and the opportunity to alter their schedules or take a leave of absence in order to complete their studies. In addition to degree programs, nurses should be encouraged to attend conferences and workshops, and in-service education programs should be strengthened. These nurses want the opportunity to grow; they do not want to remain at their present level.

These nurses were not well satisfied with their pay, fringe benefits, working conditions, or opportunities for promotion and advancement. They need not only to be supported and encouraged to seek opportunities to develop their skills and abilities but also to be rewarded for doing so. A nurse who has invested time, energy, and money into developing her skills will not be satisfied if her job responsibilities remain static. Salaries need to be made commensurate with the responsibility and educational preparation necessary for the job.

This study tends to support the work of Burton and

EXHIBIT 4.
JOB SATISFACTION

	Mean Rating	Standard Deviation
Pride and respect from my family	3.45	.56
Opportunity to use past training and education	3.43	.60
Importance and challenge	3.33	.66
Progress toward work you'll be doing at age 30	3.27	.67
Security and permanence	3.25	.66
Opportunities for developing new skills	3.19	.69
Job as a whole	3.18	.57
Working conditions	2.98	.68
Pay	2.96	.62
Opportunity for promotion and advancement in this work	2.96	.72
Fringe Benefits	2.90	.66
Supervisors	2.86	.75
Opportunity for promotion and advancement with this employer	2.85	.68

Burton who found that new graduates could be attracted by increasing the tangible and intangible rewards offered by the institutions[34]. For the nurse who has been out working for three to five years, it is also important that pay and benefits be attractive. In addition, these nurses are also looking for responsible, challenging jobs and the opportunity to continue to grow and develop.

References

1. National Commission for the Study of Nursing and Nursing Education, Jerome P. Lysaught, director. *An Abstract for Action* (New York: McGraw-Hill, 1970). p. 35.
2. C. Emory Burton and Dorothy T. Burton. "Job Expectations of Senior Nursing Students." *The Journal of Nursing Administration* 12(3):11–17. 1982.
3. James L. Price and Charles W. Mueller. *Professional Turnover: The Case of Nurses* (New York: S.P. Medical & Scientific Books, 1981).
4. C. Emory Burton and Dorothy T. Burton. "Job Expectations of Senior Nursing Students," p. 11.
5. Diane Cronin-Stubbs, "Job Satisfaction and Dissatisfaction Among New Graduate Staff Nurses," *The Journal of Nursing Administration* 7:(10)44–49. 1977.
6. Frederick Herzberg. "One More Time: How Do You Motivate Employees?" *Harvard Business Review* 46(1):53–62. 1968.
7. William H. Mobley et al. "Review and Conceptual Analysis of the Employee Turnover Process." *Psychological Bulletin* 86(3):493–522. 1979.
8. Lyman W. Porter and Richard M. Steers, "Organizational Work and Personal Factors in Employee Turnover and Absenteeism," *Psychological Bulletin* 80(2):151–176. 1973.
9. James L. Price and Charles W. Mueller. *Professional Turnover: The Case of Nurses*, p. 56.
10. Carol S. Weisman, Cheryl S. Alexander, and Gary A. Chase. "Evaluating Reasons for Nursing Turnover," *Evaluation and The Health Professions* 4(2):107–127, 1981.
11. David A. Whitsett and Erik K. Winslow. "An Analysis of Studies Critical of the Motivation-Hygiene Theory," *Personnel Psychology* 20(4):391–415. 1967.
12. Diane Cronin-Stubbs. "Job Satisfaction and Dissatisfaction," p. 47.
13. Marjorie A. Godfrey, "Job Satisfaction— or Should That Be Dissatisfaction? How Nurses Feel About Nursing," Part 3. *Nursing '78* 8(6):81–95. 1978.
14. Frederick Herzberg. *Work and the Nature of Man* (Cleveland: World. 1966).
15. Marlene Kramer. "Collegiate Graduate Nurses in Medical Center Hospitals: Mutual Challenge or Duel." *Nursing Research* 18(3):196–210. 1969.
16. Joanne McCloskey. "Influence of Rewards and Incentives on Staff Nurse Turnover Rate." *Nursing Research* 23(3):239–247. 1974.
17. Barbara H. Munro. "Job Satisfaction Among Recent Graduates of Schools of Nursing." *Nursing Research,* in press.
18. Catherine Harmon White and Maureen Claire Maguire. "Job Satisfaction and Dissatisfaction Among Hospital Nursing Supervisors: The Application of Herzberg's Theory." *Nursing Research* 22(1):25–28. 1973.
19. Douglas A. Benton and Harold C. White. "Satisfaction of Job Factors for Registered Nurses, *The Journal of Nursing Administration* 2(6):55–63. 1972.
20. Diane Cronin-Stubbs. "Job Satisfaction and Dissatisfaction, Graduate Staff Nurses." p. 47.
21. Frederick Herzberg. *Work and the Nature of Man.* p. 115.
22. Barbara H. Munro. "Job Satisfaction Among Recent Graduates of Schools of Nursing." p. 24.
23. Mabel A. Wandelt, Patricia M. Pierce, and Robert R. Widdowson, "Why Nurses Leave Nursing and What Can Be Done About It." *American Journal of Nursing* 81(1):72–77. 1981.
24. Catherine Harmon White and Maureen Claire Maguire. "Job Satisfaction and Dissatisfaction Among Hospital Nursing Supervisors." pp. 27–28.
25. Janet P. McMahon. "Factors Associated with Registered Nurse Employment in Connecticut." unpublished master's thesis, Yale University School of Nursing. 1982.
26. Patricia M. Schwirian et al. *Prediction of Successful Nursing Performance,* Part 3 and Part 4. (HRA 79–15, U.S. Dept. HEW Publications, 1979). pp. 1–138.
27. Charlotte Theis and Helen Harrington, "Three Factors that Affect Practice: Communications, Assignments, Attitudes." *American Journal of Nursing* 68(7):1478–1482, 1968.
28. C. Emory Burton and Dorothy T. Burton. "Job Expectations of Senior Nursing Students." p. 11.
29. Barbara H. Munro. "Job Satisfaction Among Recent Graduates of Schools of Nursing, p. 20.
30. Carol S. Weisman et al., "Employment Patterns Among Newly Hired Hospital Staff Nurses: Comparison of Nursing Graduates and Experienced Nurses." *Nursing Research* 30(3):188–191, 1981.
31. M.E. Reres, "Personnel Management." *The Journal of Nursing Administration* 6(8):55, 1976.
32. John W. Seybolt, Cynthia Pavett, and Duane D. Walker, "Turnover Among Nurses: It Can Be Managed." *The Journal of Nursing Administration* 8(9):4–9, 1978.
33. John Riccobono et al. *National Longitudinal Study: Base Year (1972) Through Fourth Follow-Up (1979), Data File Users Manual,* vol. 1. Prepared for National Center for Education Statistics (Research Triangle Park, N.C.: Research Triangle Institute, 1981).
34. C. Emory Burton and Dorothy T. Burton. "Job Expectations of Senior Nursing Students," p. 17.

CHAPTER 2

PACE: A Unique Career Development Program

by Lin Carney Weeks and Katherine W. Vestal

Career development programs are increasingly recognized as the answer to retaining nurses in nursing, and more important, at the bedside. In the face of economic constraints facing health care, it is imperative that such programs benefit both the nurse and the hospital so that the ultimate goal of improved patient care delivery can be met in a cost-effective and creative way. PACE, Practice Alternatives for Career Expansion, a successful career development program designed to achieve these results, is described in this article. It has some unique features which benefit both the nurse and the hospital.

The task

Designing a career pathway or a career development program is not as simple a task as it may at first seem. Although a successful career pathway program can contribute enormously to job retention and job satisfaction, a poorly designed or poorly executed program can become a major source of dissatisfaction among the staff, with widely echoing reverberations for nursing administration.

Equally important as a criterion for success is whether the program will stand the test of time and can be developed further as it matures. Realistically a career development model should be flexible enough to respond to organizational demands without compromising the basic philosophy of the program.

Lin Carney Weeks, R.N., M.S., is Director of Medical Nursing, Hermann Hospital, Houston, Texas.

Katherine W. Vestal, R.N., Ph.D., is Associate Executive Director, Hermann Hospital, Houston, Texas.

A retrospective view

Career pathways and development programs are no longer news in nursing. Many settings have implemented such programs during the past decade. Unfortunately, not all of the programs were well thought out prior to implementation, and resulted in significant organizational confusion in the institutions where they were tried. Experience has shown that the cost of a career pathway failure can be infinitely higher than that of no program at all. An unsuccessful or problem-ridden program can raise serious doubts about the leadership capabilities of nursing administration. Program failure can generate negative perceptions among the nursing, administrative, and medical staffs about nursing's ability to plan and manage a large labor force effectively. The resulting loss of credibility and confidence in nursing management can be detrimental to the hospital at large as well as to the nursing administrative team. Thus it behooves us all as nursing administrators to share our successes and failures so that we might benefit and move toward an ideal program.

As early as 1972 Zimmer explored the concept of clinical advancement[1,2]. Since that time many large metropolitan hospitals such as University of California in San Francisco, Rush Presbyterian Memorial and University of Virginia have also reported career ladder models[3,4,5,6,7,8]. Each hospital had its own approach to building such a program. Often smaller hospitals found the models from larger hospitals impossible to implement within their resources and proceeded to design a type of advancement system that would meet their own needs better. In the development of the PACE program, described in this article, we were fortunate to be able to benefit from these earlier programs, adopting the best aspects of many of them in formulating our own.

The traditional purist clinical and administrative advancement program, which often causes overlap and blurring of roles and responsibilities between nurse managers, clinicians, and educators was adapted to fit a strong decentralized nursing division in the design of Practice Alternatives for Career Expansion (PACE). The format of the program was intended to encourage flexibility while maintaining organizational consistency and practicality.

The PACE experience

In 1980 Hermann Hospital in Houston, Texas, implemented the PACE program. As a large teaching hospital, Hermann wanted to provide formal recognition of nurses, both professional and technical, through a graduated promotion and compensation plan.

Within a decentralized nursing organization that utilized a primary nursing delivery system, the PACE program was designed to combine the four basic nursing components, clinical, administration, research, and education, with a six level progression system. Registered nurses can progress through six levels or they may elect to remain at any level of responsibility indefinitely. The number of positions at each level is determined by organizational needs and financial resources.

All professional nurses are responsible for clinical patient care in levels I–III. Although all nurses are placed at level I until they have completed one year's experience in nursing, Levels II and above are earned only through promotion, not automatically. Nurses share in the responsibility for progression by making application for promotion and being formally approved by their head nurse and director. Level III has proved to be a particular asset to the hospital, because the nurse at that level has an increased degree of freedom to pursue special interests. The level III position is designed together by nurse and manager and must include a contribution to the organization beyond the normally expected patient-care activities. These contributions have included such activities as serving as unit preceptor, leading a family group, participating in the nursing practice committees, and designing a special project on a specific unit.

The enormous amount of creativity shown by the level III nurses has led to a greatly increased standard of practice in the hospital. Many of the "extras" that were heretofore not done, have been enthusiastically assumed by this group of nurses. Not only has the hospital benefited, but the nurses themselves have found the opportunity to diversify their role and include some activities related to their own interests.

At levels above III, positions are differentiated by an increased percentage of job time spent in the major track. For example, level VI nurses in the educational track are masters prepared nurses who spend the majority of their time teaching, but are also expected to actively participate in clinical, administrative and research activities. The mas-

ters prepared clinical specialist functions primarily as a level VI clinician, but also shares in activities related to education, research and administration. Thus, it can be seen that the combined track system does allow the differentiation needed to build in a recognition and reward system while maintaining the practicalities demanded by organizational contraints.

Moving laterally from track to track is quite easy, and a basic premise of the program is that no nurse is a *purist*. No matter what track they are in, all nurses have some functions that span the other tracks, the difference between tracks being the percentage of time spent on each function. Hence, clinicians may practice, teach, manage, and participate in research, although perhaps 75 percent of their time is spent in clinical practice. Instructors may spend 75 percent of their time in education. This expectation is reflected in the performance evaluations which clearly define expectations related to each area (See Exhibit 1).

An introspective look

Because the PACE program was developed by groups comprising managers, educators, clinicians, and staff nurses, it is characterized by some unique features. These have proven to be the most successful aspects of the program and are worth sharing with others.

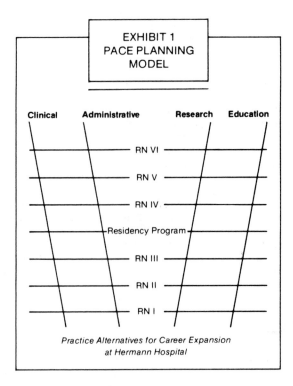

EXHIBIT 1
PACE PLANNING
MODEL

Clinical   Administrative   Research   Education

RN VI

RN V

RN IV

Residency Program

RN III

RN II

RN I

*Practice Alternatives for Career Expansion
at Hermann Hospital*

Contribution to the organization

The PACE program is unique in that it combines a fairly traditional four-track model with a new concept: contribution to the organization. The basic expectation is that nurses will successfully participate in patient-related services. In addition, the higher the nurse advances up a track, the greater the obligation to contribute to the nursing organization. This contribution can take many forms. Based on the interests of the individual nurse and the needs of the organization, particular and meaningful activities can be designed. Examples include serving on nursing practice committees, participating in the quality-assurance program, leading family support groups, and designing unit orientation booklets. The creative instincts of the nurse are thus fostered—to the ultimate benefit of nurse, hospital, and patient.

The residency program

One of the most valuable aspects of PACE is its residency program. A residency is composed of a quarter time commitment for a three-month period, in which the nurse pursues increased preparation in the track of her choice. Any level III registered nurse may apply for a residency, but it is mandatory for promotion to level IV. The residency is planned through the staff development department and includes both didactic instruction in regular, scheduled classes and self-designed learning activities. The nurses may acquire different skills depending on the track selected.

A nurse is selected for a residency program after making application. To make application the nurse must prepare a statement of both short and long-term goals for the residency and must obtain the approval of the head nurse and director. Although participation is voluntary, the nurse who begins a residency is expected to complete it.

Besides the additional knowledge and skills gained during residency, another asset has been the exposure of the nurses to different areas of the hospital and to staff from different clinical specialties. The nurses frequently report they learned things about the hospital and its operation that they never knew existed. This has great value for the hospital as well as for nursing, becuase the nurse with a broader view of the organization will likely make better decisions for the good of the hospital.

The nurses in the residency program have also been enthusiastic about having the opportunity to exchange ideas and concerns with nurses from other areas of the hospital. Many innovative programs have resulted from residents' interests and activities.

The residency program requires the completion of a project by the nurse. This project is designed by the resident and her instructor and must benefit both the resident and the hospital. Projects such as family brochures, orientation guides, cost-saving programs, and specific clinical activities have resulted.

The popularity of the residency program attests to its benefits. Nurses may take more than one residency in different tracks, when the time and space permit. This flexibility is particularly valuable when nurses are contemplating changing career directions and may want to explore other opportunities. The shared responsibility of the residency between the nurses and the hospital results in enormous benefits to both.

Pace consultation team

In an effort to provide an ongoing educational program for PACE that would address the specific issues of the staff, a PACE consultation group was formed. This team responds to an invitation by a unit for a consultation. The team is composed of five nurses including a director, a head nurse, and three staff nurses. Prior to the unit meeting, a questionnaire is distributed to the staff to assess knowledge of the PACE program from the staff. The questionnaire covers criteria for promotion, influence of transfers upon levels, and other common questions related to PACE. The PACE team then goes to a unit meeting and discusses issues about PACE and answers questions about the program.

The staff nurses on the team have proven invaluable as they can respond to issues and questions from the same perspective as the nurses on the unit. They give suggestions for promotion, clarify misconceptions, and foster enthusiasm for the program. PACE consultation visits have been a consistently positive experience for both the team and unit staff.

PACE performance appraisal

In order to maintain the proper perspective between the tracks and levels, the inception of PACE required new job descriptions and performance appraisal systems. The PACE committee developed a series of job descriptions that defined the expected behaviors for each track at each level. The nurse is given a copy of the job description appropriate for his or her position, and this also serves as the evaluation tool. There are no surprises, and expectations are clear.

Prior to the evaluation meeting with the head nurse, a self-evaluation is also completed by the nurse. They negotiate merit performance percentages and together they prepare a written developmental plan for the nurse in each of the four track areas. This developmental plan clearly outlines the goals for the coming year and can be utilized later to measure progress. Although self-evaluations require considerable guidance the first time, the benefits of performance appraisal have made the commitment of time worthwhile. The outcome, in addition to pervasive behavior change, has been increased accountability, since the nurses are held accountable for developing their own careers in concert with the organization.

While the features just described are not the only unique features of PACE, they are clearly the most successful. Implementation has not been problem-free, and it is anticipated that the development of this program will continue for several years. At the present time PACE work groups representing all levels of nurses are striving to refine and expand the program in several areas.

Evaluation

All too often when career ladder programs are implemented, no provision is made for evaluation. This results in changes being made in the program intuitively that may have little or no effect on the needs of the nurses. As PACE was implemented, a group of head nurses, directors, and staff nurses was formed to be the PACE evaluation committee. Its task was to design and conduct a research study at the end of the first year of the program that would provide empirical data on the feedback from the staff nurses. This study was designed as a four-part questionnaire that surveyed data demographics, opinions on PACE itself, job satisfaction, perceptions of leadership, and self-image. The questionnaires were distributed to all nursing staff and collected in confidential envelopes by the PACE evaluation committee members.

The return was approximately 33 percent which was lower than anticipated but proved demographically to be representative of the total group. It is surmised that the length of the questionnaire may have been a factor in the low return and that the nurses' fear of reprisal prevented many from participating. The study is now being analyzed by an independent researcher to eliminate any bias that might have been interjected by the PACE evaluation committee.

Preliminary data clearly show a problem that has been apparent since the inception of PACE. Some of the staff continue to have misconceptions about the program, remain somewhat unclear about all of its options, and worry about the "fairness" of grading nurses according to level. Despite monumental efforts to educate the staff about PACE, ongoing education about the program remains a priority.

Evaluation of any career ladder program is essential. Empirical data about such programs can benefit all of nursing, and it is important to share results. As a consequence of the findings on the residency program, a similar program will be started for licensed vocational nurses.

Conclusion

It is clear that career ladders are not the panacea for all problems in nursing. However, they are the tangible results of efforts to improve the contemporary environment for nursing in hospitals. Career ladders are the first step in acknowledging that creative solutions to long-expressed problems can be found. Many hospitals have created innovative programs for nursing recognition. PACE is one hospital's attempt to mesh the recognition needs of the nurses with the productivity needs of the hospital. It has accomplished some of the intended results and will be strengthened to meet even more. PACE is a building-block program for progress in nursing.

References

1. Marie Zimmer. "Rationale for a Ladder for Clinical Advancement," *The Journal of Nursing Administration,* 6(2):10, February, 1972.
2. Margaret Ives Anderson and Mary Jean Deynes, "A Ladder for Clinical Advancement in Nursing Practice," *The Journal of Nursing Administration,* 2(5):16, May, 1975.
3. Ruth A. Calavecchio, "Clinical Ladder for Nursing Practices," *The Journal of Nursing Administration,* 5(4):17, April, 1974.
4. Harold A. MacKinnon and Lillian Eriksen, "C.A.R.E.-A Four Track Professional Nurse Classification and Performance Evaluation System," *The Journal of Nursing Administration,* 4(7):45, July, 1977.
5. Florence L. Huey, "Looking at Ladders," American Journal of Nursing, 82(10):1521, October, 1982.
6. Julie A. Wine and Sara J. Mapstone, "Clinical Advancement," *Nursing Administration Quarterly,* 6(1):65, Fall, 1981.
7. Patricia Casey, "Up the Ladder: Development of a Clinical Series Job Description," *Nursing Administration Quarterly,* 6(4):28, Summer, 1982
8. Mary K. Kleinknecht and Elizabeth A. Heffering, "Assisting Nurses Toward Professional Growth: A Career Development Model," The Journal of Nursing Administration, 12(7 & 8):30, July August, 1982.

CHAPTER 3

Fostering Professional Nursing Careers in Hospitals: The Role of Staff Development, Part 1

by Margaret D. Sovie

In addressing issues of job satisfaction and nursing reten-tion, staff development programs and activities hold the potential for significant positive influence. This two-part article will explore responsibilities and structures for execu-ting expanded staff development functions that facilitate professional careers in hospital nursing. In Part 1, the author outlines a career employment model for hospital nurses and addresses the issues and challenges in the orien-tation and inservice education component of the model. Next month in Part 2, the author will address the redistribu-tion of staff development resources in attending to the second and third components of her model. The discussion provides a forward view of staff development that will foster retention of professionally oriented nurses and delivery of quality care at controlled costs.

Professional nurses comprise the largest group of patient care providers in the country and one of the most valuable resources of the hospital health care industry. Yet hospital nurses do not perceive themselves as *valued* health profes-sionals. Professional recognition, career mobility, and advancement opportunities were consistently identified as needs in 35 of 41 nursing manpower studies conducted across the United States. Nurses in state after state have articulated their desire for career opportunities in hospital nursing practice—opportunities that will help them achieve professional and personal satisfaction and recognition, pro-fessional growth, advancement, and increasing economic rewards based on their contributions to health care services.

Margaret D. Sovie, Ph.D., R.N., F.A.A.N., is associate dean for nursing practice and associate professor of nursing, University of Rochester, Rochester, New York.

This two-part article is based on a presentation at the Staff Education Conference for Hospital-Based Nurse Educators, sponsored by the Con-sortium of Staff Education of Beth Israel Hospital, Brigham & Women's Hospital, Children's Medical Center Hospital, Massachusetts General Hospital, and New England Deaconess Hospital, January 18–19, 1982, Boston, Massachusetts.

Several studies have shown that hospital nursing practice faces a major challenge if it is to meet the needs professional nurses have identified and address the hospital nursing shortage problem[1,2,3]. Staff development can play a major role in this effort. We must seize the opportunity to create and demonstrate an expanded role for staff develop-ment—enabling and facilitating professional careers in hospital nursing. This article describes the responsibilities such a role entails and the structures that may be required to execute the functions of the expanded role.

Defining a satisfying career

Exhibit 1 is a model of a professional career pattern in hospital nursing that can be dynamic, challenging, and rewarding. This embryonic schema includes three major components: professional identification, professional mat-uration, and professional mastery. The entire professional nursing staff participates in the professional identification component, commonly called orientation and inservice education. This has traditionally received most of the staff development department's resources, time, and effort. Because they must assure the clinical competency of staff and the achievement of nursing practice standards, orienta-tion and inservice education are indeed a critical staff devel-opment responsibility, warranting a substantial allotment of available resources. If nursing administrators are to be successful in promoting professional careers in hospital nursing, however, we must also shift significant resources to the professional maturation component. Resource invest-ment for career advancement may provide the highest return to health care institutions in cost-benefit terms. Qual-ified, career-oriented nurses who can achieve personal and professional objectives in the hospital setting will want to stay in that setting. Experienced nurses, enriched by contin-uing clinical practice and education experiences, will be available to deliver quality care at controlled costs. An ever-enlarging body of nursing expertise will be available to address and solve problems of patient care, and nursing practice as well as institutional issues. If the hospital nursing career model proposed here is pursued, eventually staff development and nursing recruitment resources will be distributed naturally in a different fashion, with increasing resource allocations shifting from recruitment, orientation, and inservice education to the second and third components of the model. Initially, however, there must be a conscious, deliberate redistribution of efforts, with potential risks.

Creating the future

Hospitals able to design and implement a successful nursing practice career plan will be the magnet hospitals of the future. They will become known as institutions where professional nurses are recognized and valued for their contributions to patient care, where professional nursing is practiced, and finally, where nurses advance in career patterns that are personally and professionally satisfying. Such magnet hospitals will have no trouble recruiting and retaining qualified nurses and will be able to assure the delivery of

high-quality patient care at controlled cost.

Each component in the hospital nursing career model includes major responsibilities for staff development educators. Each component also includes significant unresolved issues demanding new approaches and creative design and development.

A systematic approach to professional career development in hospital nursing is absolutely essential. Staff development educators must work in concert with other nursing leaders. Formative and summative evaluation should be integrated into the basic program formulation.

Experiences in designing, implementating, and evaluating programs should be published in the professional journals for sharing and criticism. A search of the nursing literature on staff development and continuing education in nursing today reveals few research results. But through individual and collective efforts in designing, studying, evaluating, and reporting programmatic approaches in staff career development, the nursing profession may be able to invent a different future for itself.

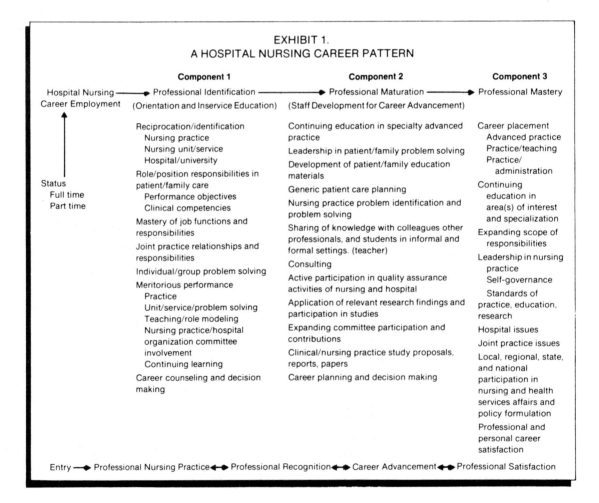

EXHIBIT 1.
A HOSPITAL NURSING CAREER PATTERN

	Component 1	Component 2	Component 3
Hospital Nursing → Professional Identification →	Professional Maturation →	Professional Mastery
Career Employment (Orientation and Inservice Education)	(Staff Development for Career Advancement)	

Component 1	Component 2	Component 3

Reciprocation/identification
  Nursing practice
  Nursing unit/service
  Hospital/university
Role/position responsibilities in patient/family care
  Performance objectives
  Clinical competencies
Mastery of job functions and responsibilities
Joint practice relationships and responsibilities
Individual/group problem solving
Meritorious performance
  Practice
  Unit/service/problem solving
  Teaching/role modeling
  Nursing practice/hospital organization committee involvement
  Continuing learning
Career counseling and decision making
	Continuing education in specialty advanced practice
	Leadership in patient/family problem solving
	Development of patient/family education materials
	Generic patient care planning
	Nursing practice problem identification and problem solving
	Sharing of knowledge with colleagues other professionals, and students in informal and formal settings. (teacher)
	Consulting
	Active participation in quality assurance activities of nursing and hospital
	Application of relevant research findings and participation in studies
	Expanding committee participation and contributions
	Clinical/nursing practice study proposals, reports, papers
	Career planning and decision making
		Career placement
		  Advanced practice
		  Practice/teaching
		  Practice/administration
		Continuing education in area(s) of interest and specialization
		Expanding scope of responsibilities
		Leadership in nursing practice
		  Self-governance
		  Standards of practice, education, research
		  Hospital issues
		  Joint practice issues
		  Local, regional, state, and national participation in nursing and health services affairs and policy formulation
		Professional and personal career satisfaction

Status
  Full time
  Part time

Entry → Professional Nursing Practice ←→ Professional Recognition ←→ Career Advancement ←→ Professional Satisfaction

The nurse's needs

The central character in the career development schema is of course the practicing professional nurse employed by the hospital. This nurse may be employed full-time, part-time, or per diem. Each employment category presents unique needs that must be addressed. In this article, I will consider together the needs of full-time and part-time nurses. Although I will not address the needs of the per diem nurse, one critical point must be made: Both per-diem nursing and part-time nursing are often necessary phases in the career patterns of professional nurses. If nurses continue to be appreciated, assisted, and supported during these career phases, they will be able to and will want to move to regular full-time staff positions as their life situations and career goals change. Hospital nursing leaders with staff educators' support and assistance, must recognize and plan for various career patterns for their predominantly female professional nursing staff.

Creating the environment

A good relationship between the person and the organization is important for fostering hospital nursing careers as well as effectively meeting institutional objectives. Levinson named this process *reciprocation,* the fulfillment of mutual expectations and satisfaction of mutual needs in the relationship between an employee and the work organization. He defines it as follows. "Reciprocation is the process of carrying out a psychological contract between a person and . . . the institution where one works. It is a complementary process in which the individual and the organization seem to become a part of each other" [4].

Another process important in fostering professional careers in hospital nursing is identification. Levinson described it as the process of learning how to behave and what to become. He points out that "identification is not simple imitation but the adoption of spontaneously selected aspects of the model which fit the person who is identifying and which will further his maturation" [5]. Levinson considers the process of identification important to the individual employee's need fulfillment and learning in the organization.

Professional nurses experience reciprocation and identification in several ways—in their experiences in the total nursing practice organization, more frequently in interactions and experiences in their particular nursing unit or service organization, and finally, in their cumulative experiences in the entire hospital or university organization. In these continuous and varying contacts and experiences, professional nurses should feel a climate, sense an ambience, that communicates how valuable they are for quality patient care and for achieving institutional goals and objectives. At the same time, they should be able to learn how the organization can help them achieve their personal and professional objectives through rewarding careers in hospital nursing.

Staff development educators share with nursing and hospital leaders the responsibility to create and maintain an organizational climate and environment that encourages and supports reciprocation and professional identification for nursing career development. No single group carries the responsibility for organizational change and dynamic renewal—prerequisites for institutional survival. However, staff development educators should play a significant role and can be influential in effecting organizational improvements and advancements.

"A systematic approach to professional career development in hospital nursing is absolutely essential."

In some hospitals, the first order of business is educating the multiple constituencies regarding nursing's present role, scope of practice in patient care, and responsibilities in unit and hospital management. Determining how this education is to be accomplished, in what sequence, and over what period of time requires strategic planning with nursing, medical, and hospital administrators. In some situations staff development educators may serve as coaches or as technical consultants to other nursing personnel who are preparing presentations for major hospital departmental or committee meetings. Or, staff development educators may make the presentations on behalf of the nursing organization with other nursing personnel serving as *their* consultants. In numerous organizational situations nursing staff can use the opportunity to inform and educate different hospital constituencies about the professional nursing role and the organizational conditions required to support nursing staff in developing a hospital career perspective. The method chosen and its success or failure depend on judicious selection of opportunity, careful preparation, and sophisticated diplomacy. To successfully influence organizational change, the nursing organization must emphasize continuous leadership development and management training for nurses through staff development programs.

Preparing leaders and managers

Conscious, deliberate allocation of increased resources to leadership and management development is critically important to the future of hospital nursing. The desired outcomes for all nursing staff members as sketched in the first component of the career model cannot be achieved effectively without well-prepared leaders and managers to guide, support, direct, lead, and encourage nurses in their career development. Effective, competent leadership staff must occupy first-line, middle, and top management positions. Because continuing self-development is usually an integral component of self-directed executive behavior, top managers probably do not require a large amount of the staff development educator's attention. However, management training and staff development programs for first-line and middle managers should be constant and ongoing. How many leadership appointees have had formal training in administration, management or teaching? Unfortunately, most are not prepared for the positions to which they are promoted. These positions usually include a whole new set of performance expectations and requirements beyond the appointees' present competencies. To compound the situation further, the vacant positions to which new leadership individuals are appointed usually are located on busy patient care units where expert leadership and direction are required to meet staff and patient needs. The common result, is that individuals are given management jobs with some harried orientation and direction, and then expected to perform to standards they are not prepared to meet.

Orientation and inservice education for leadership staff require the same attention and planned approach as do other staff education activities. Staff development educators are responsible for designing programs to meet the needs of nursing managers as they enter new positions and for assuring, through program planning and evaluation, that those already in such positions have continuing opportunities to master their job functions. Periodic educational programs designed for continuing growth and development must also be offered.

Many issues and problems must be resolved to integrate regular leadership development and management training programs into the calendar of staff development activities. Included are the usual questions of needs assessment, objectives formulation, curriculum planning, teaching methodologies, faculty resources, and time scheduling. But most essential is top management's enthusiastic backing. Without that support, leadership development and management training can easily lose priority status; the organization will revert to drifting, rather than planned renewal in which a new psychological contract for hospital nursing careers becomes woven into all parts of the organization. Nursing leaders and managers must be expert role models with whom staff identify. They must demonstrate the realities of reciprocation and its resulting need satisfaction for individuals and the organization. They must be committed to helping their staff become all they are capable of being and to demonstrating the support, providing the guidance, and engendering the trust to help this happen.

Leadership development and management training program requirements are fertile ground for reciprocation between nursing service and nursing education personnel. If there is expertise in the school of nursing to help staff development educators achieve program objectives, it should be sought. Conversely, staff development educators and other nursing service personnel have equally important expertise they can offer to faculty and students. The exchange of services is an appropriate bridge for increasing collaboration between practice and education.

Professional identification: orientation and inservice education

Component 1, *Professional Identification,* presents significant challenges for hospital staff development educators. For all organizational positions in nursing, mastery of job functions and responsibilities includes the development of identified clinical competencies and the ability to meet delineated performance objectives effectively. Staff development educators have a major responsibility in helping nurses successfully meet these requirements. Professionals need to view themselves as mature and competent. Mastering job functions and being able to make significant contributions while executing one's job are vital to feeling professionally and personally satisfied and wanting to continue association with a particular organization and setting.

Testing new approaches

Planning, coordinating, executing, monitoring, evaluating, and reporting both core and unit learning activities in the professional identification phase of career employment are important staff development functions. Because these functions can be accomplished in various ways, they afford great opportunity to create and demonstrate different approaches that will help the nursing organization and the hospital maximize resources to meet objectives in the most cost-effective way. The process of inventing and testing new approaches should identify additional resources that will complement and augment staff development functions—thus assisting the redistribution of resources to meet leadership and management development requirements as well as challenges of the professional maturation phase of career advancement. For example, selected staff nurses who have decided to pursue a practice and teaching career track may experience job enrichment through preparation and responsibility for the orientation and inservice education of new staff members. A cadre of nurses who have been promoted to an advanced practice level might rotate periodically to a practice/teaching function. During these periods, they would be part of a matrix design relating to and working with their assigned unit or service as well as the staff development department. Once such a group has been developed—and this can be a formal part of the clinical advancement program—staff development educators could actually be freed for a portion of time from their component 1 career training activities.

Another area that warrants careful study by staff development educators and experimentation in approach is the preparation of nurses for intensive care nursing. The demand for nursing staff in intensive care units continues to grow, as evidenced by the increase in the number of ICU beds over the 1970s. In 1971 there were 3,200 ICU beds; by 1979 this number had expanded to 62,000[6]. Furthermore, major medical center teaching hospitals have multiple ICU's. How can these essential nurses be most effectively and efficiently prepared to achieve mastery of job functions and responsibilities? Should there be a core ICU training program with tracks for each of the specialty areas? If not, why not? Can we afford to repeat identical basic content to different groups of nurses in multiple ICU settings in the same institution at the same time? What difference would a change in approach make in the achievement of clinical competencies? How should we adjust orientation and clinical training activities to accommodate the learning needs of the experienced ICU nurse versus the relatively new graduate? Is there a relationship between learning experiences in the professional identification career phase and longevity in a specialty area, such as ICU nursing?

Other areas of nursing that demand study and new approaches to career development are operating room nursing and emergency nursing. Preparing nurses for successful career employment in all three areas is critical for effective hospital functioning. Are there better ways to do it? Questions abound and the literature provides insufficient answers. Staff development educators must vigorously develop and test different program approaches, evaluating and publishing their findings for sharing within the profession.

In most hospitals, staff development educators probably devote their time and attention almost exclusively to orientation and inservice education of new staff members and to education of all staff members in the use of new patient care technology. Because these activities usually use traditional teaching methods, staff development educators must try to remain enthusiastic and interested while repeating the same programs time after time. This limited approach to staff development not only affects the careers of staff development nurses, but also hinders the redistribution of staff development resources to support career progression and advancement.

How much required orientation and inservice education content can and should be assembled in mediated learning packages for individual or group instruction? Are these learning packages effective? What content areas lend themselves particularly well to instructional television, which to slide and tape presentations, and which to self-study manuals? How much and what can be done in individual versus group instructional formats? Finally, do staff development educators reinvent the wheel in every hospital nursing organization? Is regional sharing of expert and scarce human and material resources being encouraged? Are consortiums used to maximum advantage?

Joining forces

An especially important question is how staff development educators can, in concert with nursing school educators, better engage in solving joint problems to facilitate both improved nursing practice and improved nursing education. For example, primary nursing is a practice approach in which the nurse receives both personal and professional satisfaction. Many say it is the practice modality of choice for professional nursing. Yet, many nurses are coming to hospital settings without a sound knowledge base in primary nursing. More confounding is the fact that many practicing nurses, experienced or not, have not integrated patient care planning—goal-directed nursing care, as described in Standard IV of the JCAH Standards for Nursing Services—into their routine clinical practice. Although the nursing process is the core of nursing practice, it is not consistently demonstrated and documented to a level of 100 percent compliance by all practicing nurses. Equally central to professional nursing practice is patient and family teaching. Yet, how frequently does a quality assurance study include significant variations that relate to patient and family teaching and its documentation? One additional concern, although many others could be iterated, relates to nurses' knowledge in the economics of health care delivery and the concept that each nurse is responsible for helping assure quality care at controlled cost. Certainly, these areas must have their foundations in basic nursing education, from which practice can then continue to build. Unfortunately, a satisfactory foundation does not always exist. For each of these problem areas, the question is how we can do our jobs in service and education in a more complementary and efficient way. Perhaps staff development educators can conduct faculty development programs to help faculty

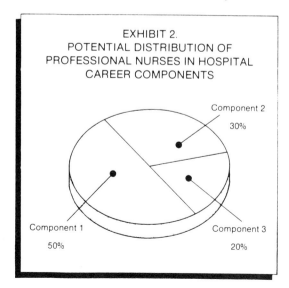

EXHIBIT 2.
POTENTIAL DISTRIBUTION OF
PROFESSIONAL NURSES IN HOSPITAL
CAREER COMPONENTS

Component 2

30%

Component 1

50%

Component 3

20%

members develop greater expertise to share with students. Or perhaps nursing practice personnel can better teach certain components to nursing students and faculty, in turn, can better teach certain content to practicing nurses.

The direction of career employment

Considering the number of new nurses starting employment every year in hospitals as well as the needs of those already employed, including the leaders and managers, the demands on staff development educators just for staff orientation and inservice are overwhelming. Even so, the challenge is not impossible—to move education program efforts from a predominant focus on component 1 to greater efforts in component 2, staff development for career advancement, and some support for component 3, professional mastery. In fact, it is essential to do so if we are to help nurses realize viable careers in hospital nursing.

Not all nurses will be interested in progressing through the different phases outlined for a professional hospital nursing career. An unknown number will be professionally and personally satisfied by continuing satisfactory or meritorious performance in the first component, as outlined in Exhibit 1. Career counseling should be available and each nurse should have the opportunity for conscious decision making regarding career objectives. It is important to emphasize that individual nurses who succeed in compo-

nent 1 and elect to remain at this level of practice are valuable professionals. Ambition in nurses is as variable as in any other group of professionals. Thus, the largest number will no doubt decide to remain in component 1, while decreasing proportions of the professional staff will move to components 2 and 3. Exhibit 2 illustrates the hypothetical distribution of staff in different career phases as it might eventually unfold if we aggressively pursue, develop, and support career employment in hospital nursing.

Next month, in Part 2 of this article, I will focus on redistribution of staff development resources to components 2 and 3 of the professional hospital nursing career pattern, identifying some challenges and issues for staff development educators.

References

1. Institute of Medicine, *Six-Month Interim Report by the Committee of the Institute of Medicine for a Study of Nursing and Nursing Education* (Washington, D.C.: National Academic Press, July 1981), p. 2.
2. Institute of Medicine, *Six-Month Interim Report,* Appendix 3, p. 3.3.
3. National Commission on Nursing, *Initial Report and Preliminary Recommendations,* NCN, Chicago, September, 1981.
4. Harry Levinson, *The Exceptional Executive—A Psychological Conception,* (New York: The New American Library, 1968), p. 56.
5. Harry Levinson, *The Exceptional Executive,* p. 166.
6. Institute of Medicine, *Six-Month Interim Report,* Appendix 2.5.

CHAPTER 4

Fostering Professional Nursing Careers in Hospitals: The Role of Staff Development, Part 2

by Margaret D. Sovie

This is the second part of an article identifying staff development educators' potential influence on job satisfaction and retention of hospital nurses. Here Sovie takes us beyond the orientation and inservice education issues she addressed in last month's JONA, to present the challenge of staff development for career advancement. Readers will benefit from her suggestions of how to meet those challenges and redistribute resources to help create "magnet" hospitals which attract both patients and excellent practitioners.

Part 1 of this article presented a model of a professional career pattern in nursing that can be dynamic, challenging, and rewarding. The conceptualization of this pattern (Exhibit 1) shows it to have three components: professional identification, which is promoted by the orientation and inservice education aspects of staff development education; professional maturation; and professional mastery. Here I will discuss the professional maturation and professional mastery components, focusing particularly on the vital role of staff development for career advancement to promote professional maturation.

Professional maturation

The term *professional maturation* is drawn from the work of H. Levinson. According to Levinson, maturation needs imply that a person has the potential for development and

Margaret D. Sovie, R.N., Ph.D., F.A.A.N., is Associate Dean for Nursing Practice and Associate Professor of Nursing, University of Rochester, Rochester, New York.

This two-part article is based on a presentation at the Staff Education Conference for Hospital-Based Nurse Educators, sponsored by the Consortium of Staff Education of Beth Israel Hospital, Brigham & Women's Hospital, Children's Medical Center Hospital, Massachusetts General Hospital, and New England Deaconess Hospital, January 18–19, 1982, Boston, Massachusetts.

expansion. The natural tendency of the human organism is toward growth, learning, and problem solving[1]. Professional maturation fostered by staff development for career advancement, is the vital component in creating careers in hospital nursing. An increasing number of career-oriented, professional nurses no longer tolerate a traditional organization in which the staff nurse is viewed and treated as the low person on the totem pole. Staff nurses are the heart of nursing practice and the central, pivotal individuals in nursing care of patients. Nursing practice is the reason they selected nursing as a career. These nurses want to develop and expand their functions in nursing practice and to have different patterns of advanced practice recognized and rewarded as legitimate career progression. Thus, staff development for career advancement is the greatest challenge facing hospital-based staff educators.

Identifying and meeting the challenge

Component 2 in the exhibit lists behaviors and functions for which practicing nurses seeking career advancement need staff development. Program content can be generated for each entry in the list. Staff development educators will need to work with staff and leadership in their respective institutions to decide which areas deserve highest priority and to choose specific content and approaches. I will highlight some of the major issues that confront staff development educators as they promote clinical career advancement for professional nursing staff.

Education for participation and growth

The concepts of career progression and promotion need to be made explicit in the nursing department and defined clearly throughout the hospital organization if nurses are to experience satisfaction and recognition as they move into advanced levels of practice. Several related staff development challenges are important.

  1. Staff nurses in hospitals as well as many members of the leadership and management staff need to learn how to

describe, illustrate, or document and evaluate excellence in nursing practice for objective review by peers and other leadership personnel who may constitute promotion review committees.

2. Many nurses need basic instruction in how to assemble a curriculum vitae or resumé that accurately reflects their individual accomplishments and professional experiences.

3. Staff nurses and others already in leadership positions need to learn more about the evaluation of nursing practice and the process of peer review. Areas of need include training in preparing objective, individual, appraisal reports and identifying strengths and weaknesses in practice. Staff members who seek career advancement can use such information in self-directed development programs.

4. Staff nurses need to learn more about group process and new program development. Skillful use of group process and knowledge of the program development process is vital to staff nurse participation in the design of clinical career ladders that delineate levels of advanced practice. Clear differentiation of advanced practice levels by specific, objective performance-based criteria is the most critical aspect of a workable clinical advancement system and the aspect in which both nurses and leaders require the most assistance and development.

5. Staff nurses need an opportunity to learn more about participative management and organizational problem-solving and decision-making processes. If nurses are to assume a more active and central role in policy and program design in nursing and hospital affairs, they must be prepared to succeed and have their potential influence realized. This goal requires a new order of staff development activities and a problem-focused approach. It also means that staff development educators must have the opportunity to function in expanded organizational settings. Consider the example of a hospital nursing practice staff charged with designing a clinical advancement system that will increase the professional and personal need satisfaction of the staff and contribute to improved quality care of patients. A special task force consisting of representative staff and leadership is appointed. A staff development educator should be appointed as an integral member of this group. Task force members will experience many learning needs as they develop the system, and the staff development educator can be central to the growth of the group and the accomplishment of the task force's charge. Describing the different levels of advanced practice is a critical component in the development of a clinical advancement system. Thus, learning to write performance criteria in terms of performance standards or expectations would be essential staff development program content to help the group accomplish its objectives. The task force's charge will generate many other learning opportunities.

Staff presentations will have to be prepared and presented. Again, in the context of the problem an opportunity exists to help prepare staff task force members in group presentation techniques and approaches. Similar situations requiring staff development expertise will be duplicated many times as a nursing practice organization moves itself into a system in which hospital nursing, as a career, is nourished, facilitated, and supported. If staff development educators are properly positioned, staff will benefit and the educators will be enriched by the expanding program opportunities and greater involvement in organizational change and renewal.

"The concepts of career progression and promotion need to be made explicit in the nursing department . . ."

Continuing education in advanced practice specialty

Staff development educator's role in continuing education for specialty advanced practice will most often be as program planners and coordinators. Nursing specialists in the specific practice areas are the content experts, along with specialists from participating, related disciplines. Although no obvious new challenge exists here for staff development educators, they can seize multiple opportunities to develop and promote new collaborative relationships with nursing educators and tap their content and research expertise as program faculty. Tradeoffs can certainly be arranged between the service and education settings to facilitate such arrangements without added costs to either institution.

Developing teaching skills

Teaching, particularly of patients and families, is considered a generic responsibility and function of professional nurses. Unfortunately, it is a function for which the majority of nurses have been ill-prepared. Most nurses meet requirements in this area only marginally. Nurses who are promoted to advanced practice levels are expected to demonstrate significantly better performance in patient and family teaching, as well as staff and student teaching. They will need staff development to meet these performance expectations. Programs that prepare nurses to be effective teachers are urgently needed. The potential rewards in both improved patient care and improved staff performance demand that this area receive high priority from staff development educators.

The problem-focused approach, with specific content directed to identified needs, seems the best. Examples abound, but only two will be given here.

Patient and family health education must be improved. Nurses need more and better patient education materials and more knowledge and skill in effective ways to influence patient and family behavior for improved health. How many nurses routinely assess available patient education materials for their reading comprehension level? How many nurses assess their patients' learning needs and styles and then plan a patient education program to meet the specific needs identified? How many nurses are able to develop resources needed to facilitate patient and family learning? Patient information booklets specific to particular health problems, slide and tape programs, and instructional television programs can all be very helpful in facilitating and supporting patient and family teaching.

Staff and student teaching responsibilities also enlarge as nurses advance in their careers. Teaching is a usual component of job enrichment, and nurses require instruction and guided experience to become more effective teachers. Preceptor training programs, which prepare nurses to act as preceptors, or mentors, to new staff members, are becoming commonplace. Every nurse promoted to an advanced practice level should have the opportunity to complete a staff development program on teaching and learning theories and methodologies. The entire organization would benefit.

Clinical problem solving and research participation

Hospital nursing career advancement will be encouraged and fiscally supported only if reciprocity is demonstrated —that is, if the organization and the professionals mutually benefit. The costs of advanced practice levels will be justified by the results achieved in improved patient care at controlled costs. All nurses, especially those promoted to advanced practice positions, must be prepared to participate in quality assurance activities designed to improve care. In addition, nurses functioning at advanced practice levels will be expected to initiate and conduct studies to improve patient care, organizational effectiveness, and cost control or reduction. Staff development educators have another critical role to play here. Most hospital nurses are not prepared to identify problems systematically, to develop proposals to scientifically study a problem, or to evaluate potential solutions. Proposal and report writing also require skills that nurses must develop.

The staff development educator, in the role of consultant, can greatly assist nursing staff members in clinical problem

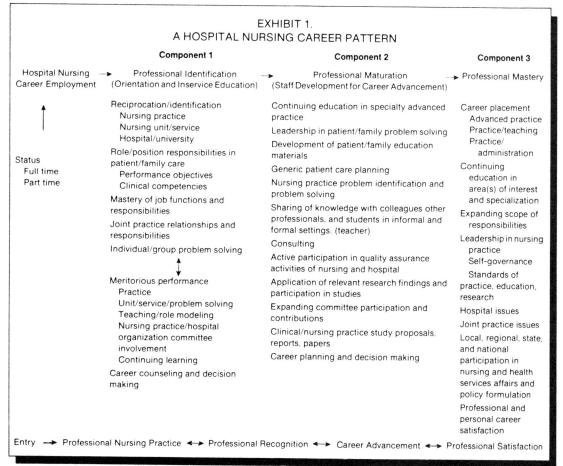

EXHIBIT 1.
A HOSPITAL NURSING CAREER PATTERN

	Component 1	Component 2	Component 3
Hospital Nursing Career Employment →	Professional Identification (Orientation and Inservice Education) →	Professional Maturation (Staff Development for Career Advancement) →	Professional Mastery

	Reciprocation/identification
	  Nursing practice
	  Nursing unit/service
	  Hospital/university
		Continuing education in specialty advanced practice	Career placement
			  Advanced practice
			  Practice/teaching

	Role/position responsibilities in patient/family care
	  Performance objectives
	  Clinical competencies
		Leadership in patient/family problem solving
		Development of patient/family education materials
		Generic patient care planning
			Practice/
			  administration
			Continuing education in area(s) of interest and specialization

Status
  Full time
  Part time
	Mastery of job functions and responsibilities	Nursing practice problem identification and problem solving	Expanding scope of responsibilities

	Joint practice relationships and responsibilities	Sharing of knowledge with colleagues other professionals, and students in informal and formal settings. (teacher)	Leadership in nursing practice Self-governance
	Individual/group problem solving	Consulting	Standards of practice, education, research

	Meritorious performance
	  Practice
	  Unit/service/problem solving
	  Teaching/role modeling
	  Nursing practice/hospital organization committee involvement
	  Continuing learning
		Active participation in quality assurance activities of nursing and hospital
		Application of relevant research findings and participation in studies
		Expanding committee participation and contributions
		Clinical/nursing practice study proposals, reports, papers
		Career planning and decision making
			Hospital issues
			Joint practice issues
			Local, regional, state, and national participation in nursing and health services affairs and policy formulation

	Career counseling and decision making		Professional and personal career satisfaction

Entry → Professional Nursing Practice ←→ Professional Recognition ←→ Career Advancement ←→ Professional Satisfaction

solving and research participation. Individual consultation and selected group learning experiences are viable approaches.

Professional mastery

The final career phase is professional mastery. At this point those who need high achievement are realizing their potential and experiencing self-fulfillment or self-actualization. (Of course individual nurses with lower needs for achievement may realize self-actualization in the professional identification or professional maturation component.) As illustrated in Part 1 of this article, only 20 percent of a hospital nursing staff will reach this level of career development. These individuals are committed, self-directed professionals who assume responsibility for their own continuing growth and development. The staff development role in the professional mastery component is responding to these nurses' ideas for new programs for themselves and other staff members. Nurses at this level will offer to initiate and conduct programs for colleagues and will be creative change agents in the nursing practice organization. Nurses functioning at the professional mastery level are the pacesetters for the profession.

Staff development structure to support hospital nursing careers

The staff development structure to support hospital nursing careers has to evolve. However, considering the burgeoning demands for education and training, it is obvious that either additional resources or a new sharing of resources for staff development is an absolute necessity. Given hospital cost constraints, the latter approach—a new sharing of resources—is undoubtedly the most viable option. It is also likely to be the option of choice. Staff development activities will be best served by a matrix design that enables a sharing of expertise. Assignments in staff development can become position responsibilities for individual nurses who elect a practice and teaching career track. Assignments can be designated for specific time periods on projects for which individual nurses have demonstrated interest and capabilities. The selected nurses gain continuing learning opportunities and also become a source of faculty for staff development program activity. Nursing administrators can create

similar opportunities for nurses who elect the practice and administration track.

Implementation of such a structure will require total nursing practice support. Staff development educators will have to sell the idea and demonstrate through pilot programs or other approaches that everyone in the organization will benefit. Program planning and evaluation of outcomes in terms of patient care, organizational effectiveness, and professional nurse satisfaction will be absolute requirements. Consequently documented results will need to be disseminated widely both inside and outside the organization.

Staff development educators must become more aggressive and creative in advertising the contributions they make to the nursing practice organization, the hospital, and the profession. If you capitalize on the opportunity to help hospitals create dynamic, challenging, and rewarding professional careers in hospital nursing, be certain to do it in a planned, programmatic approach and study and report the results to the profession at large. What differences do you expect and what actually happens? The hypothesis of this article is that those hospitals that succeed in creating exciting career opportunities for professional nurses will not have a nursing shortage. They will have quality nursing care at controlled costs, excellent joint practice relationships between physicians and nurses, and a reputation in the community and among health service professionals as magnet hospitals where patients want to go for care and professionals want to practice.

Although the career model outlined here is for nurses practicing patient care, the concept of career progression, with professional identification, maturation, and mastery components, can be applied to other hospital nursing career patterns, such as nursing administration and staff development education. The responsibility for developing and supporting career advancement in the latter two areas rests with top nursing administrators. These opportunities and challenges also must be aggressively pursued as the nursing profession assumes its central role in hospital health care delivery and management.

Reference

1. Harry Levinson, *The Exceptional Executive—A Psychological Conception,* (New York: New American Library, 1968), p. 205.

CHAPTER 5

Joy D. Calkin, RN, PhD

A Model for Advanced Nursing Practice

What is advanced nursing practice? How can the nurse administrator decide when to employ advanced nurse practitioners? The author suggests a way for differentiating basic from advanced nursing practice. She also identifies conditions that may influence decisions about employing advanced nurse practitioners. Examples of application to situations are provided.

Nurse administrators and advanced nurse practitioners (ANPs), such as nurse practitioners with the master's degree and clinical nurse specialists, often talk about the tasks these practitioners can do. Some defend spending money to hire advanced practitioners because they contribute quality through tasks such as maintenance of standards, staff development, new program development, care of patients with complex problems, consultation, and nursing leadership. It can be argued that there are other staff who can do these tasks. Hence, administrators and advanced practitioners have been confronting the difficult question, Why pay more for this expert? Too often the answer is unclear.

It is important to think about the essence of advanced nursing practice. The lack of a simple explanation of this practice can limit thinking about the appropriate use of these advanced nursing practitioners within the profession and in the delivery of nursing care. It is also a basis for the difficulty of explaining to nurses and others what we mean by advanced nursing practice. I propose a way of differentiating basic from advanced nursing practice and

of identifying conditions under which advanced practice skills increase nursing effectiveness.

Using Experts

The effectiveness of nursing and other organizations is influenced by the "fit" between the work to be done and the structure of the organization.[1,2] The major elements of structure are

1. The number and enforcement of policies and procedures
2. The mechanisms for nursing care and management decision making
3. The extent of specialization or division of labor
4. The types of nursing expertise available (education and experience).

Nursing expertise is the focus of this article.

Most nursing departments have three groups of employees (*i.e.*, three general types of expertise): practical, technical, and professional. Professional nurses are further subdivided into basic and advanced practitioners. The latter have clinical specialization at the master's level.

Hiring professional staff is not simply identifying tasks and employing someone to do them. Professionals bring to an organization the results of a *process* of formal education and socialization. They assess and intervene more from their preemployment prepara-

Joy D. Calkin, RN, PhD is an Associate Professor of Nursing and Health Services Administration at the University of Wisconsin—Madison. She works with a variety of health care organizations as a management consultant.

tion than do practical and technical nurses. Indeed, that is a hallmark of professionals. As a result, it is important to grasp the *nature* of professionals' expertise in addition to determining the specific tasks they are competent to perform. The literature for nurse managers does not provide a rationale for fitting work with the types of professional expertise available. A first step in deciding when to employ ANPs is to differentiate the nature of advanced from basic nursing practice.

Differentiating Advanced Nursing Practice

"Nursing is the diagnosis and treatment of human responses to actual or potential health problems."[3] This definition suggests nurses deal with a *population* of human responses to existing or possible health problems. For example, the population of pain responses to extensive burns may range from "negative" responses, such as immobility and total rejection of relief, to "positive" responses, such as seeking appropriate relief and maintaining range of motion. Usually these responses exist on a continuum from very negative to very positive (Fig. 1) in terms of the person's adaptation, self-care skills, or other goals relevant to nursing practice goals. Note that *positive* and *negative* do not mean good and bad responses, but rather those that are helpful or unhelpful to the patients' growth or health or other goals. These goals often arise from the nurses' conceptual frameworks. The model is based on the notion that the population of human responses to an actual or potential health problem exists as a distribution. (For this article, the populations of response were assumed to take the form of a normal distribution though this is not necessarily the case.)

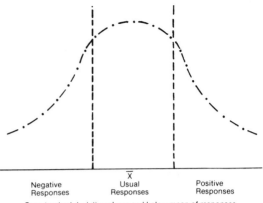

One standard deviation above and below mean of responses.

Figure 1. Population of human responses to health problems.

With the knowledge and skill they bring from their formal educational program, novice nurses are prepared to deal with a narrow range of usual or average responses of individual patients or groups. Through practice experiences with human responses, they broaden both their diagnostic and treatment skills. Their knowledge of the nature and extent of responses and their skill in diagnosis and treatment are, however, limited (Fig. 2). Under some conditions, it might be argued that the knowledge and understanding of responses by novices actually *exceeds* their practice skills.

Nurses who excel in analysis and insight when diagnosing and treating human responses are generally known as experts.[4] Although they may not be able to name the cognitive and affective processes underlying their actions,[5] they are able to treat skillfully a broader and deeper range of responses (Fig. 3).

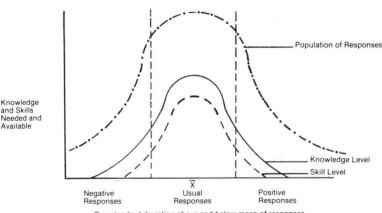

One standard deviation above and below mean of responses.

Figure 2. Beginning practitioners.

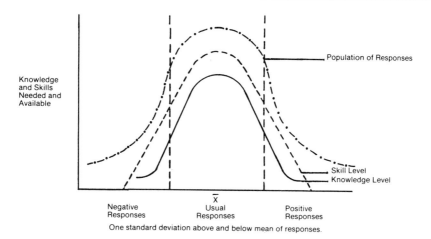

Figure 3. Experienced nurses.

Some practitioners have a capacity to sense the nature of a problematic response that goes beyond the conscious analytic diagnosis of the novice. This capacity is not often accompanied by deftness in talking about the cognitive processes that guide their actions.[5] Experts-by-experience generally earn their reputation by having greater or more rapid intervention skills than their colleagues.

It may be argued then that expertise gained through experience is sufficient for the provision of nursing services for human responses to real or potential health problems. This argument is valid to the extent that

1. Clusters of responses to these problems, including those arising from medical interventions, are relatively static
2. The knowledge bases for the diagnosis and treatment of responses changes slowly or the number of responses is relatively limited
3. There is little need to articulate or defend the basis for diagnostic statements or the rationale for treatment strategies used by nurses
4. Practicing nurses dealing with selected populations of human responses have less need to talk with students, novices, researchers, and others about the nature and extent of actual or anticipated responses
5. There is little need for patient care program development or redevelopment within the nursing department.

These statements may be characteristic of health care delivery institutions or agencies with fairly stable and readily analyzable human responses to actual or potential health problems (for example, a small community hospital that refers medically complex patients to a regional center).

Advances in nursing practice are developed by those at the cutting edge of identifying or dealing with health-related human responses. They may be experts through experience who are analytic and complex thinkers motivated to improve care and who are articulate in describing this thinking to others. They may be researchers developing basic and applied knowledge for advancing nursing practice. They may be clinicians with master's degrees who have formal preparation in using conceptual and analytic tools applied in practice settings.

In general, the largest group of ANPs is among nurses in the latter group—clinical nurse specialists and master's-prepared nurse practitioners. In contrast to novices and the majority of experts-through-experience, ANPs should understand and have the practice skills represented in Figure 4.

Figure 4 portrays several characteristics of advanced practice: (1) the population of human responses to actual and potential health problems generally exceeds nursings' present knowledge and skill; this is less true of ANPs (Fig. 4) than of the experienced nurse (Fig. 3) and the novice (Fig. 2); (2) the direct care skills of most nurses, including the ANP, exceed their conceptual and analytic frameworks for diagnosing and treating the responses of patients (hence the need for art and intuition to supplement the science of practice); (3) where responses are more frequent or usual, the levels of ANP knowledge and of skill should be virtually the same; (4) the level of ANP awareness and knowledge of the extremes of patient responses is higher than the levels of experts-

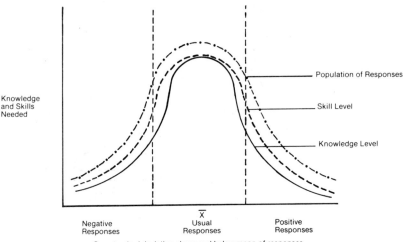

Figure 4. Advanced nurse practitioners.

by-experience and novices. This characteristic is a significant one. The identification of these extremes in responses is important to nursing research (*e.g.*, why do these positive responses occur in some people or situations and not others?), for practice (*e.g.*, how can we intervene with these negative extremes to effect changes in patient responses?), and for education (*e.g.*, what are a range of responses for which undergraduates and graduate students should be prepared?).

Although the rationale for including negative patient responses as a focus for practice is evident, it may not be as obvious why the diagnosis and treatment of positive responses is important for nursing. A number of writers describe the necessity of identifying, analyzing, and capitalizing on patients' strengths or positive responses in providing care.[6] Secondly, advancing the effectiveness of practice will rely, in part, on nurses' ability to analyze those factors associated with positive responses and to generalize those factors to other patients confronted with similar situations. Thirdly, the identification of positive responses to actual and potential health problems provides nurses with high-quality outcomes or goals for nursing interventions. Finally, the failure to identify positive responses in patients may result in using interventions that actually impede a particular patient's ability to maintain those responses.[7] For these reasons, understanding positive human responses is an important element of nursing practice and a focus for advancing practice.

The contrasts in the knowledge and skill levels of novices, experts-by-experience, and advanced practitioners were described in relation to the range of human responses to health problems. The key contrasts were in expectations of the ANP to be cognizant of a full range of possible responses, to use conscious processes to analyze and intervene in these responses, and to be able to articulate those processes to others.

Advanced Nursing Practice Defined

Advanced nursing practice is the deliberative diagnosis and treatment of a full range of human responses to actual or potential health problems. Advanced practitioners can provide a rationale for choosing diagnostic and treatment processes. Advanced practice is accompanied by specialized knowledge and skill in dealing with a human response that cuts across health problems (*e.g.*, pain) or with a cluster of human responses to an identifiable actual or potential problem (*e.g.*, diabetes mellitus) or a cluster of age-specific human responses to health problems (*e.g.*, infants) or a combination of these (*e.g.*, changes in self-concept in pregnant adolescents).

Management Decisions

The model of advanced nursing practice in Figure 4 can assist managers in making decisions about the hiring and deployment of ANPs. It should help clarify the conditions or contingencies for the use of these resources. It may assist managers and advanced practitioners in *thinking about* the nature of their functioning, in addition to what they *do*, as a basis for resource allocation. Some examples are provided to promote discussion.

Example 1

The most traditional use of ANPs occurs where the health problems may elicit a wide range of human responses with continuing and substantial unpredictable elements. The unpredictable or unfamiliar elements may arise from cultural differences, family characteristics, changing medical technology, individual differences, the sheer magnitude of the health problem itself, or other factors. Figures 2 and 3 represent visually the knowledge of staff nurses on the unit relative to knowledge required by a number of patients. The nurse manager and ANP agree that over time the picture is not likely to change because of constant changes in medical treatment or treatment of unusually high-risk patients/families or other factors. These factors are often the case in tertiary and university medical centers, even with moderately low staff turnover.

Under these conditions, the ANP functions (1) to identify and develop interventions for the unusual by providing direct care; (2) to transmit this knowledge to nurses and in some settings to students; (3) to identify and communicate needs for, or carry out research related to, human responses to these health problems; (4) to anticipate factors that may lead to the presence of unfamiliar responses; and (5) to provide anticipatory guidance to nurse administrators when the changes in the diagnosis and treatment of these responses may require altered levels or types of resources (*e.g.*, staff skills).

A decision must be made about whether to use the ANP in a consultation or line management position. Depending on the location of patients with these responses and other institutional factors, the ANP may be placed in a line position on one unit or in a staff position from which the ANP consults throughout the organization.

The use of the model in Figure 4 assists the ANP and manager in determining the focus of the ANP's functioning. Conceptually, the ANP must focus on clusters of human responses at the extremes of the response continuum. The relevant boundary spanning of the ANP is directed to those extreme environments (*e.g.*, in medical technology, relevant research in areas such as physiology and social psychology, and basic research in nursing about those responses) that are most likely to enhance the practitioner's ability to anticipate, analyze, discern, and communicate possible interventions for nonroutine human responses. For example, ANPs may use library resources and specialty nursing and medical

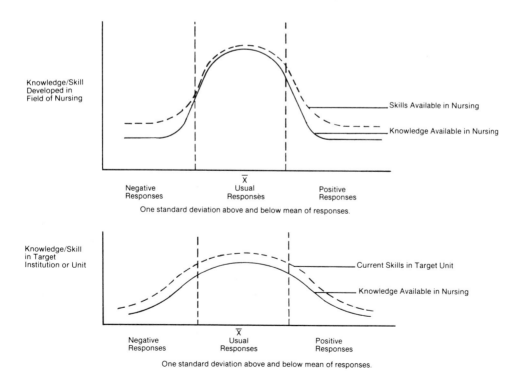

Figure 5. Field of nursing and target institution.

organizations to expand their knowledge of unfamiliar responses.

Example 2

A second use of the ANP occurs where the patient population or problem is perceived as new and different by nurses, but care is expected to be less difficult over time. This is often the case with a new program such as hospice care or adding a primary care clinic to a tertiary care hospital. With the current attention to new markets for income generation and to making greater use of existing resources, these conditions are occurring with greater frequency and in a variety of health care delivery settings.

In this example, the ANP is assigned to "translate" or transfer innovations from other settings. Innovations are changes in structure or practice that are perceived by those in the setting as substantially different from existing practice. The ANPs do not generate new knowledge regarding the care requisites resulting from a population of human responses but rather adapt programs from other settings. The difference between Figures 5A and 5B represents the gap between knowledge and skill used elsewhere in the field of nursing and that available in the target unit or institution.

The ANP and nurse administrator can use the figures to identify the objectives for the ANP's interventions. Figure 5A can represent the objectives for the nursing staff (B) with whom the ANP is to work. That is, the ANP assumes responsibility for assisting the staff nurses in improving their diagnosis and treatment of responses or cluster of responses with which they are currently unfamiliar in order to implement the new program or care for a type of patient new to the setting. The ANP must be active in identifying and learning from colleagues in other settings where this type of program is effectively established. For example, the ANP may go to a setting that has a well-developed program to learn what parts of it can be adapted to the ANP's own setting. For example, a clinical nurse specialist in a general pediatrics unit might be assigned to coordinate the planning and implementation of a new bone marrow transplant program. This would include contacting other hospitals with well-established programs and developing staff in the unit to provide patient care.

This is an instance when the advanced practitioner may not be an expert in the anticipated responses. Rather, the manager is relying on several other capacities of an ANP. First, the ANP is expected to have the analytic skill to gain new, pertinent information and to do so quickly. Second, the practitioner is expected to have a knowledge of processes by which

innovations are adapted for use in a new setting.[8] Finally, the ANP is expected to work appropriately with nurse managers to identify resources needed for the new program and, usually, to implement its initial phases. When the systems to support the program are established and staff nurses have become effective in dealing with them, the ANP's skills are no longer needed on a continuing basis—if at all.

From a structural view, the ANP in this situation would have a staff or project position. In some settings the ANP may have line responsibility on one unit or clinic interspersed with project assignments. Nurse consultants may also work in this way.

Example 3

In some situations, advanced practitioners are employed as "specialist generalists." In this instance, the patients may have a wide variety of health problems requiring nursing and medical care. If the practitioners have sufficiently advanced knowledge and skill, they *perceive* a particular patient's responses to a problem as an example of a general case and adapt their care on that basis. Practitioners who specialize as generalists may be most useful in circumstances where patients have many different medical and health problems. The ANP generalists must have skills in the nursing diagnosis and treatment of responses to a wide range of existing or potential health problems. In addition, these ANPs usually require medical diagnostic and treatment skills for dealing with the health problems themselves, often with the use of protocols. Their ability to diagnose and treat a variety of noncomplex medical problems assists ANPs in anticipating patient responses to health problems and to treatment as well as reducing costly nurse-physician coordination time when this will not benefit the patient. Family nurse practitioners and pediatric nurse practitioners are examples of those who have specialized as generalists.

The nurse manager may consider employing the generalist ANP when there is a need for extending physician resources required to diagnose and treat common health problems as well as when there is a need for providing proficient nursing care, such as in a primary care clinic. Alternately, the ANP may function in settings where primary care physicians are also being trained in nursing. For example, in a family practice teaching clinic, when family practice residents anticipate working in areas without professional nurses, the ANP may assist them in gaining skills in diagnosing and treating less complex human responses or referring patients who need more specialized nursing care.

Mastery of broadly based triage and referral functions is essential for generalist ANPs. They must keep up to date with a number of general resources related to nursing and with medical resources on current practice for the type of patients seen. For example, high-school nurses must keep abreast of nursing, medical, and other literature on common adolescent health problems and their responses to them.

In the model of advanced practice, the ANP in this example has skill in the diagnosis and treatment of human responses to health problems within the usual range. Also, this practitioner is often facile in identifying and using unusual strengths or positive responses of patients. The ANP generalist is necessarily sensitive to unusual negative responses and will consider consultation with or referral to nurse colleagues who specialize in those responses to problems (*e.g.*, sexual dysfunction).

Is the Model Useful?

The model (Fig. 4) and definition of advanced practice are intended to provide a basis for communicating about advanced nursing practice. Advanced practitioners are expected to have competence in dealing with unusual responses as well as the more common ones. I maintain that advanced practitioners tend to rely more on deliberation and reason (versus intuition) in diagnosis and treatment processes than do basic practitioners. Hence, the former should be expected to be articulate about the nature of nursing practice, to use reasoning to deal with practice innovations, and to develop or contribute to newer forms of practice. This perception and definition of their practice is the starting point for decisions about using ANPs' skills in organizations, rather than beginning with a focus on tasks and skills.

Is the model useful? That question will ultimately be answered by advanced practitioners, nurse managers, and others who apply it. In talking with a group of clinical specialists and a mixed group of specialists, nurse practitioners, and nurse managers, I have used Figures 2, 3, and 4 to compare and contrast the expected behaviors of novice and expert-by-experience nurses with those of ANPs. The practitioners were able to use the model to discuss the educational needs for advanced practice, other prac-

tice issues, and the similar styles of clinical nurse specialists and master's-prepared nurse practitioners. The managers found the model helped them think about the ANP as a resource in service settings. A director of nursing in a skilled and intermediate nursing care facility used the underlying notions to articulate the conditions under which she would want external consultation and the kind of advanced practitioner needed. She also noted how she would base her budget commitment on the approximate frequency of patient responses that staff had difficulty managing.

The nurse manager's ability to analyze the need for expertise and to establish expectations of basic and advanced practitioners is essential for sound resource management. An overall view of what nursing practice is and how advanced practice fits within that view is a necessary prerequisite for this analysis. The model and definitions of practice appear to be useful for maintaining this view. If, after analysis, the decision is made to use advanced practitioners, then the model can help in explaining to others the rationale for using ANPs' knowledge and skills, identifying the nature of their relationship to the unit or department (*e.g.*, line or staff), establishing expectations for their performance, and clarifying the kinds of continuing knowledge development required for such positions. I would appreciate readers' comments about the usefulness of this model.

References

1. Woodward J. Industrial organization: theory and practice. London: Oxford University Press, 1965:72.
2. Calkin JD. Effect of task and structure on nurse performance and satisfaction: a part-replica experiment [dissertation]. University of Wisconsin—Madison, 1980.
3. American Nurses' Association. Social policy statement. Kansas City: American Nurses' Association, 1980:9.
4. Tanner C. Research on clinical judgement. In: Holzmer W, ed. Review of research in nursing education [in press].
5. Benner P. From novice to expert. Am J Nurs 1982;82:402-7.
6. Blake F. Open heart surgery in children: a study in nursing care. DHEW Children's Bureau Publication #418-1964, 1965.
7. Calkin JD. Are hospitalized toddlers adapting to the experience as well as we think? American Journal of Maternal Child Nursing 1979;4:18-23.
8. Delbecq AL. Contextual variables affecting decision making in program planning, Decision Sciences 1974;5:726-42.

UNIT TWO

SUSAN G. SHEEDY

Managing Others

1950—1960

In the 1950s and 1960s, many hospital nursing departments managed their own personnel functions. These functions usually involved position control, salary recommendations to administration for nursing, initial interviewing, and nursing personnel policies. Nursing, then as now, was such a large department, that personnel departments generally felt it appropriate for nursing to do its own personnel functions. This posture also represented the personnel departments' unfamiliarity in dealing with professionals. These were also the times when the main function in the hospital was nursing care and many of the ancillary departments did not exist. As hospitals became larger, employing more people and a variety of professionals, it seemed more reasonable to include nursing in the overall personnel department.

1960—1970

In the late 1960s and early 1970s more nursing departments merged their personnel departments with the hospital personnel department. About this time, hospital personnel departments were being renamed Human Resources. The transferral of nursing personnel functions to the Human Resource Department was positive for the institution, nursing staff, and nurse executive. The positive effect was the broad education nursing management (vice president through head nurse) received from their association with experts in human resources and other hospital managers. This education occurred usually in educational sessions with management from across the hospital, and in discussions or problem-solving sessions conducted and sponsored by the Human Resource Department for all the hospital's managers. Such topics as motivation, disciplining, how to interview, how to counsel, the disciplinary process, how to negotiate, new and improved performance appraisal systems, how to do manpower planning, and legal implications of dealing with personnel were common issues for all department heads.

Similarly, the nurse executive and nursing organization provided expertise on nursing trends, changes in nursing education, the projected need for specialized nursing professionals, successful staffing and scheduling policies, national study results on vacancies, turnover, causes for dissatisfaction in staff nurses, and so forth. This combined expertise of human resource professionals and nursing management professionals produced a more aware and responsive working environment for the nurse.

The emphasis for Human Resources Departments continued to be hiring, orientation, terminating, payroll, and benefits sign up; in addition, Human Resources Departments became responsible for advising hospital administration and department heads on employee concerns and how to manage and retain their human resources. Human Resources Departments gave more emphasis to employee attitudes, unionization and its affect on an organization, performance appraisals, seeking employee input by way of quality circles to improve efficiency and patient care, and communication mechanisms between management and employees.

1980

Another major thrust since the late 1970s and early 1980s has been a concentration on educating, supporting, and caring about a major human resource—the manager. The nursing journals during this period are representative of articles that try to sensitize upper-level management to the burdens and problems of the middle managers. The problems of how to choose middle managers, the type of education they need to be effective, the follow-up support needed by middle managers, the trauma of promotion and how upper-level management can decrease the trauma and how to evaluate a middle manager fairly, are some of the areas these articles address.

All of the changes described are not necessarily operating in each hospital. Each institution may be at different evolutionary stages as they strive to stay abreast in a changing health care environment. For the most part, however, the changes do describe the "movements" that have taken place in the past 25 to 30 years.

The Future

More merging of the nursing personnel function with the overall hospital personnel function will occur in the future if this has not already occurred. More corporate arrangement will also occur with vice presidents of nursing in a multi-hospital system discussing, comparing, compromising, and agreeing to a personnel philosophy for several hospitals. This will be very different from the vice president of nursing being the only input for one stand-alone hospital and its nursing personnel policies. Thus, vice presidents of nursing in hospitals who are a part of corporate arrangements or multihospital arrangements will need to become comfortable with negotiating with their peers on issues such as: When is centralization versus autonomy needed in nursing personnel policies? How does one continue to be creative in this corporate or multisystem environment? When is strategic planning a corporate issue versus a single hospital issue? In the future hospital vice presidents of nursing may direct alternative health delivery systems *in addition* to hospital nursing and thus manage a different set of employee issues. As the number of vacancies remains low, many corporate or hospital administrators may decide that, because the vice president of nursing is not managing the numbers of hospital personnel that she/he once did and also because she has management expertise in the patient care environment, application of these skills to home health care, one-day surgeries, long-term care, day care, and so forth is appropriate. This broadened responsibility could give the vice president of nursing a rare opportunity to control, direct, and organize a true continuum of care driven by one philosophy and one level of excellence.

There will also be a higher expectation that thorough financial feasibility studies be done by nursing for any new program being proposed. In addition, the financial implications of changing operations, such as scheduling and staffing options, will need to be presented by nursing and justified by improving expenses. It will be a usual expectation in nursing to know the cost of nursing care. In many instances, although the institution or finance department may not be initiating a project to study the cost of delivering nursing care, the nursing department will need to initiate such a project with finance. This information is necessary in making sound operational decisions in the DRG environment.

Lastly, the nurse executive will be needed more at the policy-making, strategic-planning level than in the past. As hospitals and corporations consider new revenue sources, and vertical and horizontal integration, nursing care will often be the product offered in a different environment. Home health, one-day surgery, long-term care, and diagnostic centers have a major component to be managed, which is nursing care. Input, debate, and discussion need to be done in the presence of the expert from nursing, the vice president of nursing.

Thus, the changes in health care are all-encompassing and not just in theory. How nursing departments are conducted and managed on a day-to-day basis will change dramatically over the next few years. Human resources functions, productivity, and some basic assumptions that nursing has held may be questioned, scrutinized, and changed. The perspective on the part of nursing management must be that these changes can be challenging, creative opportunities and can benefit patient care.

CHAPTER 6

Nursing Administration and Personnel Administration

by Harold C. White and Michael N. Wolfe

This article proposes that the personnel department could be of far greater assistance to nursing directors and hospital administrators than is commonly perceived. Although many of the nursing directors, hospital administrators, and personnel directors polled by the authors expressed a desire for more support from the personnel department, their priorities concerning the degree of increased involvement differed. Analysis of the respondents' answers to questions regarding specific areas of administrative responsibility are discussed. Managers at all levels will find this article to be a fruitful basis for discussing those areas within which the personnel department could play an expanded role.

As the senior manager of nursing, the nursing director has responsibilities for planning, organizing, staffing, directing and controlling the nursing unit. The staffing function concerns obtaining, retaining, and developing employees. Staffing duties typically are associated with the personnel administration department. The personnel department is created to assist the managers in carrying out their staffing responsibilities.

For all organizations, personnel administration has received increased attention as a result of increased labor costs, greater demands for skilled employees, growth of labor unions, and expanding legislation affecting employment. There is also a growing awareness of the applications of the behavioral sciences in the work place.

Personnel administration is especially challenging in the hospital because of the high proportion of hospital expenses going directly to payroll. The benefits package, such as retirement, medical–hospital insurance, and vacations, comprises approximately one-third of total payroll.

Harold C. White, Ph.D., is Professor, Department of Management, Arizona State University, Tempe, Arizona.

Michael N. Wolfe, Ph.D., is Assistant Professor, Department of Management, Arizona State University.

The study

A survey was conducted of all hospitals within the state of Arizona to determine how key members of management perceived the role of the personnel department as it was and as they desired it to be[1]. Of the 81 hospitals surveyed, 39.5 percent responded. Exhibit 1 classifies the hospitals from which responses were received. Nonprofit hospitals made up fifty percent of the responding hospitals; the balance were almost entirely government hospitals, mainly federal installations.

Exhibit 2 indicates the size of the responding hospitals according to their number of employees. Half of the hospitals employ less than 500 persons, with no hospital employing under 100. There are 2,000 or more employees in six percent of the responding hospitals.

An example of the survey instructions and questions are shown in Exhibit 3.

Responses from the nursing directors, hospital administrators, and personnel directors are presented in Exhibit 4. The left hand column lists the twenty-four personnel administration duties included in the survey. To the right are the activities performed by the personnel department: Policy, Advice, Service, and Control. The numbers indicate the mean (average) responses for each activity; "1" indicates the minimum response and "5" the maximum response for those areas in which increased levels of personnel department support is desired. The column labeled "rank" on the right of the table indicates the relative importance given to each activity by the respondents. The personnel duties are listed in order of the nursing directors' preferences. Numbers at the bottom of the columns are means for those columns.

Results

Emphasis

Of the personnel administration activities, nursing directors rated Advice first, followed closely by Policy and Service.

EXHIBIT 1. CLASS OF HOSPITAL	
Class	**Percent**
Nonprofit-Voluntary-Charitable	50.0
Private-Proprietary	3.1
Government:	
Federal	28.1
State	3.1
County	12.5
Other	3.1

EXHIBIT 2. SIZE OF HOSPITAL	
Number of Employees	**Percent**
Less than 100	0.0
100-249	21.9
250-499	28.1
500-749	9.4
750-999	9.4
1000-1999	25.0
2000 or more	6.3

Control was given least emphasis. Hospital administrators ranked Advice and Control in highest priority, followed by Policy, with Service a distant fourth. Personnel directors ranked Policy and Advice first, followed closely by Control, and then Service. Overall, the administrators ranked the personnel administration duties higher, on the average and for each activity, than the other two groups of respondents ranked them. While the differences between groups are important, there was little overall difference in the emphasis placed by the respondents on the four activities. Indeed, with the exception of Control, there was little difference between the three groups of respondents. In regards to Control, hospital administrators indicated the desire for considerably more control than did either the nursing directors or the personnel directors.

Results indicate a strong support for increased levels of personnel department involvement. Regarding Policy, nursing directors rated 92 percent of the twenty-four duties at 3.0 or higher on the five point scale. Administrators rated 87 percent at 3.0 or higher. Personnel directors rated Policy at 3.0 or higher for 83 percent of the duties.

Similar patterns occurred for Advice. Ninety-two percent of the duties were rated at or above 3.0 by nursing directors and administrators, and 82 percent were rated at or above 3.0 by personnel directors. For Service, nursing directors rated 96 percent at 3.0 or higher, while administrators and personnel directors rated 79 percent in a similar fashion. Under Control, the figures are 92 percent for nursing directors, 84 percent for administrators, and 79 percent for personnel directors.

Priorities

Of the six duties considered most important by the nursing directors, three of the six so designated were agreed to by the administrators, and two by the personnel directors. The two duties identified by all groups as being most important were Grievances and Affirmative Action. Administrators and personnel directors were in agreement with each other concerning three additional duties: Discipline- Discharge, Wage and Salary Administration, and Performance Appraisal.

Among the six least important duties identified by the

nursing directors, four were agreed to by the administrators and personnel directors. These duties were Community Service, Employee Newsletter, Recreation- Social, and Food Service. Respondents generally agreed with the conclusion that it is an "illogical connection" to place cafeteria service and recreation councils, along with receptionists and typing pools, under the control of the personnel department[2].

Nursing directors placed substantially more emphasis than did the other respondents on Retirements, Wage Surveys, Medical- Hospital Insurance, Morale- Opinion Surveys, and Safety. Nursing directors, as opposed to personnel directors, also placed more emphasis on Collective Bargaining.

Substantially less emphasis was placed by nursing directors on Wage and Salary Administration, Performance Appraisal, and Orientation than by administrators and personnel directors. They also placed substantially less emphasis than did administrators on Promotions, and less than personnel directors on Employment Selection.

Changes

Part of the study measured how many of the personnel administration duties were actually being conducted in the same manner in which they were perceived as being conducted by the respondents. In comparison, the nursing directors indicated that the greatest desired increase among the activities was for Advice, followed by Control, Service, and Policy. The greatest increase desired by the administrators and personnel directors involved Control activity. Administrators agreed with the nursing directors that Policy should be fourth in order of increased emphasis. The personnel directors desired that the personnel department increase its policy making role to a much greater degree than was desired by the other two groups. The nursing directors wanted the personnel department to be relatively more involved in Service.

For all activities of all duties, nursing directors desired increased personnel department involvement. However, the nursing directors perceived that the personnel department is less involved in activities than is perceived by either the administrators or personnel directors. This suggests a lack of communication between the personnel department and the units they service and between the administrators and the managers who report to them. Nursing directors may not have received a clear explanation of the role of the personnel department.

Professionalism

Of the twenty-four duties included in the survey, six can be classified as "professional" in nature: Human Resources Planning, Training and Development, Wage and Salary Administration, Performance Appraisal, Morale-Opinion Survey, and Affirmative Action. Each of the responding groups indicated that they desired to have the personnel department substantially increase its involvement in Human Resources Planning. In addition, nursing directors also wanted substantially more in Morale-Opinion Surveys. Administrators also called for substantially more involvement from the personnel department in Wage and Salary Administration, Performance Appraisal and Morale-Opinion Survey.

However, of these "professional" activities, only Affirmative Action was identified among the top six most desired activities by all groups. Only the administrators and personnel directors included Wage and Salary Administration and Performance Appraisal among the six activities requiring increased personnel department involvement, while administrators also included Morale-Opinion Surveys.

Conclusions

There is a need to avoid over-generalizations from this study of a single group of respondents in a specific group of

hospitals. Nonetheless, valuable guidance for the directors of nursing can be obtained from the results.

All those who participated in the survey requested that the personnel department be more involved in each activity for each of the twenty-four duties. The increasing importance of personnel administration is recognized within the hospital.

Nursing directors are in relative disagreement with the administrators and personnel directors as to the priorities and the increased emphasis that should be given to the various duties. It may be that the needs of the nursing department differ from those of other hospital units. The most notable examples of this divergence involve Retirements, which nursing directors placed number one but which administrators and personnel directors placed fourteenth and sixteenth, respectively; and Performance Appraisal, which was ranked seventeenth by the nursing directors, but fifth by administrators and sixth by personnel directors.

It appears, therefore, that if the nursing directors wait for the personnel department to proceed with programs they consider most important or to respond to directives from the hospital administration, the nursing department may not receive the type of support desired. For the personnel department to serve effectively, conscientious work on the part of nursing directors will be called for to make their wishes known. Improved communication is required.

There is also the question as to whether or not the nursing directors are aware of the relative needs of their units. In a study of the importance of sixteen job factors, registered nurses listed both Promotions and Training in the top quarter in order of importance[3]; in the present study, however, nursing directors listed both items quite low, with

---

EXHIBIT 3.
QUESTIONNAIRE INSTRUCTIONS AND SAMPLE QUESTION

Please circle the number that best represents the level of responsibility of the personnel department for each of the following activities. More than one responsibility (Policy, Advice, Service, or Control) may be circled for any personnel activity.

Indicate current involvement for the responsibility the personnel department has right now for each activity. Indicate desired involvement for the responsibility you would like the personnel department to have for each activity. Definitions of activities are:

Policy: Assisting in the making of policy statements for the activity
Advice: Making suggestions or counseling managers who carry out the activity
Service: Actually performing the activity
Control: Measuring and evaluating the performance and results of the activity.

Scoring Instruction: 1 = No Involvement   2 = Little Involvement   3 = Moderate Involvement
4 = High Involvement   5 = Very High Involvement

Personnel Administration Duties	Personnel Administration Activities			
	Policy	*Advice*	*Service*	*Control*
Human Resources Planning	1 2 3 4 5	1 2 3 4 5	1 2 3 4 5	1 2 3 4 5
Current Involvement	1 2 3 4 5	1 2 3 4 5	1 2 3 4 5	1 2 3 4 5
Desired Involvement	1 2 3 4 5	1 2 3 4 5	1 2 3 4 5	1 2 3 4 5

Promotions eighteenth and Training and Development twentieth.

Nursing directors may be inadequately informed as to the contributions to be provided by a professional personnel department. A well run personnel department can provide knowledge and skills to aid the nursing unit to upgrade its personnel oriented programs by working with the nursing director and other members of the nursing unit. For example, Training and Development was listed a low twentieth by nursing directors for personnel department involvement. While it might be argued that training and development of nurses on a continuing basis can be best provided by nurses,

---

EXHIBIT 4.

DUTIES AND ACTIVITIES OF THE HOSPITAL PERSONNEL DEPARTMENT DESIRED BY NURSING DIRECTORS, HOSPITAL ADMINISTRATORS AND PERSONNEL DIRECTORS

Mean Responses: 1 = minimum; 5 = maximum

Duties	POLICY			ADVICE			SERVICE			CONTROL			RANK		
	Nurs. Dirs.	Hosp. Adm.	Pers. Dirs.	Nurs. Dirs.	Hosp. Adm.	Pers. Dirs.	Nurs. Dirs.	Hosp. Adm.	Pers. Dirs.	Nurs. Dirs.	Hosp. Adm.	Pers. Dirs.	Nurs Dirs.	Hosp. Adm.	Pers. Dirs.
Retirements	4.1	3.8	3.6	4.3	4.0	3.6	4.2	3.8	3.3	4.0	3.8	3.4	1	14	16
Grievances	4.2	4.4	4.1	4.4	4.6	4.3	4.1	3.9	4.2	3.9	4.4	4.2	1	3	2
Recruiting	4.0	4.3	4.0	4.0	4.4	4.0	4.3	4.3	4.0	3.9	4.4	4.0	3	1	7
Wage Survey	4.1	3.8	3.9	4.0	4.2	3.8	4.2	3.9	3.9	4.0	4.3	3.8	3	10	9
Affirmative Action	4.1	4.3	3.8	4.0	4.3	4.2	3.9	3.9	4.1	3.9	4.3	4.0	5	5	5
Med.-Hosp. Insurance	3.6	3.4	3.4	4.0	3.6	3.3	4.1	3.4	3.3	3.7	3.7	3.3	6	19	17
Discipline-Discharge	4.0	4.5	4.4	4.3	4.6	4.5	3.6	3.8	3.8	3.6	4.4	4.0	7	2	3
Job Analysis	4.0	3.8	4.4	3.9	4.4	4.4	3.8	4.0	4.2	3.7	4.3	4.3	8	7	1
Morale-Opinion Surveys	3.8	4.0	3.4	3.9	3.9	3.5	3.7	3.7	3.5	3.4	4.0	3.7	8	14	14
Human Resource Planning	3.9	3.9	4.2	4.0	4.2	4.2	3.5	4.1	4.0	3.4	4.0	3.9	10	7	7
Vacation-Leaves	3.8	4.4	4.0	3.9	4.4	4.0	3.4	3.8	3.3	3.3	4.3	3.5	11	7	12
Wage Salary Admin.	3.8	4.2	4.0	3.6	4.6	4.1	3.6	4.1	4.0	3.4	4.5	4.0	11	3	4
Employee Counseling	3.6	4.0	3.9	3.9	4.3	3.9	3.5	3.7	3.6	3.4	4.0	3.8	13	13	9
Safety	3.7	3.5	3.4	3.6	3.6	3.3	3.7	2.9	3.1	3.6	3.6	3.1	13	20	19
Collective Bargaining	3.3	3.7	2.4	3.7	3.8	2.4	3.6	3.5	1.9	3.3	3.5	2.2	15	18	23
Performance Appraisal	3.7	4.4	4.2	3.8	4.4	4.3	3.3	3.6	3.5	3.3	4.3	4.0	15	5	6
Employment Selection	3.5	3.9	4.2	3.9	3.7	3.9	3.3	3.8	3.7	3.2	3.9	3.8	17	14	9
Promotions	3.6	4.3	3.8	3.7	3.9	3.7	3.2	3.9	3.7	3.0	4.2	3.6	18	11	14
Orientation	3.5	4.2	4.0	3.4	4.1	3.8	3.4	3.9	3.7	3.0	3.9	3.7	19	11	12
Training-Development	3.1	3.9	3.4	3.4	3.7	3.2	3.4	3.6	3.2	3.2	4.1	3.4	20	17	17
Community Service	3.3	2.8	2.4	3.3	3.0	2.4	3.3	2.6	2.5	3.2	2.7	2.4	20	23	22
Employee Newsletter	3.0	3.4	2.8	3.1	3.1	2.8	3.1	2.5	2.7	2.9	2.9	2.9	22	21	21
Recreation-Social	2.8	2.7	3.3	3.1	3.2	3.2	3.2	2.9	2.8	3.0	2.8	2.8	23	22	20
Food Service	2.0	2.2	1.8	2.1	2.5	1.9	1.9	1.6	1.6	1.9	2.5	1.6	24	24	24
Mean	3.6	3.8	3.6	3.7	3.9	3.6	3.6	3.5	3.4	3.4	3.9	3.5			

such training could be facilitated by the personnel department. For instance, through designing policy statements, by performing various housekeeping functions, and by proposing means to measure training results, the personnel department may play a significant role in nurse training. Performance appraisal is another example of a duty important to the manager and the personnel department, yet one which the nursing directors rated no higher than fifteenth. Specialized assistance should be available to the nursing department from the personnel department in developing and administering appraisal forms and appraisal interviews.

There is rather close agreement between the administrators and personnel directors as to the desired role of the personnel department. This agreement, coupled with the strong expression of support for the personnel department by the administrators, suggests that the status and influence of the personnel department is growing in the hospital. The personnel department appears to be in an excellent position to make increasingly positive contributions to the hospital.

Differences between responses by the nursing directors and those of the administrators and personnel directors call for improved communication by all involved.

It is of considerable importance that nursing directors, as well as administrators and personnel directors, be able to differentiate between the various duties of personnel administration and the various activities within those duties.

Certainly a study such as reported here can be conducted within any hospital to determine the views of key management personnel concerning current and desired personnel administration practices.

It is unrealistic to combine all personnel duties and conclude that directors of the various hospital units desire the same personnel department involvement. Each duty requires separate consideration. Similarly, it is necessary to identify which activities—Policy, Advice, Service, or Control—are desired for each duty.

These distinctions, and the proven ability by the respondent to make these distinctions, provide a strong base for more effective planning and implementation of personnel administration practices within the nursing unit.

References

1. This study is adapted from the method for business firms reported in Harold C. White and Michael N. Wolfe, "The Role Derived for Personnel Administration," *Personnel Administrator* 25 (June):87–98, 1980.
2. Frank O. Hoffman, "Identity Crisis in the Personnel Function," *Personnel Journal* 57 (March):126–132+, 1978.
3. Douglas Benton and Harold C. White, "Satisfaction of Job Factors for Registered Nurses," *The Journal of Nursing Administration* 2 (November–December):55–63, 1972.

CHAPTER 7

Managing By Behavior And Results—Linking Supervisory Accountability To Effective Organizational Control

by JoAnn Johnson and Kathy Luciano

Of all the components of the management process, control has received the least attention in nursing. These authors present a performance management program that provides nursing administrators with an effective control system, yet maximizes individual professional accountability.

Of all of the components of the management process—planning, organizing, coordinating, staffing, directing, and controlling—the latter has received the least attention in nursing. This has been partially due to a perceptual bias on the part of nurses that control should be an internalized process rather than an external process instituted by nurse administrators. This bias has been reinforced by nursing's move towards greater professionalism. In an extensive review of the literature to distinguish among the concepts of responsibility, authority, autonomy, and accountability, Lewis and Batey emphasized autonomy and accountability as critical elements of professionalism[1,2]. They defined accountability as "the fulfillment of a formal obligation to disclose to referent others the purposes, principles, procedures, relationships, results, income, and expenditures for which one has authority," and control as "the application of sanctions, both positive and negative, in an effort to coordinate interorganizational effort to facilitate movement toward organizational goals"[3,4]. Although, they recognized the legitimacy of control structures, they did not emphasize the relationship between accountability and control.

Sherwin supports Lewis and Batey's distinction between accountability and control. He defined control as "action which adjust operations to predetermined standards, and its

JoAnn Johnson, R.N., D.P.A., is a Professor of Nursing, California State University at Los Angeles, California.

Kathy Luciano, R.N., M.S., C.N.A.A., is Vice-President for Nursing Services at Presbyterian Intercommunity Hospital, Whittier, California.

basis is information in the hands of managers"[5]. His perception of control meaning action is consistent with Lewis and Batey's use of control as decision making and evaluation. Likewise, Sherwin's recognition that control is based upon information in the hands of managers is congruent with Lewis and Batey's concept of accountability in terms of disclosure of information pertinent to one's responsibilities. However, Lewis and Batey added a new dimension by establishing that one who acts autonomously and uses his or her authority to meet assigned responsibility concommitantly accepts that one has as obligation to disclose and to be "answerable for what one has done, to stand behind one's decisions and actions"[6]. Building on that concept, we believe that control responsibilities clearly rest with the nursing administrator and accountability resides with his or her subordinates in nursing services.

Given that premise, the question then raised is how to effectively put the concepts of accountability and control into practice within a nursing services department. One strategy identified in personnel management literature, and utilized by Presbyterian Intercommunity Hospital's Nursing Services, is that of Managing by Behavior and Results (MBR). This strategy was created by Brumback to describe "a hybrid of behaviorally-oriented performance appraisal and results-oriented MBO"[7].

Management by objectives (MBO), a results-oriented evaluation process, has enjoyed great popularity since its introduction by Drucker in the 1950's[8]. However, according to Levinson, experience with MBO has resulted in the recognition of some major limitations: (a) MBO involves a process that needs frequent contacts between a subordinate and superior, even day–to-day contacts; (b) It is difficult to incorporate and reward creativity and innovation; (c) It ignores the interdependence aspect of work and may inhibit teamwork[9]. The latter two criticisms are especially important in the delivery of cost-effective nursing service. Schneier and Beatty recognized that "a 'results at any price' philosophy often rewards behaviors which can be harmful to an organization in the long run but which may facilitate short run attainment"[10]. They recommend that a more effective approach would be to ask "how do we use MBO to set goals *and* develop specific information on how to attain them"[11].

Brumback and McFee's MBR approach to performance appraisal addresses this question by integrating performance appraisal into a performance management process in which *both* an individual's behavior on the job and the results achieved are considered important. Their rationale for the MBR focus is that human performance is a result of two interactions: (a) personal factors such as knowledge, skill, abilities, and motivation; and (b) situational factors such as forces in the internal work setting or external environment which assist or hinder performance. The interaction of these two variables (personal factors and situational factors) results in outcomes that can be identified as either behaviors or results[12]. Thompson also saw human performance as an interaction between a person who brings aspirations and capabilities to the situation and the organizational environment which offers both opportunities and constraints[13]. This rationale for human performance "tells us not to neglect behaviors at the expense of results, or vice versa, and not to look only to the performer or only to the environment for answers to performance problems"[14].

Shifting the focus of attention from performance appraisal to performance management enables a nursing administrator to incorporate all of the following functions: "performance planning, performance monitoring, performance appraisal, performance reinforcement, performance prediction, and development"[15]. It provides a conceptual framework for the nursing service department to integrate administrative responsibility for organizational control with subordinate accountability, a need advocated by Lewis and Batey[16].

Presbyterian Intercommunity Hospital (PIH) is a 358-bed, JCAH accredited hospital that serves six Los Angeles County communities. In addition to a commitment to quality patient care, PIH serves as a clinical facility for the University of Southern California School of Medicine and for community college, baccalaureate, and graduate nursing students. Since her arrival in 1975, the Vice President for Nursing Services has made major process and structural changes within the nursing department: the percentage of RN's to LVN/aides was increased fro 30 percent RN's and to 70 percent LVN/aides/clerks to 65 percent RN's and 35 percent LVN's/aids/clerks; all nursing units converted from team nursing to a complete patient care system or primary nursing; the department was reorganized to decentralize authority; a performance evaluation system for supervisory level personnel was implemented to measure the management process; and a Performance Indicator Program* was utilized to gather current statistical data on

operations from each nursing unit. These changes are all elements of a performance management program that is designed to meet the organizational control needs of the nursing administrator. At the same time, it provides her management staff with the freedom to exercise authority to meet responsibilities.

We present the following not as a perfect model but as our willingness to share with colleagues the process, achievements, and struggles experienced in introducing a performance management program, as well as to identify gaps which still need to be addressed.

Performance planning

Initially, the organizational structure of PIH's Nursing Service was changed to reflect the desire of the nursing administrator to decentralize authority for the management process, utilize a higher percentage of RN staff, and meet the demand by nursing unit supervisors (head nurse level) for greater autonomy, status, and salary in exchange for carrying out increased charges. Simultaneously, job descriptions identified new responsibilities for unit supervisors and department heads. These structural changes were prerequisites to beginning performance planning. Then goals and objectives could be developed to identify realistic areas of accountability for the supervisory staff. Brumback and McFee consider the planning phase as the most critical phase of a performance management program "because having goals and objectives provides the performer with initial direction and a source of motivating challenge"[17]. This phase also includes determining resources, setting priorities and establishing standards[18].

Developing agreed upon performance standards for unit supervisors was an essential element in our planning phase and represents an area which still needs refinement. Exhibit 1 shows five (out of the nineteen) current Standards for the Nursing Unit Supervisor. These standards incorporate behavior and results and attempt to discriminate outstanding, very good, and satisfactory performance. Any behavior that falls below that described as satisfactory is unacceptable. Indicators of unsatisfactory behavior were deliberately not specified in the Standards because (a) all Standards reflect acceptable to desired behaviors, so they provide positive direction, and (b) unacceptable behaviors must be identified as they occur and corrective action taken quickly.

In 1978, we wrote Standards for the Nursing Unit Supervisor. At that time, some supervisors were unclear about the meanings of terms listed in the PIH Management Performance Summary (Exhibit 2). Because unit supervisors requested written job expectations for meeting the management activities of forecasting, budgeting, developing poli-

*The Performance Indicator Program was developed by Steven S. Cohn, President, Medical Management Planning, Inc., 21241 Ventura Blvd., Woodland Hills, California 91364.

EXHIBIT 1
PRESBYTERIAN INTERCOMMUNITY HOSPITAL
Whittier, California
Management Performance Summary
Standards for the Nursing Unit Supervisor

*A sample of five Standards for the Nursing Unit Supervisor out of a total of nineteen standards

ACTIVITY	STANDARD	SCORE
Forecasting	Outstanding Performance (9–10 points) 1.1 Consults with directors about predicted changes in unit operations based upon knowledge of: (a) trends in nursing practice (b) medical care technology (c) changing patient population. Very Good Performance (8 points) 1.1 Seeks clarification from directors about changes in unit operations when trends are new or unfamiliar to supervisor. Satisfactory Performance (6–7 points) 1.1 Expects that new visions for nursing practice will originate from directors while supervisor maintains the status quo.	
Programming and establishing the sequence and priority of action steps to be followed in reaching objectives	Outstanding Performance (9–10 points) 2.1 Is able to verbalize basic theory about change, including (a) factors causing resistance to change (b) methods for reducing resistance to change (c) steps in the change process (per Lewin). 2.2 Reviews strategies for implementing unit changes with directors. 2.3 Maintains positive, enthusiastic postures during periods of confusion and uncertainty from unit or organizational change. Very Good Performance (8 points) 2.1 Is able to verbalize that most changes will lead to staff resistance but does not delineate specific factors in the change process. 2.2 Asks directors for assistance in developing strategies for unit changes. 2.3 Maintains positive verbal and non-verbal postures during periods of unit or organizational change and may consult with directors about managing staff confusion. Satisfactory Performance (6–7 points) 2.1 Recognizes that change is a process and asks directors to delineate factors that will impact on unit changes. 2.2 Requests from directors strategies to be used during unit changes. 2.3 Maintains positive verbal and non-verbal postures during periods of unit or organizational change and seeks frequent assistance for managing own and staff confusion.	
Scheduling	Outstanding Performance (9–10 points) 3.1 Posts employee monthly time schedules at least 2½ weeks in advance. 3.2 Assures that daily staffing ratios (number of people on duty) are equitable.** 3.3 Is able to motivate staff to work different shifts to cover vacancies or holes in the schedules. 3.4 Keeps time sheets in Nursing Office updated with changes, and without any reminders to do so.	*continued*

	EXHIBIT 1 *continued*	
ACTIVITY	**STANDARD**	**SCORE**
	Very Good Performance (8 points) 3.1 Posts employee monthly time schedules at least two weeks in advance. 3.2 Assures that daily staffing ratios (number of people on duty) are equitable** and may seek assistance for managing vacation requests. 3.3 Manages vacancies or holes in other shifts by working some shifts herself, thus sparing the 7–3 staff from shift rotation. 3.4 Keeps time sheets in Nursing Office updated with changes, and without more than two errors/month. Satisfactory Performance (6–7 points) 3.1 Posts employee monthly schedules at least ten days in advance. 3.2 Requests assistance for developing equitable** scheduling and for managing vacation requests. 3.3 Asks directors to manage vacancies or holes in shift schedules. 3.4 Keeps time sheets in Nursing Office updated with changes, and without more than three errors/month. **"Equitable" means similar numbers of staff (quality and quantity) on duty from one day to the next, especially Monday to Friday.	

Establishing relationships	Outstanding Performance
	(9–10 points)
	4.1 Is cordial and hospitable to patients, families, staff, and physicians at all times, including periods of stress and unit confusion.
	4.2 Demonstrates active listening skills as evidenced by either positive employee/director feedback or by ability to present a situation(s) from another person's point of view.
	4.3 Is supportive of hospital administration and nursing administration and demonstrates this by:
	  (a) seeking clarification about new or unfamiliar policy changes, renovation projects, wage and salary program, etc.
	  (b) portraying to staff an informational and highly positive posture toward administrative programs, policies, and changes.
	  (c) informing staff (verbally and in writing) of administrative responses to employee requests or gripes, (e.g. new benefits, positions, equipment, social events, recognition, etc).
	4.4 Utilizes formal channels of communication to report unit problems, employee status changes, and significant unit operations.
	4.5 Resolves interdepartmental and intradepartmental problems through positive confrontation and negotiation as reflected by an absence of complaints about supervisor's conflict management.
	
	 Very Good Performance
	(8 points)
	4.1 Is cordial and hospitable to patients, families, staff and physicians at all times, except during periods of stress and unit confusion.
	4.2 Demonstrates active listening skills and is empathetic in most instances or with specific employees as reflected in employee feedback.
	4.3 Is usually supportive of hospital administration and nursing administration and demonstrates this by:
	  (a) asking directors to clarify to employees about new or unfamiliar policy changes, renovation projects, wage and salary programs, etc.
	  (b) portraying to staff a posture of "everything will work out" toward administrative programs, policies, and changes.
	  (c) posting information (without verbal reinforcement) of administrative responses to employee requests or gripes.
	4.4 Reports unit problems, employee status changes, and significant unit operations when requested to do so by directors.
	4.5 Requests assistance from director for managing interdepartmental and intradepartmental problem solving and is an active participant in confrontation and negotiation sessions.
		continued

| | EXHIBIT 1 | |
| | *continued* | |

ACTIVITY	STANDARD	SCORE

	<u>Satisfactory Performance</u>
	(6-7 points)
	
	4.1 Is cordial and hospitable to patients, families, staff, and physicians when unit is functioning under optimal circumstances (good staffing, "nice patients, compatible physicians) and is free of stress. Is usually abrupt and rushed during periods of unit confusion.
	4.2 Listens to employees and offers advice/criticism from only supervisor's point of view or personal experiences.
	4.3 Supports hospital administration and nursing administration when requested to do so, and demonstrates this by:
	  (a) referring employees to written information posted about new policies, renovation projects, wage and salary programs, etc.
	  (b) Portraying to staff an attitude of "wait and see" toward administrative programs, policies, and changes.
	  (c) informing staff of new benefits, positions, equipment, social events, recognition, etc., without giving credit to administration responding to employee needs.
	4.4 When reminded to do so, utilizes formal channels of communication for reporting unit problems, employee status changes, and significant unit operations.
	4.5 Asks director to manage interdepartmental and intradepartmental problem solving and either does not participate in the confrontation/-negotiation sessions or plays a passive role in the sessions.	

Personnel development	<u>Outstanding Performance</u> (9-10 points) 5.1 Develops *and* utilizes an up-to-date written, unit-specific orientation program. 5.2 Provides a means for all staff to share with each other the content gained from attendance at seminars. 5.3 Has a staff development plan for each unit RN 5.4 Reads and posts relevant nursing literature on contemporary issues of nursing practice. 5.5 Consults with inservice educators on a frequent basis about learning needs of staff. <u>Very Good Performance</u> (8 points) 5.1 Develops a written unit-specific orientation program that is general in nature; supplements program with verbal information. 5.2 Provides a means for 75% of the staff to share with each other the content gained from attendance at seminars. 5.3 Has a staff development plan for half the unit RNs. 5.4 Reads and posts relevant nursing literature after receiving articles from directors or instructional staff. 5.5 Responds to unsolicited recommendations of inservice educators about learning needs of total staff. <u>Satisfactory Performance</u> (6-7 points) 5.1 Provides new employees with a unit-specific orientation that is verbal and based on a buddy system exclusively. 5.2 Provides a means for 50% of the staff to share with each other the content gained from attendance at seminars. 5.3 Has a staff development plan for new employees (RN) only. 5.4 Posts (but may not read) relevant nursing literature after receiving articles and being requested to post them. 5.5 Utilized inservice educators on a fairly frequent basis, and usually to manage learning needs of *poor* performers.	

cies, and sixteen other factors, the vice president developed job performance standards that described each managerial activity.

In 1979, the vice president recognized that the standards were mere descriptions of managerial behaviors and did not describe *levels* of performance. Therefore, the unit

EXHIBIT 2
Presbyterian Intercommunity Hospital
Whittier, California
MANAGEMENT PERFORMANCE SUMMARY

Name	Dept. No.	Job Title	Hire Date	Last Review

MANAGEMENT FUNCTIONS AND ACTIVITIES

Planning   (Predetermine course of action for departmental services and procedures through the following activities)

1 2 3 4 5 6 7 8 9 10

- Forecasting
- Establishing critical and specific objectives
- Programming and establishing the sequence and priority of action steps to be followed in reaching objectives
- Scheduling
- Budgeting
- Establishing procedures
- Developing policies

Organizing   (Arrange and relate departmental work so that it may be performed most effectively by people)

- Developing organization structure
- Delegating
- Establishing relationships

Leading   (Cause departmental personnel to take effective action)

- Decision making
- Promoting effective communication
- Motivating
- Personnel selection
- Personnel development

Controlling   (Assess and regulate departmental work in progress and work completed through the following activities)

- Establishing performance standards
- Performance measuring
- Performance evaluating
- Performance adjustment

TOTAL POINTS:

supervisor job performance standards were revised to describe the requirements for outstanding, very good, and satisfactory performances. A 19-page draft of the new standards received rigorous reviews by both supervisors and department heads. Revisions to the standards occurred more frequently with such quantitative appraisal factors as the acceptable percent for budget variance, than with qualitative factors. Our current standards were implemented in early 1981.

All job factors are weighted equally. Each managerial activity is scored on a 10-point scale; the maximum number of available points is 190. Once the Management Performance Summary is completed and the points are totaled, the score is converted to a percentage by dividing the number of points the supervisor receives by 190. A supervisory performance grid determines the overall rating of outstanding, very good, satisfactory, or unacceptable performance. Currently, a score of 90–100 percent is outstanding, a 80–89 percent score is very good, a 60–79 percent score is satisfactory, and a score below 60 percent is unacceptable.

Weighting job factors equally can be a limitation for both the supervisor and his or her evaluators. A supervisor who receives a low score (below 6 points) for "establishing relationships" can still achieve an overall very good or outstanding rating because of accomplishments in other areas. However, we see a lack of interpersonal competence as reason to discipline, counsel, and possibly terminate a supervisor.

For this reason, we need to reevaluate the standards in light of their ability to distinguish critical behaviors, as well as to determine an appropriate weighting for each behavior. Another need is to decrease the weight on the forecasting activity at the unit supervisor level and weight more heavily quality assurance elements. This change would be more congruent with unit supervisors' charges and authority.

Performance monitoring

Performance monitoring includes tracking progress, performance feedback, and making adjustments[19]. Monitoring involves identifying "interim indicators of results, observations of behaviors if they are at the top or bottom levels, and any situational interferences"[20]. Such data provides a basis for the nurse administrator to plan with the appropriate subordinates a modification of situational factors or behaviors.

The Performance Indicator Program provides at specified intervals a mechanism for unit supervisors to provide formal disclosure on nine aspects related to their responsibilities. The Performance Indicator Program (PIP) was implemented in 1981 by a hospital administration mandate. The executive management team, which includes the nursing administrator, recognized the need for tighter organizational control as one response to the dilemmas of contemporary health care management. Challenges in quality assurance, financial reimbursement, staffing shortages, and consumer expectations dictated that accountability for managerial responsibility needed to be more formalized and visible. A consultant with expertise in hospital management systems was hired to develop a program for monitoring departmental performance, with performance factors and standards to be identified by the department managers (Exhibit 3).

Nursing Services department heads and supervisors selected those indicators that could possibly reflect the level of nursing unit performance and department management. The PIP was not designed as an autocratic scheme to enforce rigid controls and reduce supervisors autonomy and authority. Rather, it has moved supervisors to more pro-active managerial behaviors and goal setting.

The PIP posed a threat to the few supervisors who were already struggling with meeting the recently revised supervisor performance standards. Counseling, coaching, and support have minimized this threat, although a floundering supervisor will continue to reluctantly respond to problems identified by the program. On the other hand, those supervisors who use the PIP responsibly find the program meaningful, and they are able to orient unit staff to department goals and the measures to achieve those goals.

The PIP is one process that enables unit supervisors to be accountable for their responsibilities as advocated by Lewis and Batey[21]. The evaluation of performance data and resultant decisions fulfill the nurse administrator's charge of effective control.

Performance appraisal

Comparing performance against expectations, determining levels of performance reached, and performance feedback are all components of the appraisal process[22]. Two years experience has shown us that approximately 50 percent of the supervisory staff receive an outstanding performance score, 42 percent a very good score, and 8 percent a satisfactory score. Those supervisors who fall within the satisfactory score category are usually new to their position and need further education and experience regarding the management process. Otherwise, they are well advised to "sharpen up their resumes."

Supervisors are able to appraise their own performance on a month-to-month basis. Formal semi-annual or annual performance reviews hold no surprises. Supervisors are able to easily evaluate their progress on a variety of quantitative factors identified in PIP and in the performance standards. Qualitative factors are manageable by department heads through frequent and relevant feedback to the supervisors. Since the managerial climate at PIH is one of openness, trust, and respect; managers at all levels in the organization are able to ask for and receive informal job-related progress reports.

Formal performance reviews are initiated and completed by a department head, the supervisor's immediate superior.

EXHIBIT 3
THE PERFORMANCE POSTER

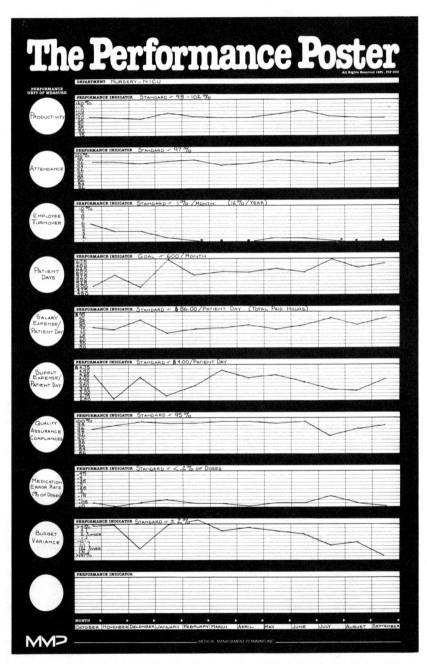

©Steven S. Cohn, President, Medical Management Planning, Woodland Hills, California. Reprinted with permission.

The written Management Performance Summary and any narrative comments are reviewed by both the department head and the vice president for nursing services. Both quantitative and qualitative data are used to support the performance appraisal.

The department head conducts the supervisor appraisal interview. While past performance is reviewed, the focus of this session is to establish new performance goals and list specific steps needed to achieve these goals. The supervisor's self-development plans and the coaching needed from the department head are determined.

Some supervisors who rate in the very good category may be there by deliberate choice, consciously having decided not to strive for the outstanding category. This decision is acceptable to the nursing administrator, although coaching the individual to a higher standard continues. Reweighting some standards will identify more specific critical managerial behaviors, and this may change the distribution of supervisors into the various score categories.

Performance reinforcement

This phase of MBR consists of both determining and applying incentives[23]. For several years, PIH has had an all merit program for staff, supervisors, and department heads. Merit increases are based upon level of achievement and not upon automatic step progression. The amount of a merit increase may vary from one review to the next as levels of performance change.

The timing of performance appraisals, and thus the formal opportunity for positive reinforcement, is based upon assumptions about the learning process. A supervisor is formally appraised six months after beginning the position and again every six months until passing the midpoint of the job salary range. Thereafter, annual reviews occur. We assume that when one is new in a managerial position or has not been in the position long enough to have reached the midpoint of that salary range, he or she is mastering the role. This individual should be expected to demonstrate progress sooner and deserve to be rewarded for that progress. As this program has matured, pay grades have been modified to avoid compression and provide economic incentive. If a supervisor is not mastering the role in expected timeframes, six-months appraisals also enable the department head and the nurse administrator to identify problems and plan prompt corrective actions.

The vice president anticipates a major problem sufficiently rewarding continuous outstanding performance in an environment experiencing increasing economic constraints. Nursing Services currently faces two major dilemmas. The first one is a decrease in operating expense budgets, and the second is a decrease in the amount of dollars available for merit increases. This tightening of the hospital budget occurs at the same time we set in motion greater expectations for managerial performance.

We think one solution to reinforcing outstanding performance is establishing increasingly challenging standards. The outstanding performer, usually a self-directed individual, will aspire to *continued* outstanding performance. Our experience shows that the distribution of supervisors into score categories remained constant even as standards increased. As fiscal controls, staff resource utilization, and quality assurance compliances increased so did the percentage of outstanding or very good performers.

Performance prediction, and development

Having progressed through the previous MBR phases, the nurse administrator, department head, and supervisor now have an adequate data base from which to develop the individual's potential and predict future performance[24]. This then brings one full circle back to the planning stage.

Supervisors have a means for frequent self-appraisal. Department heads can utilize unambiguous standards to measure and monitor a supervisor's performance. Since newer supervisors are evaluated formally every six months, development plans are more timely and specific to identified learning needs.

Supervisory development and coaching must relate to job performance standards. Continuing education programs should be directed towards learning new behaviors that upgrade the supervisor's ability to meet job expectations. A supervisor who controls his or her budget may not need to attend a class on financial management; however, this same supervisor may need to attend an assertiveness training program if he or she has difficulty in establishing relationships.

Conclusion

The MBR process provides a systematic approach for coupling nursing management accountability to effective organizational control. It ensures that sufficient data is generated in a timely manner for necessary decision-making. This approach keeps outstanding performers on their toes. At the same time, a month-to-month self-appraisal gives clues about anyone who is resting on past laurels. Both the nurse administrator and her subordinates share the data base and the creation or modification of standards, thus assuring an open decision-making process.

References

1. Francis M. Lewis and Marjorie V. Batey, "Clarifying Autonomy and Accountability in Nursing Service, Part 1," *The Journal of Nursing Administration,* 12(9), pp. 13-18.
2. Francis M. Lewis and Marjorie V. Batey, "Clarifying Autonomy and Accountability in Nursing Service, Part 2," 12(10), pp. 10-15.
3. Francis M. Lewis and Marjorie V. Batey, "Clarifying Autonomy and Accountability in Nursing Service, Part 2," p. 10.
4. Francis M. Lewis and Marjorie V. Batey, "Clarifying Autonomy and Accountability in Nursing Service, Part 2," p. 12.

5. Douglas S. Sherwin, "The Meaning of Control" in Harold Koontz and Cyril O'Donnel *Management: A Book of Readings,* (New York: McGraw-Hill, 1964), p. 426.

6. Francis M. Lewis and Marjorie V. Batey, "Clarifying Autonomy and Accountability in Nursing Service, Part 2," p. 11.

7. Gary B. Brumback and Thomas S. McFee, "From MBO to MBR," *Public Administration Review,*42(4):365, 1982.

8. Peter F. Drucker, *The Practice of Management,* New York: Harper & Bros., 1954, pp. 121–36.

9. Harry Levinson with adaptations by Elaine L. La Monica "Management by Whose Objectives," *The Journal of Nursing Administration,* 10(9), pp. 23–24, 1980.

10. Craig Eric Schneier and Richard W. Beatty, "Developing Behaviorally-Anchored Rating Scales (BARS)," *The Personnel Administrator,* 24(8), pp. 59, 1979.

11. Craig Eric Schneier and Richard W. Beatty, "Developing Behaviorally-Anchored Rating Scales (BARS)," p. 59.

12. Gary B. Brumback and Thomas McFee, "From MBO to MBR," p. 364.

13. James D. Thompson, *Organizations in Action,* (New York: McGraw-Hill, 1967), pp. 101–102.

14. Gary B. Brumback and Thomas McFee, "From MBO to MBR," p. 364.

15. Gary B. Brumback and Thomas McFee, "From MBO to MBR," p. 364.

16. Francis M. Lewis and Marjorie V. Batey, "Clarifying Autonomy and Accountability in Nursing Service, Part 2," p. 12

17. Gary B. Brumback and Thomas McFee, "From MBO to MBR," p. 364.

18. Gary B. Brumback and Thomas McFee, "From MBO to MBR," p. 365.

19. Gary B. Brumback and Thomas McFee, "From MBO to MBR," p. 365.

20. Gary B. Brumback and Thomas McFee, "From MBO to MBR," p. 368.

21. Francis M. Lewis and Marjorie V. Batey, "Clarifying Autonomy and Accountability in Nursing Service, Part 2," p. 10.

22. Gary B. Brumback and Thomas McFee, "From MBO to MBR," p. 365.

23. Gary B. Brumback and Thomas McFee, "From MBO to MBR," p. 365.

24. Gary B. Brumback and Thomas McFee, "From MBO to MBR," p. 365.

CHAPTER 8

The Causes and Costs of Promotion Trauma

by Lu Ann W. Darling and Loraine G. McGrath

Minimizing the stress that nurses experience after a promotion requires an understanding of the dynamics of fledgling managers. Middle roles such as theirs are inherently difficult. We need to be aware of what can happen in moving up the ladder—factors such as loneliness, other unmet needs and unclear job descriptions evoke unique stresses. Knowing these factors, nursing administrators can plan their programs to better support their managers in transition.

For the past three years, we have been interviewing nurses in metropolitan areas and in small towns in the United States and in Canada about their experiences of moving into management. We have also conducted workshops to assist nurses in managing their upward moves and to ease the trauma of that transition[1]. Of the nurses we have talked to, some have bailed out of management, some even out of nursing. In time others make the transition successfully but carry scars. Few manage the transition with ease. All talk about the needless frustration, and most describe the experience with deep feelings about the trauma associated with the change.

The frustration and pain of these nurses have led us to explore more fully the nature of the transition process into nursing management as it is experienced by nurses. From these explorations, we have identified causes of these traumatic experiences and developed strategies to help nurses caught in the transition process. Although growth of any kind is often painful, the trauma of the transition into nursing management experienced by many nurses appears to exceed healthy growing pains.

Lu Ann W. Darling, Ed.D., is Consultant in Leadership and Organizational Development and the principal of Lu Ann W. Darling and Associates, 11414 Albata St., Los Angeles, California. She has consulted extensively in the health care field.

Loraine G. McGrath, R.N., M.S., is Senior Consultant in Human Relations and personal effectiveness for Effective Management Consultants, San Diego, California.

Helping individual nurses manage their upward moves addresses only one part of the problem. The problem will not be corrected until nursing administrators are more aware of the causes and costs of promotion trauma and initiate programs to stem it.

Many of the facts about the transition process are known to nursing administrators, but this information does not appear to be widely used. Since retaining top quality nurses and achieving optimum performance are important management goals, the causes and costs of promotion trauma must be addressed.

In this article, we plan to focus on what we see as the four major causes and costs of promotion trauma: the unawareness of the transition process, unclear role descriptions and expectations, unmet needs, and unplanned programs of followup. In a subsequent article, we will outline actions nursing administrators can take to manage the promotional process and ease the trauma of transition.

The unawareness of the transition process

We identify three factors that make promotion a traumatic experience for nurses: the extent to which the change is experienced as cutting important social and professional ties; the extent to which the change is accompanied with decreased need gratification; and related to the first two, the extent to which change results in feelings of isolation and lack of support.

A promotion, like any transition, starts with an *ending;* and endings require giving up and letting go of things that have been[2]. What has ended in a nursing move to a higher position are aspects of professional identity and social relationships. In assuming management responsibilities, nurses end an exclusive concentration on the patient and the bedside, peer relationships with coworkers, and an exclusively clinical focus.

Where previously they were responsible only for themselves and the care of patients assigned to them for a shift, they now are responsible for a total work group and for overall patient care. They have exchanged a relatively care-free status for responsibilities and burdens that often extend beyond the end of their shift. They find that supervisory work is rarely ever completed. Their promotion means giving up the immediate rewards in patient care for uncertain and unknown long-term rewards. They give up an acknowledged and accepted role in the work group and move into a position separate and apart, with only infrequent contact with new peers. Our informants were surprised by the aloneness they experienced in the transition. They felt they could handle things as long as their support system remained intact. When that was disrupted, they encountered serious difficulties.

The promotional change also brings greater visibility and prestige. Although this is exciting at first, nurses tell us they often wish for the blessed anonymity of their old job. Former coworkers are now employees keeping an eye on the bosses, often trying to "psych" them out. Everything new managers do becomes the subject of conversation. The eyes of nursing administrations are on them, anxiously appraising and judging their progress. Envious staff members watch to see if they will stub their toes.

The managers have a difficult period of adjustment especially when being liked and being of service are important needs. They meet frustration instead of satisfaction in their need to be of service. They receive complaints instead of appreciation from their staff. Under these conditions, it is easy to feel guilty and inadequate, nurses tell us, because no matter how they try they cannot satisfy everyone. In fact, working long hours in order to make things "right" can even boomerang on their personal lives; both the personal and professional aspects of their lives become unfulfilling.

After about six months of this experience, new managers either bail out or make an adjustment. They conclude that if they are to survive in their new role, they must accept that their job is not finished at the end of the shift. They no longer stay late every night, no longer feel guilty about going home, and are now ready to settle for respect from staff rather than being liked.

The move into management is a move into a middle role in the organization. Middle roles are inherently difficult. In Oshry's study's[3], he finds that persons in middle positions tend to work at a hectic pace; they see their role as insignificant yet feel a heavy responsibility for keeping the system together and making it work. They receive very little support, reinforcement, or gratitude from people either at the top or bottom of the organization. They find themselves confused and ambivalent on many issues in their attempts to be responsive both to the top and the bottom. And, not surprisingly, they feel isolated and lonely.

Middle-group members do not experience the same closeness, intimacy, and usual respect of bottoms. The solidarity of the work group is in sharp contrast to the lack of group feeling, isolation and antagonism among middle group members. Although work-group members disagree with each other, fight and quarrel, an overriding sense of family intimacy exists among them that is absent from the middle group.[4].

Persons in middle positions also tend to personalize their experiences, attributing whatever difficulties they are having to their own personal failings. Oshry finds that this experience is common for all persons in middle positions, regardless of their ability or competence. Interestingly, this holds true even in experimental workshops where executives are randomly assigned to middle positions.

"It is easy to feel guilty and inadequate . . ."

In addition to self-blame, which is common among middles, there is a tendency for other people to see them as hard working but not very competent. Oshry maintains that this is a disease of middleness when it is not managed, but he maintains that the disease is treatable. Indeed, he stresses the great potential of the middle position when the dynamics of middleness are managed. Nurses in middle roles can have a broader perspective of the nursing organization than others: a more detailed picture than the people in upper management and a more global perspective than staff nurses at the unit level[5]. As nursing middles tap this potential, they can be a tremendous positive force for organizations.

The hazard, however, is that nurses in the middle are caught in the conflict between those at the top of the organization and those at the bottom, each pulling or pushing in an attempt to have their own needs met. Many middles resolve the conflict by becoming "telephone wires," not having an opinion of their own but simply transmitting messages back and forth from the top to the bottom. They lose the respect of both tops and bottoms when they act in this manner. Others resolve the conflict by becoming "stuck down," that is, by identifying with the work group rather than with management and allying themselves with the group as *us* against the *them* of management. Still others resolve the conflict by aligning themselves with the top of the organizations and become in Oshry's words "stuck up."

None of these three common ways of eliminating the inherent conflict in the middle role taps the potential of the role for enhancing the problem-solving ability of the organization. The middle role needs to be a role separate from top and bottom while providing links up and down the organization[6].

The middle role is a difficult role regardless of the profession or setting. By acknowledging this difficulty and reminding ourselves of the personal needs of persons who tend to enter the nursing profession and of the difficulties inherent in the transition to a nursing management role, we can begin to see the magnitude of the problem. We can begin to appreciate why the transition is traumatic for so many nurses. The problem is unnecessarily complicated by the next major factor we will address, unclear job descriptions and expectations.

Unclear role descriptions and expectations

Too often what passes for negotiation with candidates for promotional positions can more accurately be described as a courtship process. The nurse is persuaded to leave her unit for the vague but shiny new position, responding to the we-need-you-more-than-they-do message. She is asked to put her faith in the nursing administration persuader and to give up her present satisfactions for some unknown future. A nurse, particularly in a first promotion, responds all too easily to those appeals that touch her ego or her pride as she is asked to consider "the good of the organization." Unfortunately, the courtship process fails to acknowledge the impact of the promotional change on the candidate—on cutting ties, on diminishing need gratification, and on moving into unknown groups.

Discussion of the promotional position commonly is not buttressed with specific information about the management position, nor are the expectations which nursing management holds made explicit. Job descriptions are inadequate. We have been surprised to hear from most of our informants that either the job description did not exist in writing or did not match the job.

In addition, how the promotional position fits in the management ranks of nursing and the hospital often is not made clear. It occurs to us that this may be because it is not clear to the representatives of nursing management who are involved in the promotional interview. Is the role being discussed a part of management, a steppingstone to management or is it a charge position only and not considered part of the management team? Undiscussed assumptions such as these on the part of management and the new promotee can impact negatively on the new manager's effectiveness if there is a marked disparity in those assumptions. Furthermore, transitional problems differ with differing roles.

For example, the role of *relief charge* is usually the first taste of management beyond the team leader position. The expressed concerns of nurses in this role have caused us to refer to this group as *the "commuters."* The relief charge nurses commute back and forth between a work group culture (as one of the staff) and the management culture (as an arm of supervision). This creates unique difficulties for the persons in the role. They must be careful not to alienate their peers on those days they are in charge or their life as staff nurses will be miserable. Yet they are expected to take charge and keep the unit running smoothly. Small wonder

that they are cautious in exerting any leadership and work to maintain their identity with the work group. This easily leads to criticism by management about their not being more decisive, not providing strong leadership.

The transition to charge nurse seems to involve little change in professional identity, perspective, and social relationships compared with the head nurse role. Although the charge nurses themselves can feel fairly unconflicted by the promotion, if they enact the role of working supervisor by identifying strongly with the work group rather than management, they are likely not to meet management's expectations.

"The job description . . . did not match the job."

The assistant head nurse role, particularly when it is used as a second-in-command on a nursing unit, is highly ambiguous. The content of the role seems to vary greatly depending on the personal desires of the head nurses. Often they are or appear to be only "gofers" or flunkies. Sometimes they are expected to be morale builders and motivators or special project persons. At no time have we found the position to be one in which disciplining employees is regularly required, nor are they held accountable for employee performance as are the head nurses. Such persons seems able to get a taste of the fun of management with little of the responsibility. They can bump sticky problems up to the head nurses for resolution and continue to have gratification from both patient care and peer relationships.

For some managerial roles, there are hidden expectations, rarely made explicit, that make the difference between job success and failure for an otherwise well-qualified candidate. We refer here to the hurdle we call the "Special Care Olympics." Special care units often have a clinical bias, and clinical expertise is an unstated prerequisite for acceptance of the new manager by the staff and by the physicians. When this has not been previously discussed with them, nurses who are later judged by these criteria feel abused and in a no-win situation.

Unmet needs

The third aspect of the causes and costs of promotion trauma relates to unmet needs. We are concerned that the rosy glow of the promotion causes nursing management and the new promotee to gloss over the disruption of need gratification that is taking place, a disruption the nurse may not be aware of until the honeymoon period comes to a close. The work of Kelley and Connor[8] helps us understand the emotional cycle experienced by the nurse involved in this change.

The authors contend that the emotional cycle is universal for any change, whether voluntary or involuntary. Understanding the cycle can alert nursing administrators to potential problems that need to be addressed.

The emotional cycle takes the form of a bell-shaped curve with the height of the curve indicating the individual's dissatisfaction with the change at a given point in time. Five stages are described. In the first stage, dissatisfaction is low and enthusiasm high; this stage is characterized by "uninformed optimism" and a feeling of sureness and certainty, a veritable honeymoon period. The new managers are bubbling with enthusiasm; they simply do not, nor can they have, sufficient information to be aware of all the problems that lie ahead. Enthusiasm serves a purpose, however, though uninformed: it is essential if the nurses are to be sufficiently energized to undertake the change at all.

The dissatisfaction level rises as reality sets in, moving the person to the second phase of "informed pessimism." This phase is accompanied with heavy feelings of doubt and dismay. The nursing managers experience the cutting of ties and the sense of aloneness and alienation. The time they are devoting to their work often causes deterioration in their personal life. They may be burning out from working long hours and from feeling unacknowledged, unliked, unappreciated, and unrewarded. These factors cause them to be at the most vulnerable stage of the change cycle and the one where bailout is most likely to occur.

As the nursing managers work through this period, they move on to the stage of "hopeful realism," then experience the confidence of "informed optimism," and finally reach the satisfying final stage of "rewarding completion."

We are particularly concerned with the vulnerability of the new person during the stage of "informed pessimism," when the full impact of the new role—the costs as well as the benefits—sinks in. Hence the significance of the fourth cause of promotion trauma, unplanned programs of follow-up.

Unplanned programs of follow-up

We have yet to talk to newly promoted nursing managers who felt they had a good systematic program of follow-up during the transition process. Intentions may well have been good; but whether due to the lack of a systematic program or the pressures of other activities, the general pattern, we are told, is a brief orientation of the new manager and then spotty follow-up. Coaching tends to be informal and on the fly; learning is trial and error.

New nonsupervisory nursing employees seem to be monitored with more consistency and concern than new managers, perhaps because of the legal ramifications for patient care. On-the-job training for nursing managers tends to be informal and often is not completed because of the pressures and priorities of other work. Few hospitals in our sample provide systematic, formal management training.

There are a few oases in this parched follow-up desert, but the common mode seems to be the sink-or-swim approach.

This approach may be the result of preoccupation with other problems or a true unawareness of the costs of promotion trauma. Whatever the reason, lack of attention to follow-up is shortsighted and costly. Too often first-line supervisors are given little attention by upper management. They tend to be taken for granted rather than welcomed and initiated into management ranks. In fact, the rites seem more similar to fraternity hazings. In the role play "Roberta's World," that we use in the Transition Seminar, we are struck with the tendency of those who play Roberta's boss, the OR supervisors, to let the nurses struggle alone. We can appreciate the attitude of not wanting to spoon feed the new managers. She must learn to stand on her own feet, but we contend that the result is too extreme in the other direction.

"The first state . . . is . . . uninformed optimism . . ."

The response we observe has been too frequent to assume that this is an isolated occurence. Typical of the comments of those who play the bosses are these:

> "Roberta will be a bit of a pain, she'll be idealistic, want to make a lot of changes, and want everything done yesterday."

> "It will take time away from our jobs to coach her."

> "We don't want her to fail so we'll help her, but there's a lot of things we won't tell her—she'll just have to find out by herself."

We have found these attitudes about Roberta expressed by nurses in both the United States and Canada. The attitudes are surprisingly consistent: that it's a relief to have the job filled, but directing Roberta will be a chore; that "we'll let her find out for herself as we did"; that "we'll watch her, see how she does, and see if she makes the grade." There is distancing behavior, not wanting to associate oneself too closely with Roberta for fear that the supervisor may have made a poor selection and that, if Roberta doesn't work out, it may reflect adversely on the supervisor's reputation. The norms revealed by these comments, in our opinion, pose serious problems for nursing management.

The new nursing manager is a fragile commodity, one that requires careful handling for the journey into management if damage and loss is not to occur. We feel that promotional trauma can be minimized and that we do not have to lose good nurses because of their experiences in the transition.

The focus of this article has been on the causes and costs of promotion trauma. We have outlined four major causes of promotion trauma: the unawareness of the transition process, unclear role descriptions and expectations, unmet needs, and unplanned programs of follow-up. In a later article, we will outline actions nursing administrators can take to lessen the traumatic aspects of promotional transitions and help promotees achieve the expected level of competence in a shorter period of time.

References and note

1. Our interviews and experiences have been almost entirely with female nurses, and the thoughts expressed in this article may not apply as readily to men moving into nursing management.
2. W. Bridges, *Transitions* (Reading, Mass.: Addison-Wesley, 1980), p. 11.
3. B. Oshry, *Middle Power* (Boston: Power & Systems Training, P.O. Box 388, Prudential Station, 1980), pp. 8–10.
4. B. Oshry and K.E. Oshry, "Middle-Group Dynamics," in W.W. Burke and L.D. Goodstein, eds., *Trends and Issues in Organizational Development* (San Diego: University Associates, 1980), p. 59.
5. B. Oshry and K.E. Oshry, "Middle-Group Dynamics, p. 53.
6. B. Oshry, *Power and Position* (Boston: Power & Systems Training, P.O. Box 388, Prudential Station, 1977), p. 53.
7. J.P. Kotter, "The Psychological Contract: Managing the Join-up Process," *California Management Review* 15(3):91–99, 1973.
8. D. Kelley and D.R. Connor, "The Emotional Cycle of Change, in *Annual Handbook for Group Facilitators* (San Diego: University Associates, 1979), pp. 117–122.

CHAPTER 9

Minimizing Promotion Trauma

by LuAnn W. Darling and Loraine G. McGrath

In the April 1983 issue of JONA, the authors identified four major causes and the costs of promotion trauma. Nursing administrators can both minimize this trauma and its unnecessary cost by building awareness of the transition process, clarifying roles and expectations, and attending to the promoted employee's needs by developing a systematic program of manager care. Such support and encouragement can help promotees achieve the expected levels of competency in a shorter period of time, with less personal anguish. This article will help nursing administrators to develop a concept of manager care buttressed with programs for orientation of new managers, skills of mentoring, and systems of monitoring.

In a previous article[1] we discussed the trauma many nurses experience in moving into nursing management because of unawareness of the transition process, unclear role descriptions and expectations, unmet needs, and a lack of planning for followup. The costs of promotion trauma are high. In an era where retaining top-quality nurses and achieving optimum performance are important management goals, the causes and costs of promotion trauma must be addressed.

In the present article we outline actions nursing administrators can take to manage the promotional process, minimize the trauma of that transition, and help promotees achieve the expected levels of competency in a shorter period of time. While we pay particular attention to the nurses moving into their first promotional transition, many comments apply to nurses making any promotional change.

Lu Ann W. Darling, Ed.D., is Consultant in Leadership and Organizational Development and the principal of Lu Ann W. Darling and Associates, 11414 Albata St., Los Angeles, California. She has consulted extensively in the health care field.

Loraine G. McGrath, R.N., M.S., is Senior Consultant in Human Relations and personal effectiveness for Effective Management Consultants, San Diego, California.

We address four action steps significant for the nursing administrator: building awareness of the transition process, clarifying roles and expectations, attending to needs, and developing a systematic program of manager care.

Building awareness of the transition process

In the typical organization, reports Frohman[2], it takes three years for professional employees to perform at 75 percent of their capacity. Such a learning curve is repeated every time a job or assignment or supervisor is changed. According to Frohman there are two sets of reasons: factors associated with the work itself and those revolving around how a person is brought into a new position and managed. Organizations that pay attention to the way a person is brought into a position have better records of job satisfaction, productivity, and length of stay[3].

For this reason the first consideration in minimizing promotion trauma is building awareness of the transition process throughout nursing management—at the top, at middle levels where supervisors are responsible for the coaching and direction of new managers, and at the new manager's level itself.

The most important factors in bringing new managers aboard effectively are the skills of their supervisors. Kotter finds that the process is facilitated if the supervisors have skills in (1) giving and receiving feedback, (2) articulating expectations and performance criteria, (3) explaining realistic decisions passed down from above, (4) coaching and helping, and (5) communicating and understanding the new manager's problems[4].

The starting point of any skill building for middle level supervisors is increasing their awareness of the transition process so they can acquire positive attitudes toward coaching, supervising, and serving as mentors to their new managers. Without such awareness supervisors easily tend to let the new person struggle through the transition by trial and error and to keep a safe, noncontaminating distance in the event the new manager should fail.

New managers need awareness, too, in order to manage their own movement through the transition process. With awareness comes more objectivity, a recognition of the commonness of the situation and less likelihood to assume personal failure and blame themselves for all the difficulties they are experiencing in the new job.

Images are helpful in building awareness. Useful for understanding the new manager's situation are analogies from the changing seasons and from the human life cycle, particularly pregnancy. In pregnancy the first trimester is recognized as being of critical importance in providing a healthy climate for the embryo. In gardening we recognize the need to protect plants, especially young ones, from abrupt weather changes. In harsh winter climes plants are often moved indoors or put into a greenhouse. Gardeners try to start new plants or seedlings in an environment where the climate can be controlled and optimal growing conditions provided.

When we transplant a growing thing, we exercise care to ensure that the plant does not suffer trauma. Unfortunately the same care is not always exhibited in transplanting people. Levinson uses this analogy:

> If we move a tree, we sever its roots gradually, adding more fertilizer, and then place it in an already prepared site. All too often executives assume people need no such attention. Then managements complain that people are resistant to change, as if something were wrong with the people [5].

Building images of trees and trimesters encourages discussion on growth, on change, on loss. It clarifies the importance of endings to prepare for new beginnings, the importance of honoring whatever sense of mourning is experienced with the change, and the need to gain a perspective on loss and change. At the same time the emotional cycle that most individuals go through with a change, whether the change is voluntary or not, can be reviewed. After the honeymoon pessimism often sets in as reality dawns, but this should change into hopeful realism and ultimately the achievement of a sense of competency in the new position[6].

Awareness of the pitfalls of transition and of ways to avoid them can begin with reading articles such as this. For both middle level supervisors and promotees awareness needs to be reinforced by educational programs affording opportunities for interaction and discussions of all aspects of the transition. An outside facilitator can often help to focus the process and maximize the time spent. The transition will be smoother if roles and expectations are clear from the start.

Clarifying roles and expectations

The decision nurses make about accepting a promotion and their movement through the transition process can be facilitated greatly by spelling out role descriptions and expectations when the possibility of promotion is first suggested. A starting point is a written job description, which should be reviewed by management for currency and relevancy before the interviewing process is begun. It is amazing how seldom this is done.

"... the first consideration in minimizing promotion trauma is building awareness of the transition process throughout nursing management..."

In view of the ambiguity of some nursing management roles, each supervisory role in nursing should be clarified as to its status in the hierarchy of hospital management and the expectations accompanying that status[7]. For example, ambiguous aspects of the assistant head nurse role need clarification, particularly the difference in content and responsibility that exists between this role and that of the head nurse.

It may seem unnecessary to state the obvious, but because of the number of reports to the contrary, we urge nursing administrators to insist on candid and honest discussions of roles and role expectations when their representatives are negotiating with candidates for promotional positions. The significance of full and candid discussions of expectations is brought home by Kotter's research on the joining-up process[8]. Often mismatches in expectations exist from the very beginning of employment or promotional discussions but are unrecognized. The cost of these unrecognized mismatches is high. After the first year on the job Kotter finds that employees tend to experience mismatches as disappointments; they then slow down their growth efforts and become only moderately productive and creative.

Mismatches occur because individuals tend to have higher expectations than the organization regarding the personal development opportunities they are likely to be offered, the amount of interesting work, and the amount of meaning or purpose in their work. On the other hand the organization has higher expectations than the individual about the person's ability to work with groups and the person's acceptance of organizational values and willingness to conform. Kotter finds that the extent to which expectations are thought through by each party, are communicated to the other, and are agreed upon has a significant bearing on job satisfaction, productivity, and length of stay of the new person. The discussion of expectations should include not only the mandatory aspects of the job but also the areas of freedom afforded the new manager to make decisions and initiate improvements.

When role negotiation discussions are full and candid the candidate for promotion and the supervisor share information about themselves and establish agreed-upon expectations. Both roles are thereby defined in relation to the other, and both persons know what is expected of each role. This understanding brings much needed commitment and stability to the relationship. Sooner or later however, disruption is bound to occur because of some violation of expectations by one of the parties or because of some external change[9]. Whenever either person feels a pinch in the relationship, it is time to review and renegotiate role expectation. A climate needs to be established that fosters open discussion and encourages the use of role renegotiation methods such as are described by Harrison[10].

Different nursing management positions vary greatly as to the extent to which the manager needs to build relationships outside the unit and to understand the broader hospital system in order to obtain needed resources. Relief charge nurses have little need to deal with what has been called "power dependence"[11]. By contrast, head nurses must be particularly sensitive to job-related dependence since they do not have control over all the resources needed to do the job effectively. Awareness of the need to develop good relationships with the people or groups on whom they depend is essential. Yet people in their first management jobs often display an insensitivity to job-related dependence that later gets them into trouble[12]. For this reason power dependence or job-related dependence should be discussed in the role negotiation process.

In our previous article[13], we discussed the problems faced by persons in middle positions in organizations, particularly the fragmentation and isolation that often occurs. We also mentioned the great potential of the middle position when the dynamics of middleness are managed[14]. Nurses in middle roles can have a broad perspective of the nursing organization, more detailed than that in upper management and more global than that at the staff level. As nursing middles tap this potential they can be a very positive force for the hospital. In order to develop this potential they need to meet together and learn to handle job-related dependence.

Anxiety often arises within the ranks of upper management, however, when middle managers get together and become a strong, effective group. Nursing administrators have to consider just how strong they want the middle managers to be. If their goal is to develop a strong group, they must encourage head nurses to build peer relationships with one another, to meet alone as a group, and to devise alternate ways of sharing their information and solving their problems. The philosophy about middle role needs to be discussed in the role negotiation process.

Attending to needs

All human beings have a basic need for a self-image that is both accurate and acceptable[15]. How we see ourselves must be a reasonable reflection of reality and must be acceptable to us. We verify our own self-image and expand the self through association with other people who are mirrors, models, and recipients of our actions. We also verify our self-image through our own purposeful activities.

"The transition will be smoother if roles and expectations are clear from the start."

In their move into management many nurses experience difficulty that stems from their need to be liked and need to be of service[16]. These needs, formerly met by direct patient care and peer friendships, are now disrupted and unmet. The new manager frequently tries to compensate by working long hours to master the work and to earn the respect and liking of others, but unfortunately often ends up feeling unacknowledged, unliked, unappreciated, and unrewarded. This is the most vulnerable point in the transition to management, and it is at this moment that bailout or burnout is most likely to occur.

We have developed a method of joint charting of the emotional cycle[17] of the promotional transition in an effort to assist promotees and their supervisors to attend to joint needs. Cycle charting makes it possible to talk systematically and comfortably about the transition process, to identify unmet needs, and to develop appropriate supportive measures or action plans. Joint charting legitimizes talking about the process. When it is done on a weekly basis, particularly during the early stages of the transition, cycle charting monitors the vital signs of the promotee's progress and permits action to be taken before the situation becomes acute.

The supervisor can play the role of coach to help the promotee in a number of ways. For example, promotees need to develop empowering strategies that will strengthen their sense of self yet be grounded in reality and competency. Here the coach can help the new manager develop confidence and a sense of authority and competence by making sure the promotee learns to solve problems and initiate actions that are relevant and visible to the unit and to nursing management[18]. Such actions tend to enhance the expertise of the manager and verify a sense of proficiency.

The new manager's power as a referent, which is based on people's liking or identification, can be transformed to relationships in the larger hospital system. A transformation is required because any previous sense of liking that came from being accepted as one of a work group is definitely disrupted with the promotion. Some of the pain that accompanies the disruption comes from a sense of alienation from former peers. In time managers who value friendships and relationships can build their referent power within their unit and in the larger hospital system. They may well need assistance in undertaking this effort.

Building good personal networks can help new leaders manage job-related dependences. Effort must be exerted to initiate contacts and build relationships that can be mutually useful. The knowledgeable coach can help promotees see that referent power is built on trust and identification and can help them devise strategies that fit the person. Some managers can more easily promote trust; others more naturally build identification. Trust is associated with the person's availability, openness, support, and developmental attitude. Identification arises between people as they realize they have something in common, are after the same things in life, or face the same obstacles. Building referent power either through trust or through identification is essential for those who want to succeed and who find themselves dependent to some degree on others for their goal accomplishment[19].

Developing a systematic program of manager care

Nursing is devoted to patient care and has programs for employee assistance and care. What is missing is a systematic program of manager care. Such a program requires a philosophy of manager care, progressive orientation of new managers, skills of mentoring, and systems of monitoring.

The concept of manager care

A philosophy of manager care has to be articulated and modeled by top nursing management. It is the responsibility of the nursing administrator to define the purposes of manager care, to embody those purposes into specific programs and to coordinate those programs.

Nursing directors must be concerned with creating a nurturing environment in order to shorten the time it takes to develop healthy, sturdy, and satisfied managers who function at peak effectiveness. To use a farming analogy: we want to maximize the harvest from limited resources of land.

In nursing, the value of special care units to meet the acuity needs of patients is well accepted; when patients' conditions improve, they are moved out of special care units and placed on routine floor care. Manager care seems to be at the place where nursing care was many years ago. Regardless of the acuity of new managers' needs, routine floor care is all that is available.

Good manager care requires the equivalent of a cold frame or greenhouse for those critical winter months when the promotee is getting established in the new job. Protection must be provided during extremes in the hospital climate and an environment created where growth is fostered,

progress is monitored, and judgments made as to the appropriate time to move the promotee out of the protected environment. The nursing administrator wants to be sure that these valuable new plants are not killed by winter frosts, by neglect, or by lack of nurturing. The administrator wants to be sure new managers do not wither or fail to sprout because of disillusionment and alienation. To produce a strain of healthy, sturdy, functioning managers, orientation, mentoring, and monitoring are needed.

"The supervisor can play the role of coach to help the promotee in a number of ways."

Orientation of new managers

Orientation programs need to be formalized and ongoing, emphasizing the nature of the transition process and building the initial skills essential to cope with the process. In transition seminars we have conducted in both the United States and Canada, we have found that new promotees benefit greatly from group learning experiences with others who are engaged in a similar process.

Since their new role involves working closely with nursing staff, new managers evince keen interest and readiness to examine and improve their interpersonal skills. During their first six months, new managers are most concerned with understanding their role and how it relates to others' roles, as well as with dealing with the testing behavior of their employees and coping with stress. Those on the job for more than six months want to know how the hospital works a system, how to find resources, how to use the system, and how to build the management skills they need.

Orientation programs can be conducted in groups either within a hospital or from different hospitals. Both formats are equally effective, but they have slightly different outcomes. Programs for managers from different hospitals are usually seen as safe by participants, who find it easier to be open with one another since there is no risk of exposure to those with whom they will have to continue to relate.

When promotees attend programs within the hospital that employs them, on the other hand, they can compensate for the loss of previous peer friendships by starting to build relationships with new peers. In addition, the group can provide supports and resources for its members.

Skills of mentoring

The dictionary defines *mentor* as teacher, advisor, or coach. A program of manager care would concentrate on two aspects of mentoring: (1) encouraging and guiding new managers to seek mentors and resources and (2) developing the supervisors of the new managers into effective coaches or mentors.

Unfortunately many nurses do not manage their nursing careers as effectively as they should, tending to drift instead from one nursing position to another without thought as to where such moves are taking them and without effective strategies or mentors to help them learn the ropes, find resources, or develop skills[20]. In orientation programs for new managers, mentoring, "resourcing," and building support networks are all important topics of discussion.

Helping supervisors build skills in mentoring is crucial in a program of manager care. With proper attention and encouragement, human beings grow—they do not diminish. An effective coach or mentor can develop motivated and productive managers. Myers[21] has found that highly motivated managers are likely to have had what he calls "developmental bosses"—supervisors who stimulated enthusiasm, maintained high expectations, recognized performance, were open-minded and approachable, provided ready access to company information, encouraged risk-taking, were sensitive to the feelings of others, and believed in people's learning from mistakes. Only 8 percent of the highly motivated managers in the Myers study had bosses who were described unfavorably in terms of these criteria. Nurses are no exception; when asked in seminars to identify from their own work experience supervisors who stimulated them most in their growth, development, and productivity, nurses describe characteristics almost identical to those found in the Myers study.

Some supervisors are more naturally developmental than others, but all can improve their mentoring skills[22]. All need to be aware of the power of the self-fulfilling prophecy in relation to the development of their managers. Furthermore, they need skills to develop a supportive and motivating climate, to delegate challenging tasks within the competency range of the individual, to provide feedback, and to help the new manager find resources and solve problems.

Formal training in coaching and mentoring is a must for those charged with the responsibility of developing new managers. We have conducted numerous seminars on these subjects for nursing supervisors. In our experience the needed coaching and mentoring skills are teachable and are highly valued by participants.

Formal training alone will not supply the impetus to sustain a program of manager care unless this is integrated into the performance expectations of the supervisors and into the performance appraisal system. This highlights the importance of developing systems of monitoring.

Systems of monitoring

An effective program of manager care must scan all aspects of the organization to see that they are operating in a coordinated, integrated manner toward the established goals of the program[23]. For example, role expectations for supervisors must include mentoring and coaching responsibilities. The performance appraisal system must function in a way that rewards the mentoring efforts of managers. Training, recruitment, and selection programs must be consistent with the philosophy of the overall program and be supported by line management. Any disagreements or conflicts over the program of manager care must be managed, and a system of monitoring must be operating to see that all aspects of the program are in place and functioning.

"To produce a strain of healthy, sturdy, functioning managers, orientation, mentoring, and monitoring are needed."

Nursing administrators and their key management staff need to develop a comprehensive method for reviewing the manager care program. The following are practical suggestions.

Administrators or their representatives can monitor the new managers by informal interviews, manager care rounds, examining the content and progress of formal training programs, and reviewing cycle charting. They can monitor supervisors by making sure the training of those charged with coaching new managers is adequate, by conducting coaching sessions with the supervisors about the progress of their new managers, by reviewing cycle charting, and by asking probing questions. They can audit for consistency and completeness the recruitment and selection system, the responsibilities and expectations stated in job descriptions, the criteria used in the performance appraisal system, and the content, methods, and effects of training programs.

By clearly delineating programs to monitor manager care, nursing administrators demonstrate their priorities and values in the development of new managers. As they see that these purposes are embodied in functioning programs, they are well on the way to helping promotees achieve expected levels of competence smoothly. The learning curves in their organizations are likely to peak sooner than the three years and at a higher level than the 75 percent reported by Frohman. The task is not easy in this time of limited resources. Creativity and ingenuity are needed to create a functioning program, but the results are well worth the effort.

References and notes

1. L. Darling and L. McGrath, "The Causes and Costs of Promotional Trauma," *The Journal of Nursing Administration* 13(4): 29–32, 1983.
2. Alan J. Frohman, "New Approaches to Old Problems: Strategies for

Managing Professional Employees," paper presented to the Organization Development Network Conference, Washington, D.C., April 4, 1973.

3. J.P. Kotter, "The Psychological Contract: Managing the Joining-up Process," *California Management Review* 15(3): 91–99, 1973.

4. Kotter, 1973, p. 98.

5. H. Levinson, *Executive Stress* (New York: Harper & Row, 1964).

6. D. Kelley and D.R. Conner, "The Emotional Cycle of Change," in *Annual Handbook for Group Facilitators* (San Diego: University Associates, 1979), pp. 117–122.

7. Clarifying ambiguous managerial roles is especially relevant as women become sophisticated in promotional negotiations. See B.L. Harragan, *Games Mother Never Taught You* (New York: Warner Books, 1977), p. 81.

8. Kotter, 1973.

9. J.J. Sherwood and J.C. Glidewell, "Planned Negotiation," in W.W. Burke, ed., *Contemporary Organization Development: Approaches and Interventions* (Washington, D.C.: NTL Institute for Applied Behavioral Science, 1972), pp. 35–46.

10. R. Harrison, "Role Negotiotion," in W.W. Burke and H.A. Hornstein eds., *The Social Technology of Organization Development* (Fairfax, Va.: NTL Learning Resources Corporation, 1972), pp. 84–96.

11. J.P. Kotter, *Power in Management* (New York: AMACOM, 1979), p. 16.

12. Kotter, 1979, p. 84.

13. Darling and McGrath, 1983.

14. B. Oshry, *Middle Power* (Boston: Power & Systems Training, 1980), pp. 8–10. B. Oshry and K.E. Oshry, "Middle-Group Dynamics," in W.W. Burke and L.D. Goodstein, eds., *Trends and Issues in Organizational Development* (San Diego: University Associates, 1980) pp. 41–61.

15. S. Putney and G.J. Putney, *The Adjusted American* (New York: Harper & Row, 1964), p. 30.

16. Darling and McGrath, 1983.

17. Kelley & Conner, 1979.

18. R. Kantor, *Men and Women of the Corporation* (New York: Basic Books, 1977), pp. 176–181.

19. P. Cuming, *The Power Handbook* (Boston: CBI Publishing Co., 1981), pp. 86–89.

20. The senior author is currently conducting research on this subject. One useful reference is L. Phillips-Jones, *Mentors and Proteges* (New York: Arbor House, 1982).

21. S. Myers, "Conditions for Manager Motivation," *Harvard Business Review* 44(1): 142–155, 1966.

22. Useful references are F.F. Fournies, *Coaching for Improved Work Performance* (New York: Van Nostrand Reinhold, 1978); P. Hersey and K.H. Blanchard, *Management of Organizational Behavior*, 3rd. ed. (Englewood Cliffs, N.J.: Prentice-Hall, 1977), pp.189–224; H.P. Smith and P.J. Brouwer, *Performance Appraisal and Human Development* (Reading, Mass.: Addison-Wesley, 1977).

23. M.R. Weisbord, "Organizational Diagnosis," *Group and Organization Studies* 1(4): 430–447, December 1976.

CHAPTER 10

Nancy Ertl, RN

Choosing Successful Managers:
Participative Selection Can Help

The attitude and behavior of first line managers can greatly influence the success of any health care organization. Managers directly affect 90 to 95 percent of the workers in a hospital. This article offers a specific description of a new process that allows staff to participate in management selection. The author shows how the process, which is a truly participative form of management, increases the success potential of new health care managers.

Historically, nurse managers were selected by their immediate supervisors. New managers thus selected may or may not have been fully aware of the intricacies of the position and the environment for which they were responsible. Consequently, new managers often found themselves set up for failure. With the pressure on health care management to be both effective and efficient during these difficult times, hospitals can ill afford failures in management.

Mercy Health Center of Dubuque, Iowa is a 425-bed acute care hospital, a division of the Sisters of Mercy Health Care Corporation of Michigan. Both the hospital and corporation encourage highly participatory forms of management. They also encourage their management teams to be creative and innovative. This philosophy of management allowed us to develop a new system for choosing new managers.

How to Choose
Successful Unit Managers

The organizational structure of the Nursing Division at Mercy Health Center includes a Vice-Presi-

dent for Patient Care who has overall responsibility for the entire Nursing Division, three Directors of Patient Care with line responsibility for several units, and Managers and Assistant Managers who have line responsibility for a given unit.

Approximately 2 years ago, as a result of the reorganization of the Nursing Division, I acquired responsibility for a nursing unit whose manager had been terminated due to unsatisfactory performance. At the time, I was one of the Directors of Patient Care. The Director who previously had responsibility for this unit and supervised the terminated manager had resigned to move out of town. Needless to say, the unit was in turmoil. It was being managed at that time by the two assistant managers.

At our first staff meeting we discussed the selection of a new manager for the unit. The staff of the unit was comprised of many long-term loyal employees. They felt that they could readily identify the needs of the unit and wanted input into the selection of a new leader.

As the Director of Patient Care, it was my responsibility to select and hire their manager, but I could understand their need for input into the process.

Mercy Health Center, like most health care institutions, had operated under the concept that the supervisor with line responsibility for a position had the responsibility and authority to hire into that position.

Nancy Ertl, RN, is the Director of Patient Care at Mercy Health Center, St. Joseph's Unit, Dubuque, Iowa.

I researched the literature in an effort to try and discover how other hospitals had accommodated staff input. I discovered methods that allowed peers (other nursing managers) to select a new manager, but I decided that this was not the answer because other nursing managers would not know the specific needs of that unit.

After discussing the staff's concerns about the selection process with the Vice-President for Patient Care, she agreed to let me develop a new process for management selection that allowed staff participation, if the following objectives were met:

- The method would not abdicate management's responsibility.
- Assessment of the candidates would be objective.
- The confidentiality of the candidate would be protected.
- The Human Resource Department would review and approve the process prior to implementation.

Participative Management Selection

The basic system that I designed allowed staff members to interview all candidates and recommend as their manager the person they believed best met the needs of the unit. The person with line responsibility for that manager (referred to as the supervisor in this article) had the right to accept or reject that recommendation.

I felt that this process did not abdicate management's responsibility, would increase staff awareness of management's role, would recognize the value of staff members to an organization, and would operationalize true participative management.

The process has been refined by staff and management over the past 18 months. We have organized the process around nine basic steps. Our experience has shown that if the process is organized around these nine steps, this system of management selection greatly increases the potential for constant performance and management team success.

The nine steps in our participative management selection process are as follows:

1. **Establish ground rules.**
2. **Select staff participants.**
3. **Select a facilitator.**
4. **Prepare the staff.**
5. **Establish the selection criteria.**
6. **Develop interview questions.**
7. **Interview each candidate.**
8. **Evaluate candidates.**
9. **Make recommendations to the supervisor.**

Time Frame for the Staff Selection Process

The timetable for the entire process should be established at the first meeting. My experience indicates that 2 weeks is about right. If the process drags on, the staff loses interest. I would recommend the following schedule:

First Monday: Organization and staff preparation time–2 hours.

First Thursday: Complete staff preparation, establish selection criteria, develop interview questions–2 hours.

Second Monday: Finalize selection criteria, finalize interview questions and evaluation form–2 hours.

Second Thursday: Interviews, evaluation, recommendation. How much time you devote to this activity depends on the quantity and quality of the candidates.

This time frame allows the staff adequate preparation time, keeps their interest level high, and avoids repetitious discussions due to intervening time spans.

Because the hospital believes that this process benefits the organization, staff members participating in the process should be either released from work time, or paid at straight time if they come in on their days off.

Establishing the Ground Rules

The supervisor must establish the rules of the process beforehand. Then he or she must communicate these rules to staff and make sure they are aware of what they are agreeing to do. In addition, staff must be comfortable with the demands that will be put on them as participants.

Our group came up with the following ground rules:

1. At the conclusion of the process, the staff will recommend one person to the supervisor of the position. The supervisor has the right to accept or reject that recommendation.
2. The supervisor has the responsibility for staff selection and preparation.
3. The staff selected to participate must attend all preparatory sessions and interview sessions or they will be eliminated from the group.
4. The staff must honor the confidentiality of all discussions and interviews. They may not share any information with other staff members.
5. The supervisor will select a facilitator for the interviews. The facilitator will not be a member of the unit staff and will attend all preparation sessions and interviews.
6. The supervisor will serve only as an observer

during the interviews. The supervisor may participate in the final evaluation or may speak at any time if there is an infraction of the rules.

7. The supervisor will participate with the staff in the establishment of the selection criteria and interview questions.
8. All working papers must be returned to the supervisor at the end of each interview. Working papers include candidate resumes, notes taken during interview, and all evaluation forms.
9. The maximum number of staff participants will be six.
10. The supervisor will explain the process to each candidate individually and will notify both the successful and unsuccessful candidates of the outcome.

The process must be organized around these ground rules if it is to be successful for all involved, as they are the basis for the entire process.

Selecting Staff Participants

Staff participants should, of course, have a direct subordinate relationship to the position being filled. They may be chosen in a number of ways:

1. The supervisor may solicit the participation of selected staff members.
2. The supervisor may ask for volunteers and select from that group.
3. The supervisor may ask for volunteers and let the staff narrow down the choice by consensus.
4. The staff may solicit volunteers, select a group and recommend them to the supervisor.

Which method should you use? The most important thing is to know your staff, decide which method will most likely lead to a successful outcome and retain a true feeling of participation. Whatever method you employ, include participants with varying lengths of service who represent all levels of staff and all shifts, and persons who have actively participated in the department's activities or projects.

Selecting a Facilitator

The facilitator's role is an extremely important component of the process. Choose a facilitator from within the organization who has some base knowledge of the department. He or she should have some experience in group dynamics, and should not be intimidating to either the staff or the candidates.

The facilitator helps the staff stay objective, maintains time limits on the interviews, assists the staff in problem solving during the final evaluation, and assures that equal opportunity is given to all candidates. During the interviews, the facilitator makes the introduction and sets the tone for the interview,

recognizing that both interviewers and the candidate are experiencing a great deal of anxiety and stress. The facilitator does not participate in the actual interview process.

The supervisor has the responsibility of orienting the facilitator to the process and communicating his or her expectations. Before agreeing to act as facilitator, the person must have the approval of his or her own supervisor and must be able to make a commitment to complete the project.

Preparing the Staff

Allow adequate preparation time during this phase of the process. It is absolutely necessary that staff participants become a cohesive group, that they establish good working relationships with each other and the facilitator, broaden their knowledge of interview techniques, and gain more in depth knowledge of the position.

The supervisor should conduct the initial meeting of the staff participants and facilitator. He or she begins by reviewing the process and indicating why the process has been selected to choose the new manager. All participants, including the facilitator, should then share their background and experience.

Prior to the first meeting, the supervisor should prepare packets of information for all participants that include at least the following items:

1. The written ground rules.
2. The current job description for the position.
3. A copy of the performance appraisal tool used for the vacant management position.
4. Additional expectations of the supervisor that are not listed in the job description. For example, this can include reports to the supervisor, civic or professional organization activities, expected communication between supervisor and manager, and any additional requirements above the scheduled hours.
5. A selection of current articles on leadership, management, and communication will assist staff in broadening their knowledge of the current trends in health care management. Their perception of management may be based solely on the behavior of their previous manager—which may or may not be satisfactory.
6. Information on the art of interviewing. It is important to realize that most of the participants probably have never been on this side of the interviewing table.

Before discussing the position, review the ground rules and make sure that all participants agree with them. A detailed examination of the job description and performance appraisal tool is the next step, with the supervisor clarifying items as necessary. Encourage the staff to review the articles on management and interviewing prior to the next meeting.

Establishing the Selection Criteria

The second meeting should begin by reviewing the information in the packet and clarifying any items that the staff does not understand. The group then begins to establish the selection criteria. The selection criteria become part of the evaluation tool, and of course, must include any qualifications listed on the job description by the institution. Here are examples of the selection criteria that we have used:

1. Education
   a) Formal—degree required
   b) Informal—continuing education (quantity and quality)
2. Experience
   a) Clinical
   b) Management
3. Skills
   a) Leadership
   b) Clinical
   c) Technical
   d) Communication
4. Management Style
5. Interprofessional Skills
6. Nursing Philosophy
   a) Health care management
   b) Patient care
7. Other Factors to Consider

In each of these broad categories, the staff can list specific requirements. In the area of Clinical Experience, for example, you may wish to see 3 years in a specific specialty or broad-based clinical experience.

In regard to Skills, the staff has generally concentrated on Leadership and Communication. Specifics listed under communication skills have included "listening," "writing," "clear and articulate," "comfortable with frequent communication," "the ability to confront," and "a positive reinforcement philosophy."

Requirements under Management Style have included attributes such as "open and nondefensive," "ability to demonstrate confidence and ability to lead," "not easily intimidated," "follow through with responsibility," and "participative."

Expectations in the area of Interprofessional Skills have included "responsiveness," "recognition of other profession's worth," and "autonomous, but collegial approach."

Under Other Factors, you may wish to consider any activity that could contribute to the growth and development of a person. Generally, specifics were not listed in this category, but were understood to refer to leadership positions in church, civic, or professional organizations.

You will probably find that the staff has much higher expectations of their manager than does the institution. It is the role of the supervisor or facilitator during this process to see that the selection criteria are realistic and attainable.

Developing Interview Questions

Having reached consensus on the selection criteria, the next step is to formulate the interview questions. Decide how long the interview should be before developing the questions because the number of questions directly relates to the length of the interview. In most cases, it is best to limit the interviews to 1 hour since the stress levels of both the candidate and the staff interviewers are likely to be high.

The staff interviewers tend to experience a great amount of stress during the interview because they know that they are responsible to perhaps 70 to 80 employees who will be affected by their recommendation. They want their unit to run smoothly and realize that the manager will strongly influence the unit's level of success. Stress levels are further increased because most of the interviewers are not experienced in interviewing techniques.

The interview questions must be structured to identify how the candidate meets the selection criteria. The staff should decide on a priority for the selection criteria and list their questions accordingly. In addition to direct questions, we have found situational type questions extremely useful.

Sample Interview Questions

Here are some interview questions that we developed:

- What motivated you to apply for this position and what do you hope to gain from it?
- Describe for us the professional goals you hope to attain in 5 years.
- How do you feel you have been an asset to your employer and your co-workers?
- Identify the strengths that you feel make you the most qualified candidate.
- Identify and discuss your limitations.
- Describe methods you would use to evaluate the competencies of your staff.
- Describe how you would distribute your time between clinical and management responsibilities.
- How would you view this position in relationship to the medical staff, other managers, your supervisor, and affiliating students and instructors?

- We are somewhat concerned about the depth of your management and/or clinical experience, how would you overcome this?

Situational questions are designed to test the candidate's leadership and management style. Because they were situational, the staff identified what they believed was the most appropriate response to the situation. Here are examples of situational questions:

A. *The situation* → Describe your interaction with Nurse Smith, who is habitually behind in nursing care, charting, and frequently requires much assistance with co-workers.

The response the staff expects → includes evaluation, counseling, coaching and education, feedback, reevaluation, and action.

B. The situation → Dr. "X" comes to you and complains about Nurse Smith, how would you react?

The response the staff expects → the manager would do an objective evaluation of the complaints, discuss them with the employee, arrange for the employee, the physician, and the manager to discuss the problem, and finally, would resolve the problem.

C. *The situation* → Give an example from your nursing career that demonstrates your ability to handle stress.

The response the staff expects → The candidate should be able to identify a significant stressor in nursing, and to demonstrate appropriate coping strategies.

It will take considerable discussion and time to develop these questions to the point that the staff feels comfortable that the questions elicit answers that address the priority concerns of the staff.

In addition to the interview, we usually asked candidates to prepare written answers to other questions. By this method we were often able to procure additional information about the candidates and also judge their writing skills.

Here are examples of our written response type questions:

- Rank the following activities in their order of importance as they relate to the manager's function, and explain in writing your top three choices:

  Budget preparation and monitoring
  Patient care assignments
  Quality assurance activities
  Attendance at management meetings
  Performance appraisal of personnel
  Staff development activities
  Self development activities
  Patient rounds
  Physician interactions

  Staff meetings
  Staff interaction.

- Can you describe a situation that displays your leadership ability? Show how you function independently, both personally and professionally?

Specific interview questions will give all candidates an equal opportunity and will assure that the staff has all the necessary information on each candidate prior to evaluation. Developing interview questions also aids the interviewing process and makes it more organized, professional, and objective.

Having drafted the interview questions, the staff must decide whether or not to let the candidates prepare answers in advance. We decided to distribute the questions to the candidates prior to the interviews. The staff believed that this was the fairest approach; it would enhance the quality of the interviews, reduce the stress and tension of the candidates, and make the candidates cognizant of staff expectations. The staff felt that they would be able to discern textbook-prepared answers.

We found that the candidates were honest in their answers, for at least two reasons:

1) Often the candidate was someone the staff had worked with before, and
2) because candidates realize that their performance, if selected, would be judged on the basis of their answers.

Designing an Evaluation Form

The next step is to design an evaluation form for the interviews. We used a numerical ranking scale *i.e.*, 1-not acceptable, 2-below average, 3-average, 4-above average, and 5-outstanding.

We used the ranking scale to judge the candidates on their answers to the interview questions, and to ascertain how close they came to meeting the selection criteria. The ranking scale is important, because it lends objectivity to the final evaluation of the candidate. We allowed space on the form for comments so that staff members could justify their rankings.

When the working documents of the committee are completed, it is the supervisor's responsibility to get them typed, copied, and returned to the staff participants. In addition, it is the supervisor's responsibility to supply each member of the group with copies of the candidates' application and vitae. Candidate information should *not* be distributed to the group until the criteria and interview questions are formulated, however. This avoids skewing of the criteria and questions.

The supervisor then meets with each of the candidates to explain the interview process and supply them with a copy of the interview questions. The time and place of the group interview also is established at this time. Although this step could be accomplished in a telephone call, we prefer a personal visit because the candidate usually has many questions to ask.

All candidates should have been screened initially by the Human Resource Department. The supervisor should provide the Human Resource Department with some basic criteria for screening, in addition to those normally used by the Human Resource Department. This helps assure that basic qualifications are met by candidates who will be interviewed. Some candidates will voluntarily withdraw during this screening process when they become aware that the interviews will be conducted by a group of staff.

Interviewing the Candidates

All the interviews should be conducted on the same day or on two successive days if the numbers of interviews indicate that it is necessary. The group meets approximately one-half hour prior to the first interview to discuss any last minute organizational problems. When the interviews begin the facilitator should meet the candidate outside of the interviewing room and again explain the process that will be used for the interview. The facilitator then makes the introductions of the candidate and the staff interviewers. We have usually preassigned interview questions to the staff participants so that they all participate in the interview. All staff is also encouraged to ask impromptu questions if they do not understand the candidate's response, or if they wish further clarification. The candidates are also encouraged to ask questions of either the facilitator or the staff. After each interview, sufficient time is allowed between appointments to permit the staff to individually evaluate the candidate. They do not discuss the candidate with other staff members on the committee until they have completed their evaluation of the candidate.

The supervisor is present during all inteviews, only as an observer. We have found it helpful if the supervisor makes specific notes about the responses of each candidate to provide feedback to the staff in the final evaluation phase.

Evaluating the Candidates

The most difficult part of the process for the staff comes during the final evaluation and recommendation phase, after all interviews have been conducted. The facilitator leads this portion of the process, which should occur as soon after the last interview as possible.

We began by listing the ranking of each specific criteria for each candidate. If staff participants dis-

agreed on a given criteria, we discussed that ranking until a resolution was reached by consensus of the group.

We proceeded to do this for each candidate until we had achieved a group ranking on each of the selection criteria. At the conclusion of this process, the facilitator totaled the points given to each candidate and distributed the numerical rankings to all participants. Some candidates were eliminated through this numerical ranking process, if their scores were significantly low. However, no candidate was officially eliminated until the group completed its final review. As the process of elimination continues, and the candidates appear to be more equal, you will have to rank-order the selection criteria to establish a different numerical ranking.

The final evaluation phase calls for a great deal of discussion about the major strengths and limitations of each candidate. Although this is less objective than the numerical ranking, it has been used successfully in three cases where the candidates have had identical numerical scores.

Making Recommendations to the Supervisor

The staff participants must all agree to the recommendation that will be made to the supervisor. This recommendation should be made in writing with signatures from all participants.

Before we terminate the meeting I have found it helpful to ask the staff participants individually how they felt about the process. If they felt favorable, it reassured me that a decision had been made by the group, and that they would support the recommendation.

The supervisor should inform staff participants at this time of his or her decision to accept or reject their recommendation. If their recommendation is acceptable, you may want to reinforce participative management concepts at this time, with a discussion of how their participation in the management of the unit is necessary to ensure success of their new manager. It is also important to stress the need for open communication between staff and the new manager, especially as it relates to operationalizing the selection criteria they established.

We used this process during the past 18 months to select ten managers or assistant managers. In every case, the recommendation made by the staff participants was accepted by the supervisor. In all cases the supervisors agreed that the correct candidate was selected. The interviews were extremely in depth, fair, and the process was equitable.

■ Improving Health Management by
Participatory Management Selection

To follow up on the selection process, I sent out five questionnaires, to the person selected by this process, the supervisor of the person hired through this process, the facilitators, the staff participants, and four staff members who were not involved in the process, but were employed in a unit where the process had been used. The vast majority of people returned these questionnaires and many of them signed their names because they felt so strongly positive about the process. Everyone agreed that we should *not* return to the traditional way of management selection in our institution.

The respondents identified the following *advantages* of the process:

- Creates strong staff support for and cooperation with the new manager.
- Increases knowledge of management's role among staff participants.
- Increases knowledge of interviewing techniques by staff participants.
- Increases management awareness of staff's concerns.
- Increases knowledge among staff of how to write a resume and prepare for interviews.

- Reduces conflicts between staff and management.
- Increases the potential for the new manager to succeed in a shorter time frame because of general staff support and strong desire by staff to assure that their selection will succeed.
- Reduces supervisor favoritism.

The following *disadvantages* of the process were also identified:

- Stress levels of the candidates and the participants were very high.
- It is a time-consuming selection process.

I am convinced that the participative selection process is effective and helps to assure the success of our health care management team. Although it is a time-consuming process, I believe this problem is overridden by the fact that the manager chosen becomes effective more quickly. Ultimately, the organization that uses participative selection can continue to be progressive and successful. The process also creates a climate of true participative management that includes both bottom-up and top-down support.

Someone once defined a leader for me as "a person who has willing followers." This management selection process helps to assure that the manager will be a leader.

CHAPTER 11

Head Nurses
as Middle Managers

by Phillippa Ferguson Johnston

The relationship between head nurses and their staff nurses influences staff turnover rates and job satisfaction. In this article the author describes the measures taken by the management of Greater Southeast Community Hospital in response to an increasing turnover rate among staff RNs. In recognition of the head nurse role vis-à-vis attrition rates and job satisfaction, head nurses were upgraded to department head status and rigorous head nurse performance standards were developed. These standards required clinical expertise, managerial competence, and accountability. It is the author's contention that clinical practice and staff morale are directly related to a clearly defined head nurse role.

The role of middle management in retention and job satisfaction should never be underestimated. Studies show that the relationship an employee has with her immediate supervisor influences how she feels about her job and her position within the organization. The department manager sets the tone of the department and is responsible for building peer support and effective relationships, involving staff in decision making, demanding accountability, and encouraging healthy competition. Employee attitudes and morale will reflect the department manager's effectiveness[1].

As a middle manager in a decentralized nursing organization such as Greater Southeast Community Hospital in Washington, D.C., the head nurse has the responsibility for all aspects of unit operations. She manages the day-to-day clinical care of the patient population. She is the planner, organizer, motivator, evaluator, educator, and in many instances the implementor of most activities that occur on her unit. She is the one person all others turn to when problems arise.

In the traditional nursing organization, the head nurse has all the responsibility of management but none of the

power. Functioning well within the managerial framework of planning, directing, controlling, organizing, and developing in the traditional context can become an impossible chore.

According to Kantor, "the position, not the person, determines whether the person has power"[2]. She states that this power refers not necessarily to "dominance, control, or oppression," but to having the capability to move the organization toward its goal. Power, therefore, means having available the resources, information, and support necessary to do a job well.

Consider the following example. A head nurse needs a store of floor-stocked drugs on her unit increased. The pharmacy director is unwilling to discuss the issue unless the head nurse's department head agrees with the head nurse. The pharmacy director tells the head nurse to have the department head make a written request. The department head is the associate director. The head nurse approaches the associate director and spends half an hour explaining the situation. The associate director then requests a meeting with the director of pharmacy and the head nurse during which they decide to increase the floor-stocked supply of drugs. This decision is made two weeks after the original request was made. Clearly, the pharmacy director would have been forced to resolve the issue immediately if the head nurse had been a department head. No intervention from the associate director would have been required. Lack of power at the management level is bad for any organization. In addition to not having the authority to get things done, powerless managers breed a staff of subordinates who discount them as leaders and for that reason are uncooperative.

Kantor believes that "the powerless live in a different world. Lacking the supplies, information, or support to make things happen easily, they may turn instead to the ultimate weapon of those who lack productive power— oppressive power—holding others back and punishing with whatever threats they can muster"[3]. Staff nurses, therefore, need to know that their leader, the venerable head nurse, has status within the organization and is capable of

Phillippa Ferguson Johnston, R.N., M.S., is Vice President for Patient Care Services at Greater Southeast Community Hospital in Washington, D.C.

effectively influencing the system. If the staff perceive their head nurse as having power, then they will have power by association. This feeling of power is crucial to their satisfaction with their role in the organization.

The head nurse role at Greater Southeast

The head nurses at Greater Southeast Community Hospital in Washington, D.C. were designated as department heads in 1975; however, they retained the head nurse title. At the same time, the organization was decentralized into four clinical divisions, with an associate director supervising four to five head nurses within those clinical divisions (Exhibit 1). The department head role, however, was not fully realized until several years later because several basic problems within the hospital's nursing division served to hamper head nurses' attempts to function as department heads:

- Nursing practice was task-oriented and directed simply at carrying out orders.
- Physician/nurse relationships were, to say the least, poor.

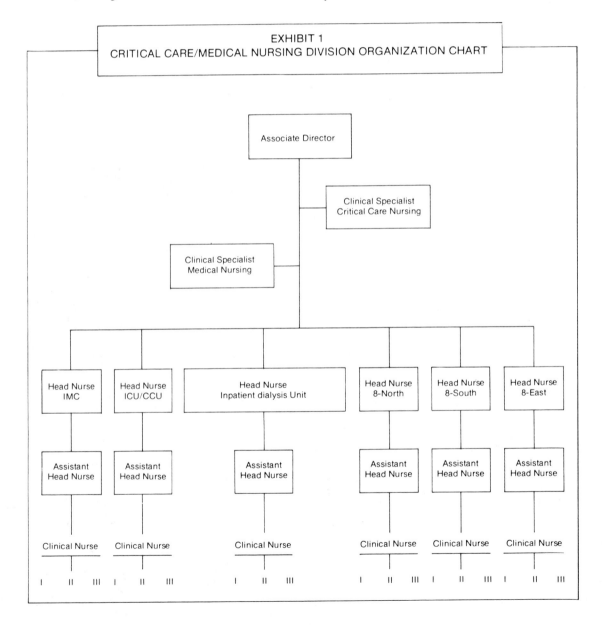

EXHIBIT 1
CRITICAL CARE/MEDICAL NURSING DIVISION ORGANIZATION CHART

- A deficit existed in role models at the associate director level.
- No clear definition of the head nurse role and practice was available. As a result, a head nurse often was caught between the opposing forces of her associate director and her staff.
- Head nurses directed the majority of their attention toward staffing only. Little administrative planning occurred, and interaction was minimal among department heads.
- Clinical and managerial skills of head nurses were found to be lacking.
- Staff RN turnover was high.
- RN staff vacancies in the entire hospital averaged between 15 and 30.

In 1979 a new management team recognized that there was indeed a problem with the effectiveness of the head nurses in the department head role. We recognized the need to close the gap in role perspectives among head nurses, associate directors, and the vice-president of patient care services. The first step was to identify roles and relationships through the use of job descriptions and performance standards. We also identified role expectations and planned to hold each level accountable for those expectations. We hoped this would encourage each level to serve as a role model for the next higher level.

With these goals in mind, the vice-president identified the following expectations for the associate directors:

- Demonstrate clinical competence and a complete commitment to patient care.
- Develop each head nurse into a highly skilled clinician and manager.
- Maintain visibility on the patient units.
- Participate in staff meetings, rap sessions, and educational programs.
- Establish a relationship with staff nurses, encourage competency, and give feedback regarding performance.
- Periodically participate in the delivery of patient care.
- Establish a visible professional relationship with physicians and serve as an appropriate role model in these relationships.

The associate directors then voiced their expectations of the head nurse:

- Encourage and facilitate the growth and learning of the nursing staff by providing relevant learning opportunities.
- Improve individual performance by means of counseling, evaluation and staff assessment of strengths and weaknesses through peer review.
- Act as a role model for staff nurses with regard to clinical competence, attitude, and enthusiasm for nursing.
- Exhibit initiative in problem identification and resolution.

- Assume hours which are flexible in an effort to be visible with all the nursing staff.
- Be fair and equitable in arranging time schedules.
- Meet with the staff at least twice monthly.
- With participation of the staff; identify objectives for the unit and outline appropriate time frames for meeting each objective, evaluate those objectives on a quarterly basis with the associate director.

The head nurse, in turn, was expected to hold registered nurses accountable for their actions. Essentially, the head nurses told their staffs that they were expected to:

- Use nursing process in the delivery of patient care.
- Develop and implement a care plan for their patients.
- Participate with physicians in the delivery of health care.
- Establish effective working relations with both physicians and peers.

The second action taken to bridge the gap in perspective among head nurses, associate directors, and the vice president was somewhat less complex. It was made clear to the head nurses and their staffs that the head nurses were to be considered part of nursing administration. This was done in order to avoid placing head nurses in the middle between staff and management; and to steer clear of the adversary relationship so often seen between the chief nurse and the head nurse group. This usually results when the head nurse is forced to administer programs or explain policies she has had no say in developing. Problems also may arise when the head nurse is not in agreement with the goals and objectives of the nursing administrator. Since it is vitally important that the head nurse identify with the nursing administration, she must be involved in developing goals and objectives, as well as in making decisions about nursing practice. The head nurse should ideally see both the associate director and the assistant administrator as role models.

Developing head nurses

Performance standards were developed by a task force of associate directors and head nurses, with the vice president serving in a consultant capacity. Each standard indicates a criterion for measurement and is evaluated as either being met or unmet. If any one standard is not met, the associate director and head nurse identify specific goals and objectives necessary to meet the standards within a specific timeframe. All standards must be met to receive a satisfactory performance evaluation.

Those nurses who failed to meet the standards were offered opportunities for management development, either by the hospital or by outside agencies. These individuals were coached one-on-one, by either their associate director or, in some cases, by the vice president.

Fifty percent of the head nurses at Greater Southeast actually sought other positions in the subsequent two years

"Clinical credibility is the basis upon which authority and respect are built."

because they were unable to meet performance standards. During this high turnover period, hospital management was forced to look at what qualities were necessary to be a head nurse with department head responsibilities at Greater Southeast. Three critical attributes were identified: clinical credibility, self esteem, and self confidence.

Clinical credibility is the basis upon which authority and respect are built. The head nurse and her staff are each accountable for different aspects of patient care. The head nurse must be able to demand and expect that the staff will communicate with her on the patient's behalf. But the head nurse also must be clinically credible so that the staff nurse feels comfortable expressing any concerns she may have. Therefore, the head nurse needs to maintain her clinical skills through inservice and continuing education. She must be capable of taking good care of patients, using a nursing process framework, identifying patient problems, and supporting her considerations by sound and appropriate documentation. The head nurse does not necessarily have to be able to do all this better than her staff, but she must have an in-depth knowledge of the process. Her authority with her staff is largely gained by expertise, not in management, but at the bedside.

Self esteem is a measure of one's attitudes about one's self image. Self esteem is a reflection of life experiences from school work to professional career. The sense of confidence and self esteem will be consistent with one another[4]. One could reason, therefore, that a head nurse with self-esteem will be competent. But the issue goes further than just competence.

Self esteem marks the difference between the head nurse who personalizes a negative employee comment, and the head nurse who can put a negative comment in perspective and move on to more important issues. Self esteem determines whether or not the head nurse can influence her staff or rely on the group for personal support. Self esteem determines whether or not a head nurse is able to laugh at mistakes or whether those mistakes will be personalized and viewed as failures. It will be self esteem that will allow the head nurse to be trusting, rather than resentful or cynical.

Self confidence is the attribute that allows one to take risks, to confront others, and to communicate effectively. A person is self confident if she knows what she can do and cannot do. The self confident person has spent time getting to know herself, and that insight is a telling characteristic. Head nurses must have a large parcel of self confidence if they are to be effective leaders capable of instituting pro-gressive change.

Summary

The organization which is successful in attracting competent, clinically credible department heads, who have self confidence and a strong sense of self esteem, will attract and retain equally competent and committed staff nurses. For the nursing administrator, the challenge lies in guaranteeing that the organization allows head nurses to be the efficient, capable, caring manager they believe themselves to be. If the organization is restrictive, the head nurse will be frustrated and unchallenged. If the organization is open and allows for creativity, the head nurse will feel supported and challenged.

Staff nurses need to work in health environments where everyone has the opportunity to give, to create, and to be resourceful; and where their leaders support and respect them and where nursing can be fun.

These goals are now being achieved at Greater Southeast. The head nurses all have the attributes of clinical credibility, self confidence, and healthy self esteem. They are planners and problem-solvers. They are enthusiastic and committed. This enthusiasm is reflected in high staff morale. They are functioning as role models not only for the nursing, but for the entire hospital.

Clinical practice, especially in comparison to just five short years ago, is greatly improved. Physician/nurse relationships have been enriched by the collaborative practice meetings chaired by head nurses on each unit. Head nurses now participate in hospital and medical staff committee meetings. They are actively involved in program planning, not only for their own units, but also for programs that cross hospital divisions.

There are two indicators of success which can be measured: vacancies and turnover. In the past ten months our average vacancy has been between zero and five. Our turnover rate has decreased by 50 percent over 1980 and is currently at the lowest level in the history of Greater Southeast Community Hospital.

Certainly, problems still exist. Head nurses will continue to need management development, help in delegating responsibility and guidance in group process, conflict management, and confrontation skills. But the challenge now is to ensure that head nurses are provided opportunities for real growth and creativity; to keep them stimulated and happy; and above all, to maintain nursing administrator, hospital administration, and medical staff support of head nurses.

In order to ensure that head nurses will be able to maintain their proven skills, Greater Southeast is developing a competency-based program for them. The program will be in two phases: phase one will be orientation, while phase two will focus on continuing education. Orientation will provide a learning structure to help head nurses acquire the knowledge, skills and attitudes necessary for the rigors of their positions. It will also provide criteria to assist the associate director in measuring head nurse performance.

Continuing education will provide a resource structure to assist the head nurse in developing additional abilities which will contribute to continued professional development.

References

1. Lynette Gerschefske, "Assessment and Development for Head Nurse Positions," *Nursing Management,* February 1982, pp. 21–25.
2. Rosabeth Kantor, "Power Failure in Management Circuits," *Harvard Business Review,* July–August 1979, p. 67.
3. Rosabeth Kantor, "Power Failure in Management Circuits," p. 67.
4. Saul Gellerman, *Motivation and Productivity* (New York: American Management Association, 1963), p. 187.

CHAPTER 12

The Clinical Specialist as Manager: Myth versus Realities

by Mary A. Wallace and Linda J. Corey

This article advocates combining administrative power and professional power in middle management roles. The usual difficulties of the clinical specialist role with staff and the administrative hierarchy are contrasted with examples of the specialist as head nurse or clinical supervisor. The authors recommend blending clinical specialist–nursing manager roles as a strategy during budgetary cuts to retain clinical expertise in the institutional setting.

Does the title *clinical specialist* denote a prescribed role or a level of preparation and expertise that can be utilized in a variety of positions, including administrative roles such as head nurse or clinical supervisor? We assert that clinical care is enhanced when clinical specialist skills and administrative authority are combined in one position. In 1967, Claire Fagin was one of the first to discuss the clinical specialist in an administrative role[1]. Since then, this combined role has been developed and implemented in many institutions. However, controversy about such a melding of clinical skills with administrative authority remains an issue among clinical specialists.

Myths

Over the years, clinical specialists and nurse administrators have exchanged numerous myths or false beliefs about their mutual roles. These beliefs are frequently characterized by animosity and mutual suspicion. The attitude of clinical specialists toward their role vis-à-vis the formal administra-

tive structure is represented in the following statements seen in the literature or made to us by a clinical specialist:

> "Clinical specialists can be change agents without having any formal power."

> "Clinical specialists are not prepared to function administratively—to do so they must abandon other pursuits to acquire administrative skills."

> "A specialist may be seduced by the ready-made power of administrative positions and forsake the slower route to professional authority."

> "Staff positions are better than line positions—line positions are beneath one's dignity and a waste of talent."

Nurse administrators characterized the clinical specialist role by statements such as these:

> "Clinical specialists are afraid to roll up their sleeves and get their hands dirty."

> "Consultant status doesn't hold enough real responsibility.

> "Clinical specialists don't understand budget constraints, staffing constraints, practicalities of providing service, or the chain of command (i.e., the real world)."

> "Clinical specialists are too expensive."

These polarized beliefs abound in nursing practice settings and, when accepted as fact, limit creative thinking about the clinical-administrative relationship. The role of the clinical specialist has occupied the nursing literature on theoretical, practical, research, anecdotal, and survey levels for the past twenty years[2–5]. Expectations of the role remain unclear and have led to difficulties in the working relationships among specialist, line managers, and staff nurses. Debate continues over parameters of the specialist role such as the method of patient case load selection; direct patient care versus indirect care via consultation; and methods of securing staff nurse trust, respect, and permission to exert influence on the daily practice of nursing. Often the staff nurse view is that the specialist role is elitist, idealistic, and not grounded in the realities of nursing practice on hospital wards. Even the more optimistic of nurse

Mary A. Wallace, R.N., M.S., C.S., is Psychiatric Nursing Supervisor, Veterans Administration Medical Center, San Diego, California. She also holds clinical faculty appointments with the University of San Diego School of Nursing and the Department of Psychiatry, University of California, San Diego.

Linda J. Corey, R.N., was Head Nurse, Veterans Administration Medical Center, San Diego, California, at the time this article was written. She is now a part-time consultant and educator.

authors acknowledge that highly refined interpersonal skill is necessary to the specialist role in addition to clinical expertise[2,3,4]. Regarding the specialist role, attitudes of those in the clinical environment range from welcoming, friendly, or curious to hostile, suspicious, and resentful. Administrators point to the unclear authority structure of the specialist role. To whom are the specialists accountable? The patient? The staff nurse? Management? Some combination of the above? The specialists wonder how to validate their role and identify the proper consumer of their services. Is success measured by changes in staff nurse performance or in improved patient outcome? Stevens summarizes these problems from a systems perspective. "The major difficulty is that the clinical specialist role was not designed to fit into the bureaucratic hierarchial management system typical of health care institutions. The role is an administrative anomaly, grafted to a system in which it does not comfortably fit"[6].

Realities

We believe solutions to some if not many of these dilemmas can be brought about by combining administrative authority with the professional authority of clinical specialization. By definition, administrative authority is derived from an organizational position. The holder of the position has authority to take action, to enforce rules, to give commands, and to make final decisions. In a line position, clear responsibility exists for the actions and management of other employees. In contrast, professional or expert authority is derived from knowledge and expertise and is granted by choice rather than fiat. When administrative and professional authority are successfully combined, the power of each is enhanced.

Middle management roles

Administration in nursing has the responsibility to both provide and improve patient care. In hospital settings, the middle management roles commonly identified as head nurse and clinical supervisor have long been recognized as critical to the provision and improvement of care. The head nurse is regarded as a gatekeeper to the subsystem of individual clinical areas where the consumers of clinical specialist services are found. Without the strong professional alliance of the head nurse, specialists have found that effecting clinical change becomes extremely difficult if not impossible.

Likewise, the clinical supervisor plays a key role. The person in this position in an inpatient setting usually selects head nurses, decides what categories of staff are needed, and decides how to deploy staff. The quality of the leader, particularly the leader who selects the rest of the staff, has a determining effect on the quality of the care provided. In any setting, the supervisor decides what modes of nursing

practice to support and by what method staff will be supervised. In many situations, the head nurse and clinical supervisor may supervise the clinical work of staff, engage in direct practice that serves as a teaching model, and function as clinical team leaders. We believe this alliance can be secured by the combining of traditional head nurse or supervisor responsibilities with the clinical/educational role of the specialist.

"A head nurse or supervisor must be viewed as competent in both the administrative and clinical arenas."

At these middle management levels, both administrative and professional authority are vital to unit function. A head nurse or supervisor must be viewed as competent in both the administrative and clinical arenas. Deficiencies in one area dilute perceived competencies and effectiveness in the other. This assertion applies primarily to the middle management levels of the hierarchy. At higher levels of administration, the relative importance of clinical to administrative competencies decreases. Likewise, in a purely clinical role, the need for administrative skill also decreases. However, at middle management levels both clinical and administrative expertise are critical.

We question the myths that "clinical specialists are not prepared to function administratively" and "specialists don't understand the real world" when we consider what administrative skills and responsibilities are called for in middle management nursing roles. Tasks of the middle manager include the provision of round-the-clock nursing care in hospital settings. The baseline competence of nursing care providers must be established and the quality of potential care privdes evaluated. The evaluation and maintenance of staff nurse performance are usually the responsibility of head nurses and supervisors. Nurses in these roles are also charged with the improvement of nursing care and are expected to make expert use of interpersonal process to channel and utilize resistance to change.

Management skills

Where does the nurse learn middle management skills? The course contents of managerial skills classes and workshops revolve around understanding human behavior, motivation, conflict and conflict management, stress theory, systems theory, and the phenomenon of change. The thrust of the current popular *participative management* methods is the involvement of those concerned in decision making. This provides for an alignment of authority and responsibility. The modern manager is encouraged to recognize good performance and creativity and utilize crisis situations to effect positive change.

Content knowledge and the skills used in good management are present in the background of most clinical specialists. For the psychiatric clinical specialist particularly, the skills of individual, group, and family therapy are readily generalized to the requirements of administrative nursing. The interpersonal expertise needed in psychiatric nursing is also a central concern of nursing administration.

Where does the specialist-manager find time to practice as a clinical specialist? The practice of participative management leads to a sharing of the responsibilities traditionally assumed by the head nurse or supervisor alone. Such delegations can free time for the clinical teaching and direct patient care for which the specialist is equipped. For example, when a subgroup of staff nurses works out a schedule for the entire month, the head nurse may find time for primary patients or leading a group.

Power and resources

The most important aspect of combining the expertise of the specialist in the head nurse and supervisor role is one nurses are just now facing straightforwardly—that of assuming power. Instead of spending countless hours courting the favor of those in power to allow them access to the setting and permission to utilize their skills, the specialist-supervisors or the specialist-head nurses *are* the ones in charge. They hire the other staff, set up the nursing policies, have the authority input on interdisciplinary executive decisions, and make long-range plans. By working with budget and staffing constraints yet designing the priorities of care, they may be the ones to make the most of the limited resources available. Indeed, with the many decisions facing clinical supervisors and head nurses on a daily basis, the clinical knowledge of their specialty is crucial to making the best choices for available resources. In this time of budget cuts, the specialist role and that of the in-service educator are often seen by hospital administration as superfluous or too expensive. Reassigning these specialists into available administrative roles is one method of retaining valuable nursing resources. The specialist as manager can then utilize methods of delegation, participative management, and task group assignments to administer the ward. This leaves significant time for consultation and clinical supervision. Finally, important decisions are made by the most knowledgeable and skillful nurses using both professional and administrative power. The reuslt can be improved quality of care through system changes.

Reduction of personnel, time and budget constraints,

along with demands for increased accountability, can evoke creative reorganization in many static systems. Perhaps the time has arrived to take advantage of the budget crises to examine the myths of clinical specialists versus administrative nurses. The blending of clinical specialist-nursing manager roles into strong leadership positions is critical to the protection of professional nursing practice in institutional settings. The option of cutting out specialist positions, with specialists leaving for private or clinic practice, will diminish institutional nursing's long-worked-for clinical leadership. More specialists need to accept and shape administrative assignments in order to retain the advances made in their clinical nursing practice.

Professional autonomy stems from the freedom to practice one's skills. Psychiatric clinical specialists particularly have long been leaving the mainstream of institutional nursing for the professional freedom of clinics and private practice. Specialists need to recognize that this autonomy can also be realized in an administrative role that has been designed to include clinical practice. The clinical specialist's skills are then utilized and appreciated over a much larger system.

In our experience as clinical supervisor and head nurse of a busy psychiatric service of a large Veterans Administration/university teaching hospital, it has been possible to combine clinical specialist skills in administrative assignments in a satisfying and effective manner. As managers with high clinical priorities, the time for clinical practice was important, scheduled, and accomplished. The high priority of clinical practice has positively affected supervision, policy making, and program planning and assisted collaborative interdisciplinary relationships. The combination of administration and clinical specialist roles has resulted in a high degree of professional autonomy.

References

1. Claire M. Fagin, "The Clinical Specialist as Supervisor," *Nursing Outlook* pp. 34–36, January 1967.
2. Sally J. Everson, "Integration of the Role of Clinical Nurse Specialist," *Journal of Continuing Education in Nursing* 12(2):16–19+, 1981.
3. J. Murphy and M. Schmitz, "The Clinical Nurse Specialist: Implementing the Role in a Hospital Setting," *The Journal of Nursing Administration,* pp. 29–31, January 1979.
4. M. Blount et al., "Extending the Role of the Clinical Nurse Specialist," *Nursing Administration Quarterly* pp. 53–63, fall, 1981.
5. L. Beebor and B. Scicchitani, "Point/Counterpoint: Should the Clinical Nurse Specialist be Free of Administrative Responsibility?" *Perspectives In Psychiatric Care* 18(6):150–268, November-December, 1980.
6. Barbara J. Stevens, "Accountability of the Clinical Specialist: The Administrators Viewpoint," *The Journal of Nursing Administration,* pp. 30–32, February 1976.

CHAPTER 13

Employee Performance Reviews that Work

by Mary Riley

Employee performance reviews can often be a frustrating, time-consuming and unproductive process for both the employee and the manager. This article outlines three steps that will make an employee performance review system more effective. According to the author, EPRs can be used to increase productivity, improve morale, and create better communication.

What does the prudent administrator do to increase productivity, improve morale and create better communication?

The commonplace Employee Performance Review (EPR) can be the single most important tool for increasing an institution's productivity; properly applied, the EPR can help determine a hospital's course. An effective Review has sometimes meant the difference between success and failure of an organization's personnel relations.

The first EPR made its appearance over twenty years ago in the U.S.; since then it has been widely modified—and vilified. However, most organizations agree that the EPR should accomplish the following *objectives:*

1. *Increase productivity by helping employees get the job done right the first time.*
2. *Put employees on management's side by instilling a team spirit.*
3. *Reduce costly turnover and absenteeism by increasing employees' commitment to the institution.*
4. *Help decrease or eliminate grievances.*

Why EPRs are often unsuccessful

Lack of structure

An EPR may fail because it is unstructured: one typical type of EPR asks the reviewer to define the employee's strengths

Mary Riley, Ph.D., President of Morgan Method, Inc., develops mutual goalsetting programs, performance review systems, and management development programs. Her Ph.D. in management was under the advisorship of Peter Drucker. She teaches nursing students at the masters degree level at the University of Southern California and University of Redlands.

and weaknesses by writing at least one long, analytical paragraph about the worker. The basic flaw here is that the reviewer must undertake two tasks that he or she may be ill-equipped to do—write a grammatically correct, meaningful statement, while accurately describing the employee's performance.

This type of EPR focuses more on the supervisor's ability to write than on the key issues related to employee performance. Organizations who use this type of faulty review often ask a personnel manager or a vice president to write the EPR. They may thus achieve a well-written descriptive analysis but one not written by the employee's immediate supervisor. Even if the supervisor does compile the information, such an unstructured report is rarely useful. How can an institution use this report to develop and encourage the employee's strengths?

One-way communication EPRs

A second type of performance review that *is* more structured asks the reviewer to rate the employee in a number of key areas. The supervisor judges the employee on a scale from "excellent" to "unfavorable" for such factors as communication, promptness, quality and quantity of work, ability to delegate tasks, willingness to take on more responsibility, etc.

The most serious flaw with this form of EPR is that it sets up a judgemental, parent-child relationship featuring one-way communication—from the reviewer to the employee. These rating review systems fail because they ask one person (the reviewer) to make negative judgements about another person (the employee). Management by intimidation may have worked twenty years ago but it doesn't work today.

In some respects, the one-way form of EPR can be more destructive than the unstructured EPR. The ratings—whether based on a numbering system of one through five, or on an "unsatisfactory-fair-satisfactory-good-excellent" system—may give the false illusion of objectivity. They are as subjective as any other kind of rating system. In addition, receiving a low score in any one area can destroy the employee's confidence and incentive.

Making EPRs more effective

A performance review should be designed to improve an employee's performance, improve the working relationship between the employee and the supervisor/reviewer, and increase employee satisfaction with the job and the institution. An effective EPR system

- does not ask the reviewer to make value judgements about the employee's "good" and "bad" performance.
- requires the reviewer to explain the priorities of the job to the employee.
- has a goal-setting apparatus that helps the reviewer and employee set goals that are specific, measurable, obtainable, realistic and mutually meaningful.
- provides a format for achieving goals built on the employee's strengths, not on perceived weaknesses.
- creates an adult atmosphere where the reviewer and employee meet as equals.

What specific steps can you take to make EPRs work for you?

1. *Discuss skills that are important to the employee's job.* Have the employee and the reviewer complete a pre-performance review form that lists various job skills *before* the review meeting. On this form the reviewer and the employee both indicate the relative importance of each skill. It is crucial that they agree on the areas that are important to the employee's job.

   One of the most common sources of low morale is when an employee spends all his energy on skill "X". Then, when promotion time arrives, another employee performing skill "Y" gets the promotion because no one ever told the original employee that Y job skill was more important! When the supervisor determines priorities, he or she will be forced to define important job activities; the employee and the reviewer both benefit in the end.

2. *Give the employee recognition for job skills the employee performs well. Recognition* is the single most important factor that motivates employees to do a good job. Build recognition firmly into your EPR. Before the review meeting takes place, have both parties consult a list of job-related skills and check those that each feels the employee performs well.

   Never discuss the employee's weaknesses—for two reasons: first, few managers or supervisors are able to see an employee's weaknesses without reflecting their own biases; second, even fewer employees are able to truly accept negative judgements.

   Remember: The goal is not to judge or criticize employees. Our objective is to improve productivity. The employee's "weaknesses" are handled in Step 3.

3. *Set realistic, attainable, measurable goals.* Both the reviewer and the employee should agree on specific goals to improve both of their jobs. Make sure the goals are time-limited.

   Goal-setting should not be a one-way street, either. If the employee does not participate in the goal-setting, he or she will feel no "ownership" in the process and will not be motivated to reach the goals. Also, goals dictated by the supervisor invariably reflect the reviewer's perceptions about the employee's strengths and weaknesses; such perceptions may be neither accurate nor shared by the employee. Finally, one-way-street goals ignore the fact that the supervisor's own role performance affects the employee's ability to operate effectively.

Conclusion

You may wish to say, "But we don't have equal roles. I'm the boss!" That may be so, but we are talking about *effective* EPRs—reviews that make employees happy and productive. Treating employees with respect works. Communicating with employees works.

We do not claim that this type of review system is the answer to all employee relations problems. But it can be a powerful first step in the right direction. A performance review method that treats employees like responsible adults and encourages them to perform and produce like responsible adults—that's the beginning of wise management . . . and a more productive workplace.

CHAPTER 14

■ Diane K. Kjervik, RN, MS, JD

Progressive Discipline in Nursing:

Arbitrators' Decisions

Nursing administrators occasionally must appear before an arbitrator during a hearing to present evidence about the disciplining or discharge of a nursing staff member. Labor arbitrators will examine the record for evidence of appropriate discipline, including progressive discipline, which gradually increases the severity of penalties. This gives the employee adequate warning about improper behavior and an opportunity to respond. The author describes progressive discipline, identifies its elements, and shows cases in which arbitrators have either upheld or overturned hospitals' disciplinary measures. Nursing administrators will discover guidelines for progressive discipline that will help them in either avoiding a demand for arbitration or convincing the arbitrator that disciplinary measures were appropriate.

N ational labor policy favors neutral arbitration for the resolution of disputes that arise during the term of a collective bargaining agreement.[1] In fact, a labor organization that does not assert an employee's rights may be legally liable to the employee for such failure.[2,3] In the health care field, the most frequent issues brought to arbitrators involve discharge and discipline.[4] Arbitrators interpret the collective bargaining agreement and apply it to the disciplinary problem presented.[1]

Most contracts in the health care field state that discipline and discharge must be for "just cause" or "proper cause."[4] Even if a contract does not include such a clause, arbitrators may imply a just cause provision.[1,5] Progressive discipline has been considered part of the just cause provision.[5] The nursing administrator carries the burden of proof for showing that discipline was given for just cause.[6,7] Therefore, it becomes imperative for an administrator to understand the meaning of progressive discipline, its purpose, and its elements.

Arbitrator Wilbur Bothwell defined progressive

Diane K. Kjervik, RN, MS, JD, is Assistant Professor in the School of Nursing, University of Minnesota, Minneapolis, Minnesota.

discipline as "the use of reprimands, written reprimands and disciplinary suspensions prior to discharge."[8] Progressive discipline encourages employees to meet minimum standards of conduct.[8,9] Common sense, reason, and a sense of fairness would demand progressive discipline even if the law did not.

■ Employer's Burden of Proof in Discipline Cases

To show that an employee was disciplined for just cause, an employer must prove three things: (1) that the employee actually breached the rule or committed the offense as charged, (2) that the employee's act warranted punishment, and (3) that the penalty was just and appropriate to the offense.[10] Progressive discipline pertains to the third point because it provides the gradual disciplining necessary to an appropriate punishment.

Arbitrators examine several elements in determining the adequacy of the employer's disciplinary procedure: (1) thoroughness of the employer's investigation of the problem behavior, (2) fairness or nondiscriminatory treatment of employees, (3) notice to the employee of the problem behavior, and (4) the effect of prior discipline on the employee. Arbitrators in nursing cases have examined each of these elements.

Thoroughness of the Investigation

Progressive discipline assumes that the nurse administrator adequately investigates the facts. This gives the employee a chance to demonstrate that minimum standards of conduct were met. An investigation is inadequate when management has not asked the grievant to provide it with a statement about the incident from the grievant's perspective. Due process rights include an opportunity to explain what happened. For instance, during a sick-out by night nurses in critical care units, a hospital failed to investigate whether all absent nurses were involved in the sick-out or were legitimately sick. Had the employer done so, the nurse's knee injury would have been discovered. The arbitrator ruled that a 2–day suspension was improper and ordered the employer to give the nurse 1 day of sick pay and reimbursement for the money lost during the 2–day suspension.[11] When there is an incident, the nurse administrator should be sure to ask the employee to describe and to explain it and should obtain a description of it from other employees who either witnessed what occurred or have highly pertinent information about it.

Fairness and Nondiscriminatory Treatment

Nurse administrators should develop fair and consistently applied personnel policies.[9] Two employees with the same backgrounds committing the same offense under the same circumstances should receive the same penalty.[6] Consistent treatment of employees serves progressive discipline. It puts nurses on notice about expected standards of conduct prior to penalties.

An RN who had been discharged for allowing a patient to take Meclamin, although he was allergic to aspirin, was reinstated by the arbitrator, in part because hospital policy regarding medication administration was not followed by other RNs in the hospital, and they did not receive severe penalties. The nurse lost no seniority, but the arbitrator denied her back pay for the time that she missed work after her discharge.[12]

Fairness can also be evaluated by the manner in which management conducted the investigation. For instance, during an investigation, a management official may not be both a judge of the facts and a witness against the employee.[13]

Notice to the Nurse

Giving notice to an employee involves a forewarning of disciplinary action to be taken should the employee engage in specified behavior. The nurse administrator can notify orally or in writing and should state the rule and the corresponding penalty.[13] By notifying, one builds the foundation for progressive discipline. Without knowing what is expected, an employee cannot be faulted for failure to conform to a minimum standards of conduct and does not have the opportunity to prepare a defense to such charges. For instance, an arbitrator exonerated a nurse whose absenteeism had resulted in a 6-month delay of her wage increase, in part because the nurse was never told that she risked this form of discipline if the absenteeism continued.[14] Nursing administrators should clearly notify their employees of expected performance and the consequences of substandard performance. Employees may be notified through oral statements during orientation or through posted or easily accessible written statements.

Effect of Prior Discipline

Arbitrators are more likely to uphold lesser penalties for first offenses than heavy penalties such as discharge. Unions consider discharge "capital punishment" because it results in the loss of one's job and one's job security.[9] However, the gradation of penalties in health care settings can be steeper than in industrial settings because of the life and death nature of the employee's activities.[15] Gradual discipline is the heart of progressive discipline. It permits the employee several opportunities to correct faulty behavior.

An arbitrator upheld an oral warning given a charge nurse for discussing work assignments with her staff in violation of her supervisor's instructions.[16] An oral warning plus a written reprimand for one offense by an RN, however, was not upheld. Two penalties for the same offense was considered a violation of the just cause provision of the collective bargaining agreement.[17] This notion of double jeopardy means that once a penalty has been imposed and accepted, it cannot be increased later.[1]

Arbitrators will uphold a more severe punishment when a lesser form of discipline precedes it. An arbitrator upheld a 2.5–day suspension of an RN for abusive language toward a patient's relative. The nurse had been informally warned 2 weeks prior to the incident to restrain her temper.[18] An arbitrator upheld the suspension and discharge of an LPN for giving the wrong medication to a patient. The LPN had been previously involved in three such incidents and had been retrained in medication administration. The corrective discipline was shown to be ineffective, according to the arbitrator.[19]

Arbitrators hold discharge to be too severe when

other methods of discipline have been minimally used prior to discharge. An RN who had been given three reprimands by her supervisors about her personal grooming, her attitude toward physicians, and transcription of orders from a physician who had no hospital privileges was discharged for improper drug administration that had resulted in a patient having suffered a severe allergic response. The arbitrator reduced the discharge to a suspension with a statement to be placed on the nurse's record specifying that any other serious professional error would result in immediate discharge.[12]

Nursing administrators should remember to apply discipline gradually, beginning first with oral warnings to the employee, then written warnings followed by suspensions and finally by discharge. They should keep a record of disciplinary measures used with a given employee so that they know whether the discipline has been applied gradually. Probationary or retraining periods give the employee a chance to improve performance and the nurse administrator an opportunity to evaluate the degree of improvement. Subsequent disciplinary measures are reasonable based upon performance during such periods.

Exceptions to the Requirement of Progressive Discipline

Arbitrators will consider the progressive discipline requirement mitigated by such factors as the gravity of the offense, the time period during which the offenses were committed, and the provisions of the collective bargaining contract. They will consider the offense grave enough to justify discharge if the nurse deliberately files false reports.[20] They also consider intentional violations of hospital rules and signing other nurses' names on charts to be unusually serious violations.[21] If a short time elapses during which a nurse commits several offenses, progressive discipline is not necessary. If the collective bargaining agreement itself specifies that progressive discipline is not necessary, management is not legally required to discipline progressively.

Conclusion

Collective bargaining agreements require nursing administrators to discipline employees only for just cause. Part of the just cause concept is progressive discipline, that is, gradual application of discipline that gives the nurse clear notice of the nature of the problem behavior and time in which to correct it. Whether or not a disciplinary matter eventually goes to an arbitrator, it is in the employer's best interest to take appropriate disciplinary steps so that all employees perceive that fairness and consistency have been observed.

Arbitrators evaluate several elements when determining the fairness of the discipline. A thorough investigation of the charges against the grievant, including the employee's own explanation of the events, is necessary. Nursing administrators should develop personnel policies fairly and apply them fairly to employees who are in similar circumstances. Administrators should give notice of policies, including ramifications for rule breaking, in a clear manner. In setting a penalty, they should consider the nature of any prior discipline, its effect on the employee, and the length of adequate service.

Although limited exceptions to the progressive discipline requirements exist, a nursing administrator should demonstrate every effort to discipline progressively. When this is not possible, an administrator should be prepared to show the arbitrator clear evidence of the reason that the progressive discipline was impossible to use for the nurse in question.

References

1. Elkouri F, Elkouri EA. How arbitration works. Washington, DC: Bureau of National Affairs, Inc., 1981:28-31, 296-7, 611, 636.
2. Vaca v. Sipes. United States Reports 1967;386:171-210.
3. Bowen v. United States Postal Service. Supreme Court Reporter 1983;103:588-608.
4. Petersen DJ, Halstead EG. The arbitration of cases involving improper professional conduct in the health care industry. Journal of the American Association of Nurse Anesthetists 1977;45(2):189-92.
5. Jackson County Medical Care Facility *and* American Federation of State, County, and Municipal Employees, Local 139. Labor Arbitration Reports 1975;65:389-94.
6. Metzger N. Hospital labor scene marked by union issues. Hospitals 1980;57(4):105-12.
7. Alabama Dept. of Mental Health *and* Public Service Employee's Union, Local 1279, Laborer's International Union of N. America. Labor Arbitration Reports 1976;66:279-86.
8. Southwest Electric Co. *and* Communication Workers of America, Local 6016. Labor Arbitration Reports 1969;54:195-6.
9. Arbitration of labor-management disputes. New York: AMACOM, 1974:232-3.
10. Metzger N. Handling grievances: guidelines for RNs. Hosp Prog 1979;60(9):69-94.
11. Kingsbrook Jewish Medical Center *and* New York State Nurses Association. Summary of Labor Arbitration Awards. Report Number 283.7, October 1982.
12. Ohio Valley Hospital Association *and* the Ohio Nurses Association. Labor Arbitration Reports 1982;79:929-34.
13. Grief Brothers Cooperage Cort. *and* United Mine Workers of America. Labor Arbitration Reports 1964;42:555-9.
14. Cottage Hospital *and* Massachusetts Nurses Association. Labor Arbitration in Government 1979;9(7):8.

15. Baderschneider ER, Miller PF, eds. Labor arbitration in health care. New York: Spectrum, 1976:XXV.
16. County of Erie (NY) *and* New York State Nurses Association. Labor Arbitration in Government 1982;12(8):2.
17. Auburn Faith Community Hospital *and* California Nurses Association. Labor Arbitration Reports 1976;66:882–99.
18. Crozer-Chester Medical Center (Philadelphia, PA) *and* Pennsylvania Nurses Association. Labor Arbitration in Government 1982;12(5):2.
19. State of New York, Office of Mental Health *and* Civil Service Employees Association. Labor Arbitration in Government 1980;10(10):3.
20. Dameron Hospital (CA) *and* California Nurses Association. Labor Arbitration in Government 1976;6(2):6.
21. Cook County (IL) Health and Hospitals Governing Commission *and* Illinois Nurses Association. Labor Arbitration in Government 1977;7(5):7.

CHAPTER 15

Improving Nursing Management and Practice Through Quality Circles

by Julie Wine Schaffner and John E. Baird, Jr.

Health care in general, and nursing in particular, is experiencing dramatic changes in worker values, economic realities, and management theory. All three areas of change move toward actively involving employees in organizational decision making. Although nursing managers have implemented a variety of systems to gain employee participation, "Quality Circles" seems to be the most promising method currently available. This article describes some techniques for effectively implementing Quality Circles within a nursing organization.

Today, more than ever before, the cliche that "we live in a changing world" is true. And nowhere are these changes seen more clearly than in the health care field in general, and in nursing specifically. During the last few years, dramatic changes have occurred in three major areas:

1. *Worker values.* Workers in every industry have developed a new set of expectations concerning how they are to be treated and what role they are to play in the organizations that employ them; and when their expectations are not met, workers often become disenchanted and nonproductive. And, in nursing, employees are demanding more input and influence in determining their own work environment, greater equality with the medical staff in decision making, and more respect from administrators be given to nurses' professional standing. Increasingly, nurses have become militant in their demands, often taking action against administration when their expectations are not met.

2. *Economic realities.* Difficult economic times necessitate that all organizations give more attention to their costs, incomes, and worker productivity. Certainly this is true in health care, as the widely-publicized reductions in governmental funding and decreases in patient census due to high unemployment in their immediate areas cause hospital administrators to seek ways in which productivity can be maximized and costs minimized.

3. *Management theories.* Increasingly, scholars writing about the "best" ways in which to manage people emphasize worker participation in organizational decision making. Theory Z, which formalizes the management approach taken so successfully by the Japanese during the past 25 years, stresses trust between workers and management. And, it suggests that the development of that trust can come about only when labor and management participate together in organizational decision making and problem solving. In turn, this trust has been shown to bring about increased productivity, increased worker morale, reduced turnover and absenteeism, improved quality of work, and enhanced organizational success.

It seems clear that all three changes are moving in the same direction. Today's nursing professional has the desire —and the ability—to participate in organizational decision making. Today's economic climate necessitates management involve employees in order to maximize productivity. Management theorists, perhaps reflecting these realities, call upon management to institute programs which involve employees in work-related decisions, and, thus, build trust between labor and management. A more participative style of nursing management seems, therefore, to be required by, and an inevitable result of, today's realities in health care.

While a variety of techniques such as task-forces, committee structures, and management-employee "rap" sessions have been implemented in an effort to meet these challenges, the most promising technique currently avail-

Julie Wine Schaffner, R.N., M.S.N., is the Director of Nursing Management Services, a division of Modern Management, Inc. She received the Bachelor of Science and Master of Science in Nursing from the University of Virginia. She was a Head Nurse and an Administrative Fellow to nursing administration while at the University of Virginia.

John E. Baird, Jr., Ph.D., is the Manager of Positive Personnel Practices, a division of Modern Management, Inc.

able seems to be Quality Circles, a system for participative management and productivity improvement. Developed in Japan nearly three decades ago and used recently in American manufacturing firms, Quality Circles now have a place in health care. Quality Circles prove an effective tool for improving the quality of patient care, increasing employee job satisfaction, reducing health care costs, and maximizing employee productivity. They involve nursing professionals in decision making and facilitate communication between the medical and nursing staff. This article describes in some detail the most effective techniques to implement Quality Circles within a nursing organization.

Quality Circles structure

Quality Circles are groups of six to twelve employees from the same department or unit who meet regularly, usually once a week, to identify, analyze, and solve work-related problems. As such, Quality Circles are not mysterious, magic, or even new. Many health care organizations have quasi Quality Circles in operation already but call them unit or departmental meetings. To be truly effective, however, a Quality Circles system—and any other problem-solving system, for that matter,—must have both a coordinating structure and members who possess specific skills. These two characteristics—structure and skills—distinguish Quality Circles and make them far more effective than usual departmental or unit meetings.

Exhibit 1 illustrates the structure of a nursing Quality Circles system. At the top of the structure is a Steering Committee, which provides direction and support for the operating circles. Steering Committee membership typically is comprised of top and middle-level administrators representing such major areas of the organization as nursing, ancillary services, support services, finance, and public relations. Members review circle proposals and ultimately determine whether those proposals will be enacted. On occasion, however, Quality Circles begin only within the nursing organization. In those situations, the Steering Committee is comprised of the directors of each nursing functional area, with the director of nursing acting either as the committee chairperson or as the program facilitator.

The facilitator may be the single most important element in the entire system. It is his or her responsibility to oversee the program, to train (usually with the assistance of an internal or external consultant) the circle leaders and participants, to coordinate the activities of individual circles with one another and with the rest of the organization, to assist each circle in obtaining the information and resources they need to complete their tasks, and to attend initial circle meetings to ensure that activities are proceeding properly. When Quality Circles are first implemented, roughly 50 percent of the facilitator's time will be devoted to circle activities. Once the system is under way, however, relatively little time will be required.

In nursing organizations, head nurses typically act as Quality Circle leaders; although charge nurses, shift supervisors, department directors, and assistant directors occasionally serve in this capacity. The functions of the circle leader are to convene circle meetings, train circle participants in problem-solving techniques during initial meetings, ensure that conflicts are resolved and decisions reached, and, above all, remain silent as much as possible so employees can do the work. This last function often is the most difficult for new circle leaders to learn, but it is vital to the success of this participative decision-making program.

Circle participants are the employees themselves: six to twelve volunteers from the same department or unit who have been trained in communication and group decision-making techniques. In very large departments or units, these people are selected from a pool of volunteers. Those not selected may be called upon at some later time to replace a participant who has left the program or to form new circles when program expansion seems warranted. In smaller departments, the entire department may act as a Quality Circle. In any case, it is desirable to confine circle membership to employees working within the same unit, and to involve all categories of employees such as RNs, LVNs, and Ward Clerks, from that unit. Since the goals of Quality Circles are improved communication and problem resolution, these goals first need to be achieved among different sub-groups within a particular unit before expanding outside that unit.

Clearly, many employees and members of management will not be directly involved in circle meetings. Nevertheless, it is important to keep these people informed of circle activities via normal departmental, supervisory, and management meetings. Non-circle employees and other management personnel naturally will be curious about circle proceedings and often will contribute their ideas or concerns to individuals who are actively participating. Again, facilitating this on-going communication ultimately is the responsibility of the Quality Circles facilitator.

Implementing Quality Circles

The Quality Circles structure must be developed and put in place through a carefully-designed and well thought-out series of activities.

1. *Set program objectives.* Before implementing Quality Circles, decide what objectives are to be achieved by the program. Directors of nursing have identified and achieved a variety of such objectives as:

   - Improved nurse retention
   - Reduced absenteeism
   - Increased recruitment
   - Improved employee morale

- Improved the quality of patient care
- Reduced costs of patient care delivery
- Improved nurse-physician relations
- Improved communications
- Alleviated staff shortages by increasing work efficiency.

Setting objectives serves a number of purposes, such as providing a foundation for building management support for the program, providing some direction for subsequent program efforts, and ultimately suggesting measures which should be taken to evaluate the program's success.

2. *Building management support.* If the program is to be successful, management genuinely must be committed to obtaining and using employee suggestions. We have observed a few instances of failure in Quality Circle programs, all of which can be traced back to managers who give "lip service" to the program, but who truly do not want employee input or participation. In these cases, employee action plans to resolve the problem were rejected by management out of hand, leaving employees with the impression that management had never intended to listen to them in the first place. The

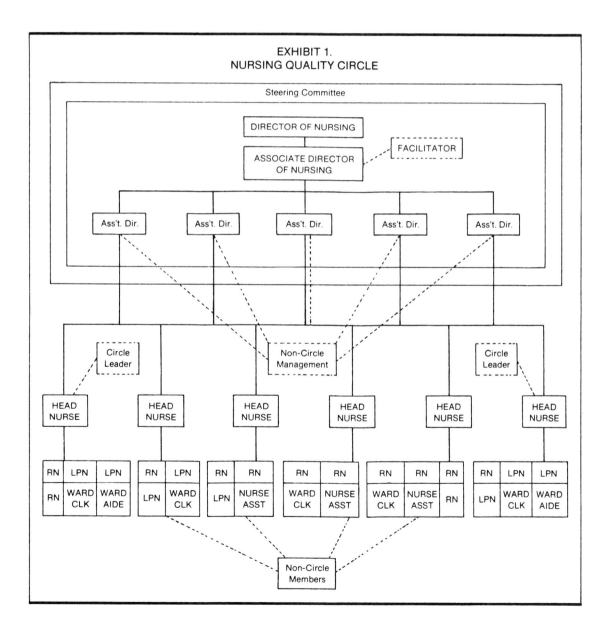

EXHIBIT 1.
NURSING QUALITY CIRCLE

resentment aroused by this impression of Quality Circles creates a destructive rather than positive force in those organizations. Certainly, top management must be committed to implementing the program. Even when Quality Circles will be initiated only in the nursing organization, it is important that members of hospital administration support the concept; otherwise, they may refuse to provide assistance to the circle participants when it is needed.

3. *Organizing the Steering Committee.* Steering Committee members should represent major functions within the organization, and express committment to making the program work.

4. *Selecting the facilitator(s).* If no one emerges as the facilitator, the Steering Committee should select one. If more than eight groups will be formed, additional facilitators should be selected. As selection criteria, the Steering Committee should search for someone who:

   - Is committed to the Quality Circles process
   - Is able to devote the necessary time
   - Understands the organization, both technically and politically
   - Is skilled as a communicator, both in formal presentations and in informal interactions
   - Is respected throughout the general organization.

Again, the director or assistant director of nursing often plays this role. However, nursing education coordinators, department heads, and shift supervisors also have performed well as facilitators. The key criterion is not the organizational level the facilitator holds, but the qualities that person possesses.

5. *Training the facilitator(s).* Facilitators must possess strong communication skills. Since they have primary responsibility for training circle leaders and participants, they also may need to learn specific concepts and skills to facilitate the group activities which occur during leader and participant training. Moreover, they must develop some skills unique to the facilitator role:

   - Involving all levels of management in the process
   - Identifying and resolving potential problems
   - "Selling" the program internally and externally
   - Scheduling and coordinating circle activities
   - Evaluating circle participants and leaders
   - Rewarding participants and leaders
   - Expanding the Quality Circles program

Facilitators may acquire these skills in three ways. First, they may be self-taught, simply reading everything they can about Quality Circles, and then based on their reading and previous skills develop any additional materials needed to implement the program. Second, they may attend seminars offered by various agencies which teach basic Quality Circles principles, but which typically do not provide in-depth instruction. Finally,

and most commonly, facilitators may hire a consultant experienced in Quality Circles health care implementation to help them structure the program and develop facilitator skills. Cost for such consultants ranges between $8,000 and $20,000, and most provide the instructional materials which the facilitator(s) will need to teach circle leaders and participants. Experienced consultants also are able to tailor the program specifically to the facilitator's organization, and to provide advice and assistance should problems in the program's implementation develop.

6. *Identifying circle leaders.* Supervisors and middle-level managers should be informed about the Quality Circles concept and process and what involvement in that process means, and then be given an opportunity to volunteer. Typically, more individuals will volunteer than can be put into the program, at least initially. The Steering Committee and facilitator should select the leaders who seem best suited to the program, whose units or departments could profit most from the program, or whose leadership style could most be improved by participation in the program. It is important to note, however, that later in this article we suggest some conditions which must be met in order for Quality Circles to be successful. One of these conditions is a reasonable level of employee satisfaction with the immediate supervisor. We have found that employees who are extremely disenchanted with their supervisor do not participate enthusiastically when that individual convenes their Quality Circle meeting.

7. *Selecting circle participants.* The Quality Circle program should be announced to the entire organization, and those individuals selected as circle leaders should ask for volunteers from among their own employees. Again, usually more employees volunteer than are needed. The circle leader should be the one to select members and should be allowed to do so with only one restriction: employees who have not completed a probationary period should not be selected to participate. This includes the employee who is new to the organization or one who transfers from one job to another within the organization. Effective participation comes about only when the participants know their own jobs well enough to analyze and improve them, and probationary employees lack that knowledge.

8. *Taking base-line measures.* As much as possible, the Steering Committee should take measures of factors relevant to the objectives of the program. If one objective is to reduce turnover, current turnover statistics should be collected; if another objective is to reduce costs, cost-related data should be obtained. These measures ultimately will be compared with later measures of the same factors to produce an index of the extent to which the program has been successful.

9. *Training circle leaders.* In approximately sixteen hours

of formal classroom content, circle leaders are taught skills in participative management, communication, problem analysis, presentation techniques, conducting meetings, and resolving conflict. They are trained in the same skills that circle participants need to learn, but also learn the skills they need to lead their groups effectively. These training sessions are usually conducted by the Quality Circles facilitator and/or an internal or external consultant.

10. *Training circle participants.* Circle participants receive two types of training. First, in formal half-day sessions conducted by the facilitator and/or a consultant, participants are instructed in effective communication techniques and are provided with an overview of the problem-solving process. Second, when the circle meetings begin, members learn specific problem-solving skills with the guidance of the circle leader by analyzing and resolving a real-life problem of their own choosing. This "learn by doing" approach has proven far more successful than the classroom hypothetical problem approach, but it places heavy responsibility upon the circle leader to train the participants effectively.

11. *Initiating meetings.* When actual circle meetings begin, the facilitator should attend as many meetings as possible to ensure that activities proceed smoothly. Generally, the sequence of meetings is as follows:

Meeting 1: Identify problems; brainstorming session
Meeting 2: Analyze work; flow-process charting
Meeting 3: Gather information; assign responsibilities
Meeting 4: Display information
Meeting 5: Select problem; fishbone diagram causes
Meeting 6: Selecting causes
Meeting 7: Brainstorming solutions; select viable options
Meeting 8: Evaluate viable solutions
Meeting 9: Select solution(s)
Meeting 10: Develop action plans

At the end of approximately ten weeks, participants will have learned specific problem analysis and resolution techniques such as brainstorming, flow-process charting, and fishbone diagramming, a brainstorming-based technique by which participants identify every conceivable cause for the problem they have identified. Also, they will have applied these techniques to each problem-solving step, and ultimately will have selected and analyzed a problem, chosen a solution, and developed an action plan by which the solution could be implemented.

12. *Presentations to Steering Committee.* After the circle develops an action plan, members meet formally with the Steering Committee to present their work and their proposal. In turn, the Steering Committee reviews the proposal, evaluates its merits, and decides whether it should be implemented. Then the Steering Committee communicates its decision to the circle, indicating either when implementation will occur (as is the decision in most instances) or why the proposal could not be accepted. In the latter case, suggestions for additional work or for proposal modifications should be given. Action plans are communicated throughout the organization, giving proper credit and recognition to the circle participants and circle leader.

"... management genuinely must be committed to obtaining and using employee suggestions."

---

13. *Review and expansion of the program.* The Steering Committee continually reviews the group's progress through the use of program facilitator's reports. After a predetermined time period, typically six to eight months the committee formally reviews the program by comparing such measures as turnover and costs with the original baseline information. Based on the results of that comparison, the Steering Committee decides whether the program should be continued in its present form, modified, expanded, or even discontinued. Usually, the decision is to expand the program to other areas.

Occasionally, the actual sequence with which organizations implement Quality Circles differs from what we have presented. However, we believe the program's success depends on each of these steps being completed at some point; and the system seems to work best when these steps occur in the order we have described.

Problems considered by nursing Quality Circles

With one important addition, nursing organizations implement Quality Circles in the manner we have outlined. Often, members of the medical staff are invited to participate, or even volunteer, as regular circle members. Such participation is highly desirable, for often many of the issues nursing circles deal with impact directly upon the physician's role in the organization.

Although the specific problems considered by nursing circles vary from one circle to the next, generally topics include:

• Improving retention
• Improving recruitment

- Improving nursing practice
- Improving coordination with other departments (for example, Laboratories, Housekeeping, Dietary)
- Improving delivery or distribution of supplies, medication, and so forth
- Improving physician-nurse relations
- Developing clinical advancement strategies
- Improving scheduling and staffing
- Increasing quality assurance in patient care
- Improving communication
- Decreasing waste, theft, costs, and so forth.

In almost all instances, nursing circles develop action plans that deal with each issue in a practical, inexpensive, easy to implement, and, above all, an effective manner. When management supports participative decision making at the outset, rarely have we observed an action plan which management has found unacceptable.

Preconditions for effective Quality Circles

While Quality Circles repeatedly have proven successful in achieving their goals, they are by no means fool-proof. A set of preconditions must be present at implementation for Quality Circles to function effectively. If these conditions are met, the program will be a striking success. If these conditions are not present, Quality Circles are likely to be a disaster. Briefly, these conditions include:

1. Moderate or higher levels of employee satisfaction. Angry employees do not contribute their ideas voluntarily to management.
2. Some value placed by management upon innovative approaches. Quality Circles are designed to produce change, and, thus, should not be implemented by people opposed to change.
3. Reasonable levels of satisfaction with the immediate supervisor who may serve as circle leader.
4. Reasonable levels of satisfaction with compensation. Employees who feel they are being cheated or under-

paid will not be anxious to contribute more effort.
5. Some trust in top management. Employees must believe that management supports the process and genuinely intends to implement employee ideas. Otherwise, employees will see the program as an exercise, and will participate reluctantly or for such wrong reasons as having an opportunity to complain and to be destructive influences.
6. Some sense of job security. Employees who are concerned that they may be laid-off, transferred, or lose their positions through some other mechanism probably will not be interested in participative problem solving.
7. Some job-related expertise on the part of the participants.
8. A desire among employees to participate.

When these conditions are met, the program probably will achieve the objectives set out at the very beginning. If they are not, administration should investigate methods other than Quality Circles for reaching those objectives.

Conclusion

We have provided an overview of the potential Quality Circles hold as a nursing management tool, the structure for such a program, the stages through which implementation is achieved, the topics often considered by nursing Quality Circles, and the preconditions necessary for circles to work well. Certainly, a great number of other factors also should be considered by anyone contemplating implementation of Quality Circles, such as how circle contributions will be rewarded, how nursing circles can be coordinated with current quality assurance programs, and what topics should be designated as "off limits" for circle consideration. Nevertheless, we hope our recommendations will assist nursing administrators in determining whether a Quality Circles system should be pursued in their organizations to enhance nursing management and practice.

UNIT THREE

SANDRA R. EDWARDSON

Quality Assurance

Nurses' traditional concern about the quality of health care has been heightened by continuing financial pressures to reduce the cost of health care. As lengths of hospital stays are reduced and services trimmed, they observe first hand how rapidly many practices have changed and worry that it may have a negative effect on their patients' outcomes and rates of recovery. For these reasons, quality assurance activities have become a major challenge facing the profession.

Quality assurance (QA) refers to being accountable for the quality of services given. In health care, quality assurance programs are the sets of activities performed by the hospital or other organized service to ensure the public that the care given is safe and in accordance with the current state of the art.

The focus of activities used to ensure quality has evolved over the years from an early concentration on quality assessment to the current emphasis on quality assurance. Quality assessment and quality assurance differ in that the former is a care review process that measures the adequacy of care given, whereas the latter involves both a review of care and procedures to change practices when deficiencies have been uncovered.

Quality assessment involves three steps: identifying standards of care, measuring actual care against these standards, and then noting when practice does not match the standards. Until the passage of Medicare and Medicaid, the most prevalent quality review methods included activities such as tissue and incident review, evaluation of credentials of the medical and hospital staff, assessment of the safety of the environment, and so forth. More recently, the chart audit method for evaluation of the care process and outcome became important. Nurses have been involved in most of these activities either as data collectors and system monitors for other care providers or as participants in studies of the quality of nursing care. Several methods for auditing nursing elements of hospital records have been developed.[1-5] At about the same time, methods for measuring nursing care quality by observation of the care process or questioning clients were also developed.[4-9]

The emphasis on quality assessment began to change in the late 1970s largely in response to experience with the quality review requirements of the Joint Commission on the Accreditation of Hospitals (JCAH) and the federal legislation that established Professional Standards Review Organizations (PSRO). A common failing of both efforts was that, although many useful quality reviews had been performed, there was little evidence that the results had been used to improve performance once problems had been identified.[10] Two of the articles (Smeltzer, Feltman, Rajki and Edwardson, Anderson) describe some of the problems encountered by nursing departments in attempting to implement meaningful QA programs.

In 1979, therefore, JCAH replaced a prescriptive QA standard that had led to a heavy reliance on retrospective chart audits with a new standard. It emphasizes an integrated (multidisciplinary) approach that focuses on identifying and analyzing direct and indirect problems in the delivery of patient care and then taking appropriate action to correct the problem and sustain the solution. Although these investigations may involve all patient care units and services, there seems to be a trend toward performing some unit specific studies based on care problems unique to that unit.[11]

These developments present an exciting, yet difficult challenge to the profession. On the one hand, the problem-oriented approach not only encourages nurses to adopt a new QA strategy, but also offers a great opportunity for exploring the scientific bases of nursing practices. It may eventually permit nurses to establish standards that are not based just on commonly accepted practice but that are derived from scientific evidence that certain processes are most likely to produce the desired outcome. The article by Larson discusses the advantages and disadvantages of integrating quality assurance and research programs. Edmunds describes how computer technology can be used to enhance QA programs.

On the other hand, nurses share responsibility for resolving the dilemma facing all professionals currently engaged in delivering health care — namely, how much quality can we afford? While future advances in nursing care and medical technology will undoubtedly make it possible for patients to benefit from more expensive care and treatment, pressures to keep costs down will force all involved to make complex trade-offs between an additional, marginal improvement for the one as opposed to more modest improvements for the many.

The challenge for the future is for nurses to demonstrate the efficacy and cost effectiveness of the services they provide. All citizens will benefit from the diligent and systematic efforts of nurses to assess and ensure the quality of health care services.

References

1. Blanche S: Nursing audit. Hosp Prog 36:67–69, 1955
2. Fischer PR: The nursing audit. Nurs Outlook 5:590–592, 1957
3. Phaneuf MC: The Nursing Audit: Profile for Excellence. New York, Appleton–Century Crofts, 1976
4. American Nurses' Association: Guidelines for Review of Nursing Care at the Local Level. Kansas City, American Nurses' Association, 1976
5. Haussmann RKD, Hegyvary ST, Newman JF: Monitoring Quality of Nursing Care, Part II. Bethesda, MD, US Department of Health, Education and Welfare, US Public Health Service, Health Resources Administration, Bureau of Health Manpower, Division of Nursing, 1977
6. Wandelt MA, Ager JW: Quality Patient Care Scale. New York, Appleton–Century–Crofts, 1974
7. Wandelt MA, Stewart DS: Slater Nursing Competencies Rating Scale. New York, Appleton–Century–Crofts, 1974
8. Weinstein EL: Developing a measure of the quality of nursing care. J Nurs Admin 6:1–3, 1976
9. Horn BJ, Swain MA: Development of Criterion Measures of Nursing Care. Springfield, VA, National Technical Information Service, 1977
10. Institute of Medicine: Assessing Quality in Health Care: An Evaluation. Washington, DC, National Academy of Sciences, 1976
11. Schroeder PS, Maibusch RM: Nursing Quality Assurance—A Unit-Based Approach. Rockville, MD, Aspen, 1984

CHAPTER 16

Hospital Nurses' Valuation of Quality Assurance

by Sandra R. Edwardson and Darlene I. Anderson

Nurses responsible for quality assurance in ten metropolitan hospitals surveyed nurses from their institutions in an attempt to understand sluggish interest in quality assurance activities. The registered nurses surveyed agreed that involvement in quality assurance is an important part of the professional nurse's role, but this belief did not often translate into positive attitudes toward nor participation in quality assurance activities.

A discouraging reality for nurses who hold quality assurance positions in hospitals is the conclusion that their nurse colleagues are ambivalent about the quality assurance process. Yet as a group, nurses guard vigorously their right to define what constitutes good nursing care; furthermore, they defend as a fundamental professional privilege and responsibility their right to regulate the quality of care. Why, then, do individual nurses show so little enthusiasm for the mandated quality assurance functions? Why is participation in patient-care audits and other quality assurance activities often little more than an exercise in compliance, when it should be an activity born of conviction?

Today's quality assurance director must determine whether these antithetical feelings are merely inherent in any activity that demands self-examination, or whether the prevailing approaches to quality assurance are intrinsically unsatisfying (if not irrelevant) in day-to-day practice. Our study reports the efforts of one group of hospital quality assurance nurses to understand just what staff and management nurses know—and how they feel—about quality assurance activities.

Background of the study

Metropolitan Nurses in Quality Assurance (MNQA) is a group of greater Minneapolis and St. Paul hospital nurses

Sandra R. Edwardson, R.N., Ph.D., is Assistant Professor of Nursing and Interim Assistant Dean for Graduate Studies at the University of Minnesota School of Nursing, Minneapolis, Minnesota.

Darlene Anderson, R.N., is Director of Quality Assurance Services at United Hospitals, St. Paul, Minnesota.

involved in quality assurance activities. These nurses have been meeting monthly for several years to share their knowledge, help one another solve problems, and exchange ideas concerning this aspect of the nursing profession.

At about the same time the Joint Commission of the Accreditation of Hospitals (JCAH) was rewriting its quality assurance standard, MNQA nurses were questioning the worth of their activities within their own hospitals. Actions resulting from audits were not correcting deficiencies, data from quality assurance activities were not being utilized by nursing management, and there prevailed a gnawing sense that staff nurses were not concerned about the quality of their patient care. MNQA members began to wonder if their expectations for quality patient care were in fact the same as those of their staff nurses and nurse managers. To test their perceptions, they needed an accurate analysis of the situation. If the problem emerged as real, then possible areas of intervention could be identified.

Thus the group appointed a task force to detail a method for turning their perceived need into a study design. With the assistance of a school-of-nursing faculty member who served as a consultant, the task force concluded that MNQA needed answers to three basic questions:

1. How do hospital nurses define and describe quality assurance?
2. How highly do hospital nurses value quality assurance activities?
3. Is there a relationship between nurses' attitudes and their participation in quality assurance activities, and if so, is it a positive or a negative relationship?

Conceptual base

Quality assurance has become an increasingly important concern for nursing. The profession is under considerable internal and external pressure to demonstrate greater accountability for the services delivered by nurses. From within there is a growing conviction that scientific accountability through expansion and ongoing verification of the body of nursing knowledge is essential for achieving full professional status[1,2], for maintaining nurse control of nursing services[3-5], and for attracting students and retaining nurses in the profession. External pressures for increased accountability come from several regulatory and quasi-regulatory sources (rate-review bodies, Professional Standards Review Organizations, Health Systems Agencies, JCAH, etc.) and from third-party payers and other funding agencies. These groups are asking for evidence that outcomes of nursing care are of good quality and represent a cost-effective use of resources.

The accountability required by external groups involves "an obligation to reveal, explain, and justify what one does or how one discharges one's responsibilities"[6]. As a profession, nursing seems to have had an unusually difficult time "revealing, explaining, and justifying" its contribution to health care. At least part of the difficulty may lie in the fact that while nurses are legally accountable for their own practice, current organizational structures in which most nursing is practiced mitigate against identifiable nurses bearing the direct consequences for inappropriate decision making. Except for flagrant malpractice or illegal and immoral acts, accountability for nursing services is likely to be diffused among a group of nurses or assigned to an administrative superior. In other words, while individual responsibility to reveal, explain, and justify what one does and how one does it is inherent in the licensure laws and professional ethics that govern the profession, the precept is often enfeebled by the arrangements of practice.

A second, but not necessarily competing, explanation for reluctance to engage in quality-assurance activities is that nurses may hold negative attitudes toward the activities. The assumption that attitudes are powerful predictors of a person's actions is widely shared. Despite decades of debate and conflicting data about whether attitudes exert a directive or dynamic influence over behavior[7] or whether a change in behavior sometimes leads to a change in attitudes[8], the notion persists that attitudes toward an activity and performance of the activity are somehow related. Regan and Fazio, for example, present evidence suggesting that the method by which attitudes are formed may affect the consistency between attitudes and behavior. Specifically, their results showed that "direct behavioral experience produces an attitude which is more clearly, confidently, and stably maintained than an attitude formed through more indirect means"[9]. Furthermore, attitudes were better predictors of behavior among subjects who had had prior experience with the situation in question than among those who had not. If these findings hold true for nurse attitudes toward quality assurance activities, they suggest an important method for increasing nurse participation in such activities.

In an attempt to explore the possibility of a relationship between prior experience with quality assurance and positive attitudes toward the activity, two hypotheses were posed.

• *Hypothesis 1.*   Staff nurses who have had experience in

EXHIBIT 1.
FREQUENCY OF SUBJECTS IN
EACH JOB CLASSIFICATION*

Position	Frequency	Percent of sample	Response rate
Staff Nurse	215	69.8	.71
Head Nurse	41	13.3	.87
Supervisor	35	11.4	.90
Director of Education	6	1.9	1.00
Director of Nursing	10	3.2	1.00
Total	307	99.6	.76

*Not all participating hospitals had a Director of Education; and one small hospital employed fewer than four supervisors and five head nurses.

the last year with at least one formal quality assurance activity performed in participating hospitals will value those activities more highly than those who have not.
• *Hypothesis 2.*   Staff nurses who have had experience with at least one formal quality assurance activity in the last year will be more likely to view such activities as part of every nurse's role and as an ongoing responsibility.

Tests of these hypotheses cannot answer the question about the direction of the influence. Those who argue that attitudes lead to behavior would argue that it is more plausible for positive attitudes to lead to participation in quality assurance than for participation to lead to positive attitudes. The collective experience of the MNQA members, however, was that some of their most enthusiastic quality assurance participants were individuals who had decided to cooperate only after considerable persuasion. Their experience is consistent with Harmon's report that an inservice education program which provided direct experience in identifying programs that interfere with care planning, coupled with discussion of the importance of evaluation, led to more positive attitudes toward quality assurance[10].

The study hypotheses were posed to test whether positive attitudes and quality-assurance experience are related. If a relationship emerges, a future step would be to conduct studies to test the order of the relationship.

Method

To obtain the required data most directly and expediently, a survey was conducted among nurses working in the representative MNQA hospitals.

Sample

The nursing service departments of ten hospitals ranging in size from 60 to 706 beds (mean = 372 beds) consented to participate in the study. Subjects were selected according to the following plan:

For each hospital, registered nurses were stratified into

categories of management and staff. From the management group, four supervisors, one education/staff-development nurse, and five head nurses were selected at random. The director of nursing was also included in the management portion of the sample. Staff nurses were sampled using proportional random sampling; one staff nurse was selected for every 12.4 operating beds. Of the 405 questionnaires distributed, 308 usable forms were returned for a response rate of 76 percent. The number and response rate of subjects in each position is presented in Exhibit 1.

Instrument

Unable to find a tested instrument that measured the areas of interest, the task force developed its own. In addition to basic personal information, the questionnaire included (1) items to measure the nurse's current level of involvement in various aspects of the hospital nurse's role; (2) questions to assess the nurse's attitudes toward quality assurance and relative preference for quality assurance as opposed to other aspects of the individual's role; and (3) items related to the nurse's choice of hospital as an employer and her or his plans for continued employment at that institution. The last set of items was included as a way of identifying nurses who were unusually dissatisfied with their work based on the assumption that highly negative feelings about the job itself might influence feelings about specific aspects of their work, including quality assurance.

After the total MNQA membership had provided reaction to several drafts of the questionnaire, the instrument was pilot tested on ten nurses from each of the participating hospitals. The two items related to the choice of the current job and plans for continuing in that job were previously used by Schwirian, et al[11]. The validity and reliability of the remaining items is unknown, although the development process supports the belief that the items have face validity and a measure of content validity as judged by a group of practicing quality assurance directors.

Questionnaires were distributed to subjects through normal in-house mail delivery and were returned to a drop box in a central location in each hospital. An MNQA member from each hospital then collected the forms and returned them unopened to the consultant to guard the confidentiality of the responses. MNQA members received only aggregate data about their own institutions.

Findings

Participation in quality-assurance activities

When subjects were asked to indicate if they had participated in typical quality assurance activities in the last year, 98 percent of management personnel and 71 percent of staff nurses said they had been involved in at least one activity (see Exhibit 2). The largest proportion of staff nurse experience had been in areas of reviewing the care given by other

nurses, reading about quality assurance, or doing nursing audits. Nurses in management roles reported a high rate of involvement (80 percent) in reviewing the care given by other nurses, although much of this may have been related to their personnel-management functions. The lowest level of participation for both groups was in serving on audit committees.

Opinions about quality-assurance activities

Most of the subjects (96 percent of management and 85 percent of staff nurses) believed quality assurance involves all levels of nursing personnel. But, as Exhibit 3 indicates, a noticeably smaller proportion viewed such activities as part of their daily work. A relatively small number believed quality assurance was a waste of time, took up time that should be spent on patient care, or was the responsibility only of supervisory personnel or of a quality assurance director. One-fourth of the total sample, however, believed that quality assurance was primarily a means of meeting accreditation requirements. It is not known if individuals within this 25 percent were responding to quality assurance as they had seen it practiced in hospitals or as one method by which a profession regulates itself. In either case this finding elicited concern among MNQA members.

In an attempt to sort out how highly nurses valued quality assurance activities in relation to other aspects of the

---

EXHIBIT 2.
INVOLVEMENT IN QUALITY ASSURANCE
BY STAFF AND MANAGEMENT NURSES

Item: In the last year I have been involved in the following activities . . .	Management personnel		Staff nurses	
	N	Percent of sample	N	Percent of sample
Reviewing the nursing care given by other registered nurses	81	80	65	32
Developing standards for measuring the quality of nursing care	58	56	30	15
Doing a nursing audit	60	59	51	25
Serving on an audit or quality assurance committee	37	36	16	8
Reading about quality assurance methods and/or findings	70	69	64	31
Using the results of quality assurance studies	53	52	40	20
Total number involved*		101		144
Percent of respondents		99		71
Number (%) of sample involved in none of the above	1	(1)		(29)

*Total number of respondents involved is less than column total because some nurses checked more than one activity.

EXHIBIT 3.
OPINIONS OF MANAGEMENT AND STAFF NURSES ABOUT RESPONSIBILITY FOR QUALITY ASSURANCE

Item: I feel quality assurance activities . . .	Management personnel		Staff nurses	
	N	Percent	N	Percent
Are for a quality assurance director	20	19	34	17
Are for a committee	37	36	86	42
Are for the supervisory-level nurses	17	17	81	15
Do not involve me at all	1	1	9	4
Are a waste of time	1	1	6	3
Take up time that should be spent on patient care	7	7	20	10
Involve all levels of nursing personnel	99	96	173	85
Are primarily used to meet accreditation requirements for the hospital	19	18	56	28
Are a part of my daily nursing activities	84	82	126	62
Total number of respondents	103		203	

nurse's role, staff nurse subjects were asked to rank order a set of activities in terms of their preference for the activity. They were also asked if they would engage in the activity if they had the opportunity. As Exhibit 4 indicates, staff nurses showed a clear preference for direct patient-care activities and ranked formal quality assurance activities and social interaction low. Kendall's Coefficient of Concordance was computed and showed a very highly significant level of agreement among the rank orders assigned by the subjects ($p < .001$). MNQA members were gratified to see that staff nurses valued direct patient-care activities so highly. However, the findings show not only that peer review and the activities experienced as part of patient-care audits rank low in relation to direct care, but also that fewer than half the respondents would want to participate in these activities if they had the opportunity.

Tests of hypotheses

Hypothesis 1

The hypothesis that staff nurses who have had experience in the last year with at least one formal quality assurance activity performed in participating hospitals (QA Experience) will value those activities more highly was tested in the following manner:

1. Nurses with QA Experience were defined as those who had participated in one or more of these activities:
   a) reviewing the nursing care given by other registered nurses

b) developing standards for measuring the quality of nursing care
c) doing a nursing audit
d) serving on an audit or quality-assurance committee.

2. The QA-Experience variable was cross-classified with whether or not the nurse *would* participate in selected elements of the nurse's role if she or he had the opportunity. The chi-square test was applied for each element.

As you can see in Exhibit 5, Hypothesis 1 was accepted for two of the three formal quality assurance elements of the nurse's role. Nurses who had had experience with quality assurance in the last year were significantly more likely to want to write nursing care standards for their specialty area and participate in peer review. But they were no more likely to want to be a member of a quality assurance committee.

Hypothesis 2

The second hypothesis was that nurses who have had quality assurance experience will be more likely to view quality assurance activities as part of every nurse's role and as an ongoing responsibility. The procedure for testing Hypothesis 2 was the same as that for testing Hypothesis 1, except that items regarding responsibility for quality assurance were cross-classified with the variable QA Experience. The findings, presented in Exhibit 6, support the hypothe-

---

EXHIBIT 4.
FREQUENCY OF "YES" RESPONSES AND RANK ORDERING OF SELECTED ELEMENTS OF THE NURSE'S ROLE BY STAFF NURSES

Item: If I could, I would...	Percent answering "Yes"	Mean rank	Pooled rank
Spend more time teaching patients and/or families	81	2.4	1
Involve patients in planning their care	78	2.8	2
Improve skill in performing nursing care procedures	80	3.3	3.5
Spend more time planning patient's care	72	3.3	3.5
Write nursing care standards for my specialty area	49	5.2	5
Participate in reviewing the nursing care given by other registered nurses	38	6.1	6
Spend more time getting to know my fellow workers	30	6.2	7
Be an active member on a quality assurance committee	18	6.8	8

Kendall's Coefficient of Concordance: W = .516 ($p < .001$)

sis. The only items for which there was a significant difference in responses were those stating that quality assurance activities involve all levels of nursing personnel and are a part of the nurse's daily activities; nurses who had had quality assurance experience were more likely to agree with these statements. There was no difference between the responses of the QA-Experience nurses and those of the group without recent experience on items that assigned responsibility for quality assurance to others or stated that such activities were a waste of time or took up time better spent on patient care. Only one other item revealed a difference that approached significance; nurses with quality assurance experience were somewhat less likely to view the primary use of such activities as a means of meeting accreditation requirements.

Fulfillment of job expectations

The findings from the first two sets of items suggest that the sampled staff nurses viewed quality assurance as an important but less compelling aspect of their role than direct-care activities. To assess what effect unmet expectations of the job may have had on this valuation, the task force examined responses to the third set of survey items. These were the questions concerning why subjects had chosen their current positions and under what conditions they would consider changing jobs. Respondents were instructed to check as many answers as were true for them.

Most staff nurse respondents chose their current job because it offered an opportunity to use their education and abilities (65 percent), because the position was in their clinical area of choice (64 percent), and/or because it provided additional learning experience (62 percent). About half (48 percent) chose the job because working conditions were favorable. Few chose the current job because it provided a good chance for advancement (10 percent), because they needed the money (13 percent), because fringe benefits were good (15 percent), or because the salary was good (17 percent). Very few chose the position because they were limited to the locality (2 percent) or because the job was the only one available (5 percent).

Response to the questions about when they would consider leaving their current job showed that one-third of the staff nurses had no intention of changing jobs. The remaining two-thirds cited reasons for considering a change divided about evenly between those related to working conditions and those related to the content of the work. The most frequently cited reason to change was the availability of another job with better working hours (44 percent). Other reasons included the availability of a job with a higher salary (30 percent), more professional independence (30 percent), a chance for advancement (30 percent), better working conditions (20 percent), and more individual status (20 percent). Reasons cited least frequently were the opportunity for a job in a better location (11 percent), outside of the field of nursing (11 percent), or in a preferred clinical

area (17 percent).

Thus the survey revealed that while most nurses chose the current position because they believed it would help them achieve professional goals, nearly half were willing to change jobs for better working hours; and nearly one-third would consider another position that offered higher salary, more professional independence, or a chance for advancement. However, further analysis revealed that those nurses who were seeking greater professional independence and an opportunity to use their education and abilities were no more likely to rank formal quality assurance activities high than were those not seeking those features ($p < .05$ using chi-square test).

Summary

Staff nurses who participated in the study tended to agree that involvement in quality assurance activities was an important part of the professional nurse's role. The majority had participated in at least one formal or informal quality assurance activity and viewed participation as a responsibility of all nurses. But when compared to direct patient care,

EXHIBIT 5.
RELATIONSHIP BETWEEN
QUALITY ASSURANCE (QA) EXPERIENCE
AND SELECTED ELEMENTS
OF THE NURSE'S ROLE

Item: If I could, I would . . .	QA Experience	No QA Experience	X^2	p
	Percent of respondents in each group answering "Yes"			
Spend more time teaching patients and/or families	84	80	.28	.60
Involve patients in planning their care	80	78	.05	.83
Improve skill in performing nursing care procedures	77	82	.61	.44
Spend more time planning patient's care	75	68	.84	.36
Write nursing care standards for my specialty area	59	39	7.71	.006*
Participate in reviewing the nursing care given by other registered nurses	46	29	6.18	.01*
Spend more time getting to know my fellow workers	31	27	.32	.57
Be an active member on a quality assurance committee	20	18	.02	.88
Total number of respondents	**115**	**100**		

*Indicates that X^2 is significant at alpha = .05

staff nurses predictably ranked quality assurance activities much lower than patient care. Not only were formal quality assurance activities such as peer review, writing standards, and serving on a QA committee ranked low: less than half of the staff-nurse respondents would choose to participate in these activities if they had the opportunity.

Both study hypotheses were fully or partially confirmed. Nurses who had participated in formal quality assurance activities within the last year were significantly more likely to want to write care standards for their specialty area and engage in peer review. They were no more likely to want to be a member of a QA committee, however. It appears that those formal quality assurance activities most obviously relevant to direct patient care are also most valued by these nurses.

Staff nurses with QA Experience were also more likely to believe that quality assurance was a responsibility of all levels of nursing personnel and was a part of the nurse's daily activities. They were somewhat less likely to view quality assurance primarily as a requirement for hospital accreditation than were their fellow nurses who had not had formal QA Experience, but the difference was not large enough to be significant.

The findings lend support to the notion that positive attitudes toward and participation in quality assurance activities are related. Furthermore, the data suggest that QA activities which are most salient to day-to-day direct care activities have the greatest support overall.

Implications

The findings of this study have two major implications for organizing quality assurance activities in acute-care hospitals. First, assuming that some type of committee structure is necessary in order to carry out quality assurance responsibilities and that QA committees are as unpopular in other hospitals as they appear to be in this sample, nursing administrators must investigate the cause of this disaffection. Subsequent to this study, for example, one hospital in the sample discovered that staff nurses were frequently unable to free up a two-hour block of time for QA committee meetings because of lean scheduling and/or unexpected urgent patient needs. Participation in and enthusiasm for the QA committee increased markedly when this hospital substituted quarterly all-day sessions for the monthly two-hour meetings. Freeing nurses for a large block of time also conveys the message that quality assurance is a highly valued activity. Other institutions may find that their own innovative scheduling changes or reward systems increase interest and participation.

At the time of the study, staff nurses in the participating hospitals had been given no particular reward for participating in QA activities. Rewards for "good performance" were given informally by offering charge-nurse responsibilities, hospital-wide committee assignments, special-project and continuing-education opportunities, and in-house kudos of various kinds. Labor contracts limited management's freedom to offer financial rewards. Clinical ladders had not yet been established in any of the hospitals represented.

A second major implication of the survey findings is that hospitals experiencing sluggish interest in QA activities may wish to target their change strategies on activities that are most obviously relevant to direct patient care. For example, findings support the change many hospitals already have made in how topics for quality assurance studies are selected. While a certain number of hospital-wide studies continue to be conducted in these institutions, a significant number of study topics are identified by the staff nurses of a single unit as problems of particular relevance to that unit. The unit then designs its own plan for studying and solving the problem. Identifying study topics at the lowest possible level in the organization seems to engage nurses' interest by giving them a sense of personal investment in the study, by fostering exploration of the scientific basis of common nursing practices, and by providing satisfaction when a relevant problem is solved successfully.

Once they become involved in meaningful quality assurance activities closely related to their practice, staff nurses

---

EXHIBIT 6.
RELATIONSHIP BETWEEN QUALITY ASSURANCE (QA) EXPERIENCE AND ASSIGNMENT OF RESPONSIBILITY FOR QUALITY ASSURANCE

Item: I feel quality assurance activities:	QA Experience	No QA Experience	X^2	p
	Percent of respondents in each group answering "Yes"			
Are for a quality assurance director	17	15	.002	.96
Are for a committee	40	46	.61	.43
Are for the supervisory level nurses	13	19	1.13	.29
Do not involve me at all	5	4	.02	.88
Are a waste of time	2	4	.30	.58
Take up time that should be spent on patient care	10	9	0	1.00
Involve all levels of nursing personnel	91	77	7.55	.006*
Are primarily used to meet accreditation requirements for the hospital	23	33	2.45	.12
Are a part of my daily nursing activities	73	51	10.45	.001*
Total number of respondents	115	103		

*Indicates that X^2 is significant at alpha = .05

predictably may develop more positive attitudes toward the process. If changes in the way quality assurance responsibilities are accomplished were to be accompanied by pre- and post-assessments of attitudes toward quality assurance, directors of quality assurance could begin to accumulate a body of evidence on how to effect an increased commitment to this aspect of professional accountability.

References

1. C.Z. Dachelet, "Nursing's Bid for Increased Status," *Nursing Forum* 17(1):18–45, 1978.
2. R.M. Schlotfeldt, "On the Professional Status of Nursing," *Nursing Forum* 13(1):16–31, 1974.
3. American Nurses' Association, *Standards of Nursing Practice*, (Kansas City, Missouri: American Nurses' Association, 1973).
4. S. Fuller, "Holistic Man and the Science and Practice of Nursing," *Nursing Outlook* 26:700–704, November 1978.
5. S.R. Gortner, "Scientific Accountability in Nursing," *Nursing Outlook* 22:764–768, December 1974.
6. S.J. Matek, *Accountability: Its Meaning and Its Relevance to the Health Care Field* (Hyattsville, Maryland: U.S. Department of Health Education and Welfare), DHEW Publication No. (HRA) 77–72, 1977.
7. G.W. Allport, "Attitudes." In C. Murchison, (ed.), *Handbook of Social Psychology* (Worcester, Mass: Clark University Press, 1935).
8. R. Abelson, "Are Attitudes Necessary?" In B.T. King, and E. McGinnis, (eds.), *Attitudes, Conflict & Social Change* (New York: Academic Press, 1972).
9. D.T. Regan, and R. Fazio, "On the Consistency Between Attitudes and Behavior: Look to the Method of Attitude Formation," *Journal of Experimental Social Psychology* 13:28, 1977.
10. D.A. Harmon, "Involving Staff in Nursing Quality Assurance," *Quality Review Bulletin* 6:26–30, November 1980.
11. P.M. Schwirian, et al. *Prediction of Successful Nursing Performance*, Parts III & IV. (Hyattsville, Maryland: U.S. Department of Health Education and Welfare), DHEW Publication No. (HRA) 79–115, 1979.

CHAPTER 17

Nursing Quality Assurance: A Process, Not a Tool

by Carolyn H. Smeltzer, Barbara Feltman, and Karen Rajki

A meaningful quality assurance program comes only with appropriate knowledge, communication, and accountability for all quality assurance functions among nurses at all levels. Describing the implementation of their quality assurance program, these authors tell of their eventual realization that, in fact, they had merely implemented a quality assurance tool that brought the nursing staff little benefit and a lot of grief. Highlighting the identified problems, the factors contributing to the program's failure, and the actions they took to develop and meet appropriate objectives, they detail their later, successful implementation of the concept and the process of quality assurance. Their experience provides readers with food for thought and stimulus for critical evaluations of their own quality assurance programs.

The problem

Are there problems with your quality assurance program? We thought we didn't have any problems, nor did we anticipate any. We believed we had all the needed components for a quality assurance program. An administrative position was allocated for coordinating the program. A systematic, valid, and objective tool (the Rush-Medicus Quality Monitoring Tool) had been chosen to evaluate nursing care. Head nurses had been delegated to collect data. And a computer was available to tabulate the results from the collected data.

But in retrospect, it is clear that we had not implemented

Carolyn H. Smeltzer, R.N., M.S.N., is Associate Director of Nursing, Quality Assurance, Foster G. McGaw Hospital, Loyola University Medical Center, Maywood, Illinois.

Barbara Feltman, R.N., M.S.N., is Quality Assurance Coordinator, Nursing Department, Foster G. McGaw Hospital, Loyola University Medical Center, Maywood, Illinois.

Karen Rajki, R.N., M.S.N., is Nursing Staff Development Instructor, Foster G. McGaw Hospital, Loyola University Medical Center, Maywood, Illinois.

a quality assurance program, but merely a quality monitoring *tool*, without attention to some other critical aspects of quality assurance.

In this article we discuss our initial implementation of quality assurance, the problems we identified, how we resolved them, and what we are now doing to maintain a true quality assurance program.

Our program began in 1976, only six years after the opening of the medical center, with the implementation of a process tool called the Medicus system. The nursing organizational chart at that time did include an associate director for quality assurance, but because of the newness of the hospital, the authority and responsibility for coordinating a quality assurance program was overridden by other administrative priorities. Our first problem therefore was that, in reality, an administrative resource was not available to coordinate or maintain the program. Quality assurance was not a priority.

Perceptions

The main thrust and emphasis of our quality assurance program was coordinated by a core group of Medicus Corporation personnel, whose principal function was training. They conducted a two-day workshop for the head nurses, staff development instructors, assistant directors, and other hospital administrative personnel. The function of the workshop was to explain the tool, the data that would be received from the tool, the data collection procedures, and the mechanism to assure systematic assignments for data collection. The workshops did not address how to use the data collected to affect the quality of nursing care. They did not show how administrators could use the information when analyzing the quality of nursing care that was being delivered. Because education focused only on the mechanics of using the tool, not on the concept or plan for the quality assurance program, nurses, including nursing administrators, viewed the tool with skepticism. Staff nurses believed that many of the criteria (expressed as questions on the tool) were inappropriate for evaluating care. They did not understand the universal nature of the tool and therefore felt that the objectives were not unit- or patient-specific enough to evaluate care. They questioned the tool development: Who had devised the criteria without their input? Lacking understanding or direction in using the data collected on the tool in conjunction with patient care data from other sources, they wanted the tool to evaluate certain measures of care that were unique to the patient populations on their units.

Communication

Our quality assurance program designated head nurses as the data collectors. A computer would tabulate the data, generating scores from 0 to 100 in 6 major objectives and 28 sub-objectives. The major objectives included (1) nursing care plan formulated, (2) patient's physical needs attended, (3) patient's nonphysical needs attended, (4) achievement of objectives evaluated, (5) unit procedures followed, and (6) delivery of nursing care facilitated.

During the implementation phase, we did not identify lines of accountability or communication for quality assurance. We did delegate functions, but no one was held accountable for their assigned functions. No procedures existed for communicating, reviewing, and discussing quality assurance reports. Head nurses were not certain about who was to receive a copy of their units' quality assurance reports. Most head nurses did not share their reports with staff, and many nurses were not aware that their care was being systematically evaluated. The confusion surrounding communication of quality assurance results generated anxiety about the evaluation process; head nurses became defensive when discussing the reports.

Data collection

Head nurses were taught the responsibilities and method for collecting data by Medicus personnel. Nursing administrators however, did not reinforce this explanation nor did they make data collection a priority. Therefore, data were not collected when assigned, and were insufficient and unreliable. Consequently, the data were not used; yet administrative authority was never called upon to improve the data-collection process.

Head nurses did recognize that data collection for the quality assurance program was a monumental task to be added to the other responsibilities of their position. They recommended changing the system by delegating their task to experienced staff nurses. Their recommendation, which was accepted, became their first input into the program.

The orientation for the staff nurse data collectors, however, was limited. They were taught only about data collection, not about quality assurance. They were not made aware of the way in which their function provided information used to measure nursing objectives. For example, the quality monitoring coordinator developed a calendar of

data assignments but failed to explain the rationale behind the assignments. The data-collection system requires that 60 percent of the data be collected on days and 40 percent on evenings and weekends. Ten percent of the patient population was scheduled to be evaluated within a month's time. This plan was developed to ensure that the quality assurance reports represented nursing staff on all shifts, excluding nights, within a month's time. However, it was not unusual for most of the data to be collected during the last week of the month, without weekend data included. Again, because data were not being collected when assigned, the data were subject to criticism and less useful.

> **"Quality assurance was a term that had little meaning and many negative feelings associated with it."**

No policies and procedures were developed concerning the mechanisms of evaluating patient care. The purpose and use of quality assurance data were not documented in writing. With the turnover of the head nurses that attended the original workshop on quality assurance, a need developed for written policies and procedures to be used as resource material. New head nurses had only a brief introduction to quality assurance and were confused as to their role and responsibilities in the program.

In summary, a system for evaluating care was nonexistent. Quality assurance was a term that had little meaning and many negative feelings associated with it. The tool and its implementation were expensive, providing little benefit and a lot of grief. It was clear to everyone that the responsibilities generated by the tool produced a large volume of work with few results.

Changes in the program

After identifying these problems, quality assurance personnel (including the associate director for nursing, quality assurance, the quality assurance coordinator for quality monitoring, and the staff development instructors) developed objectives for the program and used creative brainstorming to determine how they could be met. We developed the following objectives:

1. Nurses would have a positive attitude about quality assurance
2. Quality assurance data would be used in management decisions to improve patient care
3. Head nurses would view the data as an asset in setting unit priorities and in making changes in the delivery of patient care.

To meet these objectives, the quality assurance department developed the following goals:

1. Educate the nursing staff about the concept of quality assurance
2. Communicate quality assurance results in a systematic manner
3. Improve the reliability of quality assurance data
4. Assist head nurses in using quality assurance as a resource for establishing change.

At the same time that we developed goals and priorities for the quality assurance program, we created an additional position for an associate director for nursing practice. Thus the associate director for quality assurance was able to focus on the quality assurance program objectives as a major administrative priority. The quality assurance department had to make changes to achieve the objectives. To begin, we felt that we must be viewed as a resource to the nursing staff.

The resource role

Our role transition from policing data collection to providing a resource, took time, support, and commitment from nursing administration. Visibility of quality assurance personnel was the first step in the transition. We enhanced our visibility by presenting inservice programs for staff nurses on the concept of quality assurance and by providing consultation to head nurses about data analysis and use of data-collection results in initiating changes in nursing practice.

We were always responsible for recording the completion of assigned observations in quality monitoring, but we needed to change the perception of our role. As our role changed from that of monitor to that of resource, staff nurses gradually became educated about the quality assurance program, eventually grew to trust us, and came to feel that our goal was, in fact, improving the quality of care.

Education

We developed formal classes and inservice programs to teach RN orientees about the quality assurance program and its importance to the staff nurse. We taught staff development instructors to use the data in planning inservice programs and developed a workshop to help head nurses and staff development instructors recognize their function in the evaluation of patient care.

We set aside a portion of the regularly scheduled monthly business meeting for head nurses to present and discuss quality assurance reports. This exchange of information provided head nurses regular opportunity to assess each other's problems and helped to increase understanding and promote problem solving. One suggestion from a head nurse—that all nurses be oriented to quality assurance—resulted in the development of two types of quality assurance classes: one eight-hour class for staff nurse observers who are chosen by the head nurse and a four-hour class for other interested staff nurses.

In educating the staff, we stressed the positive aspects of quality assurance data. A unit that excelled in a particular objective or made a significant improvement in an individual quality score was commended. We made positive comments to head nurses who sent most of their staff to quality assurance classes, and we gave feedback about the quality of nurse-observers who consistently completed data-collection assignments on time.

"To improve reliability of data collectors, we created a mentor or preceptor role...."

Areas identified for improvement were always specific to the objectives evaluated. If a unit received a low score in documentation, the appropriate administrator might make comments to the head nurse suggesting the use of flowsheets, supplementary audits by nursing staff or staff development instructors, or the institution of an inservice program. We always stressed positive aspects of the quality assurance data, and attempted to focus attention on one or two quality issues that could be improved. We also compared quality assurance reports with staffing reports.

Improved communication and coordination

We developed a system for communicating quality assurance reports and other information in a more systematic manner.

Our communication included specific time frames, (for example, all quality data had to be in by the first Tuesday of the month, and all quality reports distributed by the following Friday). We instituted a mid-month audit to assist both ourselves and the head nurses in keeping track of completed observation assignments. Quality-monitoring calendars sent to head nurses two to three months ahead of schedule assisted them in preparing their staff assignments.

We developed a master schedule of observation assignments, inter-rater testing sessions and orientation classes to enable the head nurses to incorporate these aspects of quality monitoring into their daily schedules. Planning and scheduling for quality assurance activities facilitated completion of tasks associated with quality assurance.

All information related to quality assurance activities, including quality monitoring schedules, quality assurance orientation class schedules, inter-rater reliability testing sessions, and quality score reports, was directed specifically to the head nurses. Quality score reports were also communicated to the director of nursing and the assistant directors. We reviewed all the reports and decided on other appropriate recipients, basing our decisions on the purpose, content, and confidentiality of the report. For example, the discharge planning coordinator received reports about discharge and family teaching; the infection control nurse received reports about protecting the patient from infection; and clinical specialists received reports about the units for which they were responsible. The head nurses were made aware of who received the reports. As a final step, we incorporated the lines of communication and the circulation of reports into the nursing policy and the quality assurance program procedures.

Data collection

Each head nurse on our 23 clinical units delegated data collection to one or two nurses. Because of the increased number of data collectors, and turnover of some of these nurses, we needed more quality monitoring classes. Besides increasing the frequency of the classes, the time allotment, and the focus of the quality assurance monitoring, we changed the orientation class to broaden the scope of its content to include the concepts of quality assurance. Research concepts incorporated into the classes therefore included methodology of data collection, practice sessions, and examples of the quality assurance program's contributions to nursing practice within the hospital.

Head nurses were made accountable for ensuring that staff collected data as assigned on the calendar. This responsibility was considered in each head nurse's performance appraisal.

As more staff nurses were learning to collect data, we noted a difference in the nurses' skills, experience, and education. Reliability of data collectors therefore became an issue. To improve reliability, we created a mentor or preceptor role in quality assurance data-collection. We also expanded the inter-rater testing sessions, both in scope and in frequency, to address questions and problems encountered in data collection, and to observe and analyze the performance of the data collectors.

Eventually, we developed a list of characteristics for head nurses to consider when choosing staff to do quality monitoring. We feel that a good data collector should:

Possess a comprehensive knowledge base in nursing
Demonstrate clinical expertise
Feel comfortable working on the unit
Be interested in the nursing profession
Demonstrate good interpersonal skills
Feel comfortable interviewing patients and nurses.

These are some of the aspects of data collection that became apparent as we refined the program.

Another factor that became immediately apparent was that chart forms and documentation differed from unit to unit. To assist the data collectors in obtaining accurate data,

each head nurse developed a fact sheet. The fact sheets contained information specific to that unit (for example, the location of chart forms and individual unit policies regarding patient care). The fact sheets served to reduce data collectors' frustration and required time and to improve the reliability of the data.

"Nurses began to realize that the information . . . could be a source of power for change."

We justified the cost of these additional resources because valid data were collected and could be used to generate changes in nursing practice. Head nurses' used the data for more efficient management decision making. The data base also provided head nurses with the means to evaluate the appropriateness of their decisions. Each nursing unit had equal responsibility and commitment for data collection; the specific unit budget absorbed the cost of staff nurses doing observations.

Changes in attitude

Approximately a year after we started initiating changes, we noted a remarkable change in attitude. Head nurses began requesting inservice programs on all aspects of quality assurance, and they wanted to increase the numbers of data collectors from all clinical units. On one or two units every staff nurse was oriented to be a data collector. Staff nurses wanted to know their quality assurance results and the criteria used to evaluate their nursing care. Because of the enthusiasm, we opened quality monitoring orientation classes to all staff nurses so that they would understand the principles and concepts of quality assurance. We felt that such understanding would also improve the staff nurses' own professional conduct and documentation.

Nurses began to realize that the information generated from the quality assurance department could be a source of power for change. Head nurses began requesting more information. They wanted to know how they could evaluate critically and objectively the quality of nursing care on their units. Nursing committees, such as the policy and procedure committee, the forms committee, and the patient education committee, were requesting information from the quality assurance program when planning and instituting changes. Committee members wanted to structure forms and policies that would enable the staff to meet standards as evaluated by the quality assurance program. It was becoming clear to us that involvement in the program and use of the data were improving. The data could be a basis for change, could stimulate intellectual curiosity, and actually could result in improvement of patient care through an awareness that care was being evaluated.

Uses of the data

As the data became more meaningful and understanding of the quality assurance concepts increased, staff and administrators used the information from the quality data to make various changes in the department.

- Head nurse members of the policy and procedure committee communicated with quality assurance personnel to determine criteria which could be used to evaluate documentation. From this information they developed several chart forms and new policies and procedures.
- Based on needs identified through quality assurance data, staff development instructors instituted inservice programs and revised the abbreviation list.
- Ad hoc committees composed of head nurses and staff nurses developed new admission assessment forms, more clearly defined policies regarding medications and emergency procedures, and changed the IV labeling policy to include specific information about the patient and the medications.
- Assistant directors and head nurses evaluated patient acuity levels and staffing in light of quality information.
- Certain units evaluated change from eight-hour to twelve-hour shifts using quality assurance results to determine the impact on patient care.

The quality assurance program provided a common ground for nursing professionals at all levels to discuss patient care. Terminology associated with quality assurance gradually became common vocabulary for all nursing staff.

Maintaining the program

Involvement, education, and use of data from the quality assurance program are the ingredients for maintaining the program. However, we cannot merely maintain it; we must constantly seek improvement. We must be continually reviewing, revising, and researching the criteria used to evaluate nursing care, for nursing practice is a changing field.

The body of data collected must be accurate and large enough to be reliable. To assure reliability further, data collectors must be selected appropriately, given adequate instructions, and evaluated through inter-rater testing sessions. Nurses' roles and responsibilities in a quality assurance program need to be clarified, communicated, and incorporated into their job descriptions so that evaluation of staff members on the performance of their assigned quality assurance functions, and will help make quality assurance a priority, instead of an unwanted addition.

"Terminology associated with quality assurance gradually became common vocabulary . . ."

Another aspect of maintenance is use of the quality assurance information. Nursing committees that use results from the quality assurance reports must be visible and effective in making changes. They must also share suggestions and actions concerning patient care appropriately and frequently with staff. As quality assurance reports become an active, forceful component in improving patient care, nurses benefit, but most of all, patients benefit.

Summary

Our experience illustrates some specific criteria common to any well-implemented quality assurance program. Nursing administrators might therefore benefit by keeping the following points in mind:

1. Quality assurance must be a priority.
2. Those responsible must implement a program, not only a tool.
3. A coordinator should develop and evaluate quality assurance activities.
4. Roles and responsibilities must be delineated.
5. Nurses must be informed about the process and the results of the program.
6. Adequate orientation of data collectors is essential.
7. Data must be reliable.
8. Quality data should be analyzed and used by nursing personnel on all levels.

CHAPTER 18

A Computer-Assisted Quality Assurance Model

by Linda Edmunds

This article describes a modular quality assurance program that was designed for computer automation. The author explains how the quality assurance model not only meets this need but also satisfies other critical objectives, including integration with the hospital's multidisciplinary quality assurance program and minimal redundancy in developing standards and measurement criteria. Readers will benefit from ideas for refining or developing effective quality assurance programs that can also use computer technology to increase productivity.

Quality assurance programs are labor intensive. The day-to-day process of developing standards of care, writing measurement criteria, compiling data, and implementing recommendations consumes a considerable amount of time and energy. If a hospital adopts a peer review program, then the bulk of the program's work will fall to the nursing staff, whose prime responsibility is patient care.

At Stony Brook's University Hospital, a new tertiary care facility, as at most other hospitals, patient care needs always seem to absorb or exceed the number of nursing care hours available. Hence the committee charged with developing a quality assurance program there faced the proverbial dilemma of developing a viable program with limited personnel resources.

A labor-saving approach to the problem was suggested by the availability of an IBM computer at the hospital. This computer supports a housewide information system that communicates patient information between clinical, ancillary, and administrative departments.

Of course the model also had to satisfy critical objectives unrelated to its adaptability for computerization. Nursing's program had to integrate with the hospital's multidisciplinary quality assurance program in order to satisfy standards of the Joint Commission on Accreditation of Hospitals

Linda Edmunds, R.N., M.S., is Systems Nurse at University Hospital, Health Sciences Center, State University of New York at Stony Brook.

(JCAH). Second, a direct link between patient care evaluation and patient care planning was perceived as essential if recommendations for change were to be implemented effectively. Third, an approach that would allow for evaluation of care provided to individual patients as well as patient groups was required. And finally, a modular framework was projected to foster expansion of the program's scope while minimizing redundancy in developing standards and writing measurement criteria.

This article describes the nursing division's model for quality assurance in relation to these four objectives. The foundation of the model rests, however, not only on the work done at University Hospital, but on many excellent ideas developed at Duke University Hospital and also at El Camino Hospital and at Rush Presbyterian Medical Center. We have drawn significantly on the methodologies, standards and concepts published by Jelinek et al.[1], Peter and the Duke Nursing Service[2,3] Mayers[4], and Gall[5].

Coordination with a multidisciplinary program

As have others before us[6], we perceive quality assurance to be a cyclic process of setting standards of care; measuring care according to those standards; evaluating data from use chart review, observation, and interview; and making recommendations for improvement (Exhibit 1).

Communication between nursing's quality assurance program and the hospitalwide multidisciplinary program proceeds in two directions. First, recommendations for improvements in care delivery stemming from completed nursing evaluations may be forwarded to the hospital's quality assurance committee, to departments external to nursing, as well as directly to groups within the nursing division itself. Second, the hospital committee or external departments may identify patient care problems requiring self-evaluation by nursing or by a multidisciplinary team when joint responsibility for a problem is indicated. If no relevant standard exists, the quality assurance cycle would begin with the development of standards of care.

Because derived measurement criteria can be written to make use of a variety of methods for data collection, the quality assurance model supports contributions to a retrospective chart audit or to a concurrent review of patient care. This allows sufficient flexibility so that nursing, without altering its own focus, can contribute to multidisciplinary studies whatever the methodological specifications of those studies might be.

A link between care planning and care evaluation

The premise of this quality assurance model is that the standards of care serve as the cornerstone for both care planning and care evaluation. Unless there is congruence between the defined standards for giving care and the criteria used for measuring care, data collected in the evaluation process will not clearly identify the achievements and deficiencies of nursing practice.

To this end, patient care standards are used as reference guides by nursing staff as they write care plans for individual patients. These standards define the outcomes expected for patients, the nursing activities required to assist the patient meet the specified outcomes, and the structural resources the institution should provide to facilitate optimal nursing care.

The patient care standards also serve as the source from which the criteria to measure care are derived. A patient care standard cannot serve as an evaluation instrument itself because, as a guide to optimal care, it must be comprehensive. In evaluating care it is not always feasible to determine if each outcome, process, or structural standard is met. Because some aspects of care are difficult to measure and because the measurement process is time consuming, it is usually necessary to be selective in determining what areas of care are to be evaluated.

Another reason patient care standards cannot be used as evaluation instruments is that they do not specify the evidence required to indicate compliance or the method to be used to collect data. For example, in the surgical intensive care unit planned admission standards of care, one outcome standard states "The patient and family are well informed post-operatively" (Exhibit 2). This outcome might be measured in a variety of ways. In the case where the option selected is question the family, the measurement criteria requires the evaluator to ask a family member, "Do you feel you were provided with adequate information regarding your relative's condition?"

The measurement criteria are derived directly from the standard. "Derived" implies that the criterion is an indicator of the standard and measures one variable. The variable measured might be one of many variables that could be included in the operational definition of the standard. In the example given, the family's subjective impression of their

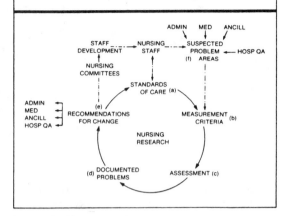

**EXHIBIT 1.
QUALITY ASSURANCE CYCLE**

informed status was selected as the variable to be measured. Alternatively, a variety of more objective measurement criteria could have been written. A family member could have been asked to state the patient's condition post-op, to describe the surgery performed, or to explain the purpose of any tubes, drains, or equipment connected to the patient.

In selecting one measurement criterion out of the many that could be written, the assumption is made that the measured variable reflects the associated variables. If the measured variable falls within defined limits, the standard has been met. This is certainly a large assumption but one that a pragmatically based quality assurance program will have to make until the reliability and validity of measurement criteria can be tested with the rigor characteristic of the work done at Rush Presbyterian by Jelinek and the Medicus Group[7].

Each measurement criterion is referenced by code to a specific outcome, process, or structural standard (Exhibit 2). This assists the quality assurance committee in determining which standards have not been met and whether the deficiency is in relation to patient outcome, nursing care, or institutional resources. Following an evaluation or at the recommendation of groups external to nursing, standards may be modified or extended to reflect suggested changes in care delivery. Because nurses use the standards to plan care, a plausible mechanism exists for communicating to staff the standards of quality that are considered acceptable.

Evaluating patient groups or individual patients

Duke University has divided its patient care guidelines into general guidelines applicable for all patients and specific guidelines applicable to patients with a particular diagnosis or therapy[8]. The five-tier framework presented in Exhibit 3 is an extension of the Duke concept. It allows the combin-

EXHIBIT 2.
MEASUREMENT CRITERIA DERIVED FROM
STANDARDS FOR THE SICU PLANNED ADMISSION

Surgical Intensive Care Unit Planned Admission

STANDARD	CRITERIA	TYPE	MEASUREMENT CRITERIA CODE
C. 1	Did a nurse from the SICU establish contact with you to let you know that your family member was out of the operating room and moved to the AICU?	IF	C1p1–IF
	Did the SICU nurse establish visiting hours for you?	IF	C1p2–IF
	Did you feel that the SICU nurse was available to you to answer questions when necessary?	IF	C1p3–IF
	Do you feel you were provided with adequate information regarding your relative condition?	IF	CO1–IF
D. 1	The progress notes include an admission note written by the admitting SICU nurse.	CHART	D1p1–C
	The admission note is inclusive of the following data: Post-op diagnosis Statement re: physiologic homeostasis Pertinent physical findings Pertinent lab findings Summary statement of status since admission *Score:* Met – 5/5 P.M. – 3-4/5 N.M. – less than 3	CHART	D1p2–C
2	Nursing orders are formulated to address the post-op diagnosis and identified post surgical problems. (Nursing order sheet)	CHART	D2p1–C
3	Interviewer is asked to either attend an intershift report or ask the patient's nurse to give the report she would give the oncoming nurse. Information should include all of the following: Post-op diagnosis Physiologic homeostasis Pertinent events since admission Review of 24 hr. flow sheet Review of current SICU orders Information regarding whereabouts of family or significant other Pertinent negatives (abnormals on PE) Review of nursing orders *Score:* Met 7-8/8 P.M. 4-6/8 N.M. less 4/8 Written by: Mary H. Hawthorne, R.N., M.S.N. Clinical Nurse Specialist/SICU/CVICU May, 1981 Accepted by the Q.A. Committee July, 1981	IN	D3p1–IN

NOTE: Measurement criteria for the process and outcome standards in Exhibit 3 are shown. The measurement criteria specify what data are to be collected on the floor. Each criteria is scored as "met," "not met," "partially met" or "not applicable." The code (D3P1–IN) in the last column indicates the specific triad that is the source of the criteria (D1), if that standard is a process, outcome, or structural standard (3P means third process standard), whether it is the first, second, third, etc. measurement criteria to be derived from the third process standard (1 = first) and finally the method for obtaining data (IN = interview with a nurse).

ing of standards of care to support care planning and care evaluation for either individual patients or patient groups. Standards are written for patient conditions organized on five levels. A set of patient care standards may apply to (1) all patients, (2) patients at a specific developmental stage or (3) belonging to a discrete social group, (4) patients with therapy or function associated needs, and (5) patients who are being treated for an identified medical, surgical, psychiatric, or obstetric problem.

Included in the first level of the patient care pyramid are standards that address the basic requirements and rights of all patients who seek health care regardless of age, social group, therapy, or medical diagnosis. At the second level are standards relating to patients' developmental status, such as toddler or aged person, which bears characteristic needs that may affect their participation, response, or reaction to treatment.

Third-level standards address needs that may be connected to the societal groups to which the patient belongs.

Membership in a religious, ethnic, or economic group may have implications in terms of a patient's compliance with a treatment modality, the psychological support he can rely on during an illness, or his ability to afford life-style changes necessary to maintain an improved health status.

Standards included at the fourth level define optimal nursing care for patients and families who are preparing for, undergoing, or responding to a treatment modality. The standards at this level are not derived directly from the medical diagnosis but deal with associated patient needs such as education and discharge planning, which must be met in order to support medical treatment strategies.

At the final level are the standards that define patient outcomes and nursing care related to the patient's medical, surgical, or psychiatric diagnosis. A pathological condition, regardless of the individual's unique characteristics, imposes on the patient actual or potential physiological and functional problems the nurse must address to assist the physician in the implementation of the medical regimen.

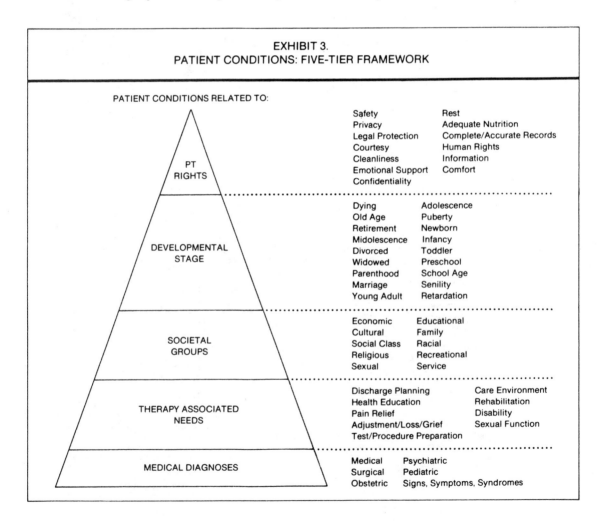

**EXHIBIT 3.
PATIENT CONDITIONS: FIVE-TIER FRAMEWORK**

PATIENT CONDITIONS RELATED TO:

PT RIGHTS

Safety	Rest
Privacy	Adequate Nutrition
Legal Protection	Complete/Accurate Records
Courtesy	Human Rights
Cleanliness	Information
Emotional Support	Comfort
Confidentiality	

DEVELOPMENTAL STAGE

Dying	Adolescence
Old Age	Puberty
Retirement	Newborn
Midolescence	Infancy
Divorced	Toddler
Widowed	Preschool
Parenthood	School Age
Marriage	Senility
Young Adult	Retardation

SOCIETAL GROUPS

Economic	Educational
Cultural	Family
Social Class	Racial
Religious	Recreational
Sexual	Service

THERAPY ASSOCIATED NEEDS

Discharge Planning	Care Environment
Health Education	Rehabilitation
Pain Relief	Disability
Adjustment/Loss/Grief	Sexual Function
Test/Procedure Preparation	

MEDICAL DIAGNOSES

Medical	Psychiatric
Surgical	Pediatric
Obstetric	Signs, Symptoms, Syndromes

Organizing standards of care into levels assists us in conceptualizing and implementing a modular approach to care evaluation and care planning. A nurse planning care for an inpatient who has just been diagnosed as having hepatitis would use the hepatitis patient care standards to update the patient's care plan. If, however, the nurse was to plan care for a newly admitted 16-year-old heroin addict with hepatitis, all of the following patient care standards would be used in developing the care plan: the general admission standards, standards for the adolescent patient, standards for the drug abuser, and the hepatitis standards. To evaluate nursing care for this same patient, measurement criteria would be derived from all of these patient care standards. These derived measurement criteria would be combined and arranged according to method of data collec-

tion into an efficient evaluation instrument. By allowing use of measurement criteria derived either from a single set of standards or from multiple standard sets, the model facilitates equally evaluations focused on individual patients with unique requirements and evaluations focused on patient groups with common conditions. Exhibit 4 is a diagram depicting the combining of multiple standards. In the exhibit patient care standards from each tier of the pyramid have been selected for evaluation. The measurement criteria, derived from each set of standards are combined and reorganized by data collection method, (chart review, observation, etc.) into an instrument to be used by the evaluator. As data are compiled, the discrepancies between established standards of care and actual care may become apparent.

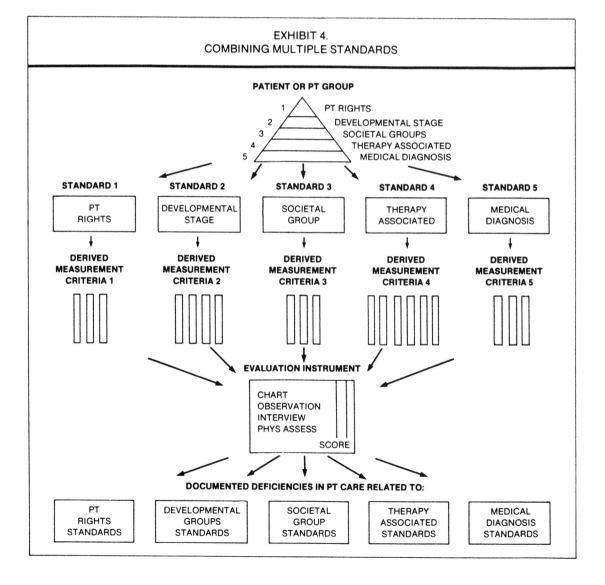

EXHIBIT 4.
COMBINING MULTIPLE STANDARDS

Modular structure to facilitate computerization and reduce redundancy

A central feature of the quality assurance model is its modular design. It is this design that allows translation of the model into a computer-based application and assists in the reduction of redundancy between patient care standards and measurement criteria.

The term *modular design* means that the model is constructed of discrete components that can be used independently, in conjunction with one another, or in new combinations to serve alternative purposes. The basic modular components of the model are (1) the set of patient care standards (2) the outcome/process/structure triad, and (3) the individual standard with its derived measurement criteria.

Modular component 1: patient care standards

A set of patient care standards consists of all the outcome, process, and structural standards for a patient group with a defined condition. A set of standards such as the one for the SICU planned admission can be used independently or in conjunction with other sets of standards. When staff begin to write new standards, they should be instructed to review existing patient care standards, so that redundancy between standards is minimized. For example, once a set of general pre-operative standards is developed, it is not necessary to define in standards for specific surgical procedures, patient outcomes, or nursing process common to all patients undergoing surgery.

Modular component 2: the outcome/process/structure triad

Each outcome standard is linked conceptually to process, and where applicable, structural standards. The outcome standard "The patient and family are well informed post-operatively" is connected to three process standards, but no structural standards are identified. The process standards include establishing initial contact with the family, communicating appropriate information to them, and providing resources for additional support as necessary. Each outcome/process/structure triad is a distinct unit that can be extracted and reused. This one might be included, for example, in a set of standards for a pediatric intensive care planned admission or in a general post-operative standard.

Modular component 3: the standard with derived measurement criteria

A measurement criteria with its parent standard or standard segment also forms an independent module. To facilitate instrument development, each measurement criteria is coded to indicate the standard from which it has been derived. The outcome standard "The patient and family are well informed post-operatively" would be coded CO1-IF. C

identifies the appropriate outcome/process/structure triad, O that the parent standard is an outcome standard, and 1 that it is the first measurement criteria written for this outcome standard. The IF indicates that the method of data collection is an interview with a family member.

Whenever an existing outcome, process, or structural standard is to be used in a new set of patient care standards, any derived measurement criteria are transferred with it. Because developing clearly written, objective measurement criteria is a process not without pitfalls, reusing tested criteria minimizes problems in interpretation that may occur in the data collection process. And if preexisting criteria have been evaluated for reliability, some measure of reliability is conferred on any instrument into which they are integrated.

In summary, a modular approach to quality assurance should increase methodologic efficiency and broaden programmatic scope by reducing redundancy between standards and measurement criteria and by supporting studies of multiple patient groups using recombinations of modular components.

Toward computerization

The quality assurance model presented here was designed with the intent of using computer technology to advance a feasible nursing program. Although implementation has been accomplished with manual procedures, in a number of areas automation is being used or will be used to improve programmatic efficiency and effectiveness. These include distribution of standards, patient identification, instrument construction, and data compilation.

Distribution of standards

Because use of patient care standards as the primary guides to patient care planning is a basic principle of this quality assurance model, up-to-date standards must be accessible on all nursing units. Standards can be made available by filing them in looseleaf notebooks at each nursing station, but this becomes cumbersome as the library of standards grows. A more convenient approach is to store patient care standards in computer memory. Standards are cross indexed in the computer three ways: alphabetically, by clinical area of origin, and according to the five-tier framework. When a nurse requires a standard it is selected from an index displayed on the computer terminal at the nursing station (Exhibit 5). A copy of the standard is immediately printed out on the unit's printer. (To print out a copy of the SICU planned admission standard the nurse could select level 4 (therapy associated), SICU (unit of origin), or the letter A (admission planned). In the case shown in Exhibit 5 "A" was probed and a list of standards displayed. By using the light pen attached to the computer terminal, the nurse can select the SICU standard that prints out immediately on the unit's printer.)

Addition of new standards and revision of existing standards on the computer is more efficient than manual procedures. Rather than typing, xeroxing, distributing, and hoping that a new or revised standard will find its way into the proper section of the appropriate manual, computer libraries can be revised and updated from a central terminal with changes immediately available throughout the hospital. Because modification of standards is a relatively simple process, incorporation of recommendations from the quality assurance committee into the care planning process is facilitated. Availability of the standards on all units is useful particularly when the census is high and patients are housed temporarily on units to which they normally would not be assigned. Nursing orientees and student nurses can print out copies of standards to take home and review at leisure. Staff developing new standards can access, review, and extract appropriate modular components from existing standards, thus minimizing overlap between standards written by different clinical areas of the nursing division.

Patient identification

The majority of patient care evaluations undertaken in hospitals are retrospective audits with the chart serving as the primary source of data about patient care. Generally charts are identified for review by clerical personnel because their discharge abstracts contain an ICD-9 (International Classification of Diseases/9th Revision) code designating a medical diagnosis within a predetermined range. The availability of a computer allows the writing of programs that scan stored abstracts and produce within a matter of minutes reports that identify appropriate charts. Furthermore,

---

EXHIBIT 5.
COMPUTERIZED INDEX TO PATIENT CARE STANDARDS

@@@TOP

PATIENT CARE STANDARDS INDEX   07/14/82   1517

BY LEVEL	BY CLINICAL AREA		ALPHABETIC	
1: GENERAL STANDARDS	AICU	MICU	A	M
2: DEVELOPMENTAL	AMB	NBN/NICU	B	N
3: SOCIETAL GROUP	BURN	OB	C	O
4: THERAPY ASSOCIATED	CVICU	O.R.	D	P
5: MEDICAL DIAGNOSIS	ER	ORTHO	E	Q
	EHS	PED/PICU	F	R
	GYN	PSYCH INP	G	S
	HEMO	PSYCH DAY	H	T
	HOUSEWIDE	SICU	I	U
	LAB/DEL	SURG	J	V
	MED		K	W
			L	XYZ

RETURN

NQAIND

@@BOT

@@@TOP

PROBE STANDARD TO PRINT A COPY   07/14/82   1517

A	SEE ALSO:	LETTER
101.Z01 ADMISSION. GENERAL		
401.U01 ADMISSION. SICU PLANNED		
200.P01 ADMISSION. PEDIATRIC PT		
410.S01 ASSESSMENT. HEAD AND NECK		

NQAAA   RETURN

@@BOT

additional data within the abstract can also be scanned to include or exclude patients with other defined characteristics, obviating the prereviewing of charts by hand. Although initial development of computer programs for patient identification may take some time, the programs once developed can be reused.

Although patient selection by ICD–9 codes may be appropriate for medical or multidisciplinary reviews, many patient conditions to which nurses address care cut across medical diagnoses. An objective of this quality assurance program is to evaluate care provided to meet the nurse-identified patient conditions, as illustrated in the pyramid in Exhibit 4. To this end some method must be used to label patient charts by condition so that they can be retrieved for review. The approach that suggests itself is to include in the discharge abstract codes specifying the patient care standards used to guide care. Computer selection of charts for retrospective evaluations could then be based on a nursing classification as well as on the medical designation. Alternatively, if the patient care plan and the codes referencing it to the standards of care used to develop the plan are stored during the course of patients' stay, then the same computer programs can be used to select patients for concurrent assessment.

Instrument compilation

As measurement criteria are written they are simply listed in parallel to the outcome, process, or structural standards from which they are derived without regard to the specified method of data collection. To provide the evaluator with an efficient tool for collecting data the criteria must be sorted according to data collection method. All measurement criteria requiring information from the patient chart must be listed in one section of the tool, all directing the evaluator to interview the patient must be in another, and so forth.

If multiple patient care standards are to be included in an evaluation, the manual process of combining, sorting, and typing measurement criteria into the evaluation instrument can be time consuming. When coded criteria are stored in a computer file, however, criteria sorting and instrument printing can be done by the computer once a list of the appropriate criteria codes is entered into the computer.

Data tabulation

The reason for deriving measurement criteria directly from the process, outcome, and structural standards is to clarify where recommendations for changes should be focused when collected data indicate deficiencies in care delivery. To do this, raw data from individual patients must be combined, percentage scores calculated, and results for each measurement criteria reorganized according to source standards. This is necessary to identify which standards are

met, which are partially met, and which are not met at all. Although tabulation is still manual, it should be possible in the future to collect data on mark-sensitive forms so that compilation, tabulation, and data reorganization procedures can be computerized.

Conclusion

The model for quality assurance implemented at University Hospital has been accepted by nursing staff with enthusiasm because it provides a logical and understandable conceptual foundation for initiating a program. It is accepted by the hospital's multidisciplinary quality assurance program because the means of integrating the two programs is straightforward.

The model, originally implemented in manual mode, is designed to use computer technology to facilitate productivity. We have taken the first steps in this direction but, practically speaking, the road is problematic for two reasons. First, with the exception of the work done by Jelinek[9], who used a computer for instrument compilation, there is little if any nursing literature to guide us. Second, bringing to fruition all of the concepts outlined requires substantial programming resources. These are a scarce commodity in any facility that has a broad-based hospital information system and multiple user groups sophisticated in their understanding of how computerization can facilitate their individual disciplines.

Nonetheless, a blueprint exists and although building may progress slowly and design will have to be adjusted in light of experience, we believe the quality assurance model described here will support a practical, efficient program, increasingly sensitive to the accomplishments and deficiencies of nursing care delivery at our hospital.

References

1. Richard C. Jelinek, R.K. Dieter Haussmann, Sue T. Hegyvary, and John F. Newman, A Methodology for Monitoring Quality of Nursing Care, DHEW Publication no. (HR) 76–25, U.S. Department of Health, Education, and Welfare, 1974.
2. Mary Ann Peter, Duke Hospital's Quality Assurance Program in Nursing—Background, Organization and Evolvement. *Nurs. Administration Quart.* 1(3):9–25, 1977.
3. Duke University Hospital Nursing Services, *Quality Assurance, Guidelines for Nursing Care,* (Philadelphia: J.B. Lippincott, 1980).
4. Marlene Mayers and El Camino Hospital, *Standard Nursing Care Plans* Vols. 1–3, (Stockton, Calif.: K/P Co. Medical Systems, 1974).
5. John E. Gall, A Patient Care Quality Assurance System. Progress Report, Grant no. HS02027-02, National Center for Health Services Research, U.S. Department of Health, Education, and Welfare, Washington, D.C., 1978.
6. Peter, 1977, p. 14.
7. Jelinek, 1974, pp. 52–77.
8. Peter, 1977, p. 14.
9. Jelinek, 1974, pp. 39–40.

CHAPTER 19

Combining Nursing Quality Assurance and Research Programs

by Elaine Larson

This article discusses the advantages and disadvantages of combining nursing quality assurance and research programs in clinical settings. The intended audiences and scopes of quality assurance and research differ, causing potential conflicts in combined programs. Such conflicts include the methods of disseminating findings, action taken on data obtained, analytic methods used, and issues of territoriality. However, advantages of combining these programs are great. Nursing research can be introduced into the clinical setting via quality assurance; resultant studies are more likely to be of direct clinical relevance; and results are more likely to be integrated into practice when programs are combined rather than separate. Combined programs are also cost efficient.

Nursing Quality Assurance Programs and Research Programs have evolved in clinical settings over the past decade. Since both quality assurance and research contain elements of evaluation and seek to improve patient care, it is not surprising that in some major healthcare institutions (e.g. Beth Israel, Boston; Stanford; University of Washington Hospital) the programs have been combined. For this reason, it would be helpful to compare and contrast definitions and functions of nursing quality assurance and research in a clinical setting (Exhibit 1) and to discuss advantages and disadvantages of combining the two within a single program (Exhibit 2).

Quality assurance plans began to form in the early 1970s as a result of governmental requirements for evaluating use of Medicare and Medicaid funds. Programs such as Professional Standards Review Organization and Utilization Review required agencies to show evidence of appropriate use of medical resources. In addition, the Joint Commission

for Accreditation of Hospitals (JCAH) established a requirement during the 1970s that a minimum number of chart audits be done to show evidence of the adequacy of care provided. There is currently no requirement regarding the number of audits. Indeed, the type of quality assurance activity in which an agency engages and the data sources used have, since 1982, been left to the discretion of each individual institution. The requirement for hospital accreditation is simply that there be a defined and functioning quality assurance program which shows evidence of solving patient care problems[1, 2]. The emphasis, then, of quality assurance is on solving identified patient care problems in the local institution. This deceptively simple standard for quality assurance requires a high level of sophistication in terms of assessing the needs of an institution and methods of data collection.

For decades housed almost exclusively within academia, nursing research also has begun to take new forms in clinical settings. Nurse researchers with masters and doctorate degrees are being hired by hospitals, health departments, and other agencies for the specific purpose of doing clinical research directed toward the general goal of improving patient care. About one-third of the hospitals surveyed in the 1970s employed at least one part-time nurse researcher [3]. Astute nursing and hospital administrators are recognizing the far-reaching as well as the local advantages of employing a clinical researcher[4–8]. Far reaching advantages include prestige for the institution, advanced knowledge for the general community of nursing professionals, and a data base for clinical nursing practice. Local advantages include improved patient care within the institution and systematic evaluation of administrative issues such as staffing, cost containment, and staff retention.

In research, new knowledge is sought about the relationship between outcome and process. In assessment and monitoring, existing knowledge of that relationship is used to obtain information about the behavior of professional personnel or of the larger system [9].

Elaine Larson, R.N., Ph.D., F.A.A.N., is the Director for Nursing Quality Assurance and Research at University Hospital in Seattle, Washington. She is also Clinical Associate Professor in the Schools of Nursing and Public Health and Community Medicine at the University of Washington.

EXHIBIT 1
COMPARISON OF RESEARCH AND QUALITY ASSURANCE

	Research	Quality Assurance
Focus	Answering questions: contributing new knowledge	Solving immediate problems
Intended audience	General, beyond study population: information public: replication of study encouraged	Usually local, within institution studied: information private: replication usually not necessary or possible
Study methods	Should be unbiased and representative population; may be descriptive or experimental	Should be unbiased and representative population: usually descriptive only
Analysis	Usually involves some form of statistical testing of significance or association	Usually reporting of summarized raw data only
Applicability	Often does, but may not necessarily change practice immediately; may contribute to theory development	Used primarily to change practice immediately: usually doesn't contribute to theory development

In contrast to quality assurance the emphasis of nursing is on identifying new knowledge for the general healthcare community. The goal is long-term advancement of nursing knowledge with an ultimate influence on clinical practice. Given these foci, definitions of quality assurance and clinical nursing research might be as follows:

Quality assurance: systematic inquiry including those activities or program components designed to evaluate patient care and identify, study and correct deficiencies in the patient care process.

Nursing research: systematic inquiry to discover and interpret new facts and add to the body of nursing knowledge for the ultimate purpose of improving patient care.

Clearly there are aspects of nursing quality assurance and research which overlap. They are both concepts which require systematic inquiry, and they are concerned with the improvement of patient care. Both require similar, unbiased methods of data collection. Their differences seem to lie in the areas of the intended audience and scope. The audience for quality assurance activities are the care givers and administrators in one particular institution; the scope is limited to the problems within that institution. This contrast with nursing research, for which the intended audience extends far beyond the study institution and study population, the scope extends to advancing knowledge in general[10].

EXHIBIT 2
ADVANTAGES AND DISADVANTAGES OF COMBINING NURSING QUALITY ASSURANCE PROGRAMS IN A CLINICAL SETTING

Advantages	Disadvantages
Links research (sometimes viewed as a frill) with a mandated process in the organization	Confusion regarding definitions and functions of quality assurance and research
Increases the probability that research will be related to patient care	Conflicts arise: Local vs. general focus Disposition of results Direct vs. sophisticated analysis Territoriality
Increases likelihood that successful quality assurance approaches will be shared with others outside the institution	
In nursing, quality assurance and the types of research needed are closely related	
Efficient use of personnel and other resources	

These differences can raise several conflicts in a program which combines nursing quality assurance and research. First is the issue of confidentiality. Whether a study is conducted primarily for quality assurance purposes or for research purposes, the privacy of participants must be insured. Individuals with a quality assurance focus may believe that everything done to solve patient care problems should remain within the institution. They may feel that it is unethical to publish or disseminate information such as incidence of patient falls, infection rates, or data regarding other iatrogenic problems. The researcher, on the other hand, may believe that it is unethical or at least unprofessional *not* to publish or disseminate such information, which could be of use to others in various health care settings.

> "When we recall that the main business of nursing is sophisticated caring in clinical practice, it is difficult to see how quality assurance and the types of research needed by the profession can be anything other than intimately linked."

A second conflict may arise when a decision regarding the disposition of results is imminent. It is often viewed as sufficient for the researcher to collect data, do a rational analysis, and publish a scholarly report of the findings. Researchers do not necessarily perceive themselves, and are not perceived by others, as implementers; rather as describers or discoverers. The process of quality assurance, on the other hand, requires that an action plan be developed as a result of data collection and interpretation; that a change in practice be implemented; and that the effectiveness of that change be monitored. This goes beyond what the researcher is accustomed to, and may cause difficulties when quality assurance and research are combined.

The study methods used by researchers and by individuals involved in quality assurance also can cause conflict or confusion. In general, data for quality assurance studies are summarized as percentages and proportions. Emphasis is on meeting a predetermined level of compliance with established standards. Research methods often require sophisticated tests of association, correlation, and statistical significance. Evaluation of complex, multivariate relationships is often necessary. The researcher may lose sight of the more direct and clear-cut needs of quality assurance in the

midst of sophisticated analysis of the data. This is one way in which the nurse scientists may feel alien, caught between two worlds[11].

Lastly, a conflict of territoriality can arise. Quality assurance personnel often are members of medical records departments, and may not approve of the researcher who attempts to change small evaluative studies into major research projects. Likewise, the researcher may find it difficult to comply with the constraints of institutional forms, and with the requirements to follow up on action plans based on study findings. Considerable interpersonal skills are necessary to a smooth integration of nursing quality assurance and research activities with those of other institutional departments.

Despite the conflicts, there are several advantages to a combined nursing quality assurance and research program. In institutions where the value of nursing research is not recognized and may be considered a frill, linking with a mandated quality assurance program can provide credibility to forthcoming research studies. A successful combined program of sound clinical quality assurance and research will soon result in improved performance of personnel, and staff will begin to recognize the relevance of research to their practice[12]. For example, the common problem of patient falls is often dealt with in quality assurance. By expanding the scope of their studies and the intended audience beyond their own institutions, several nurse investigators have developed research projects which grew out of quality assurance studies of patient falls[13–15].

By combining quality assurance and research one also increases the likelihood that nursing research priorities, as in the patient falls studies cited above, will be more directly related to patient care[16]. The need for increased collaboration between clinical and academic nursing has been identified[17,18]. The marriage of practice oriented quality assurance and academically oriented research is an ideal way for this gap to be narrowed.

When we recall that the main business of nursing is sophisticated caring in clinical practice, it is difficult to see how quality assurance and the types of research needed by the profession can be anything other than intimately linked[19–21]. For this reason, the most efficient use of personnel and other resources could be made with a combined program. In terms of cost containment this is an important consideration.

Nursing administrators concerned with the direction and focus of their clinical methods of inquiry must weigh the advantages and disadvantages of combining or segregating quality assurance and research. For instance, it is necessary to continually assess the combined program for an appropriate balance of practicality and scholarship. Despite the greater administrative workload such assessment entails, there is increased opportunity for enhancing both programs and bringing nursing staff into a mode of systematic inquiry and clinical investigation.

References

1. C.P. Schlicke, "American Surgery's Noblest Experiment," *Archives of Surgery* 106(4):379–385, 1973.
2. Editorial staff, "J.C.A.H.'s New Quality Assurance Standard: Requirements Aired," *Hospital Peer Review* 4(9):113–128, 1979.
3. Janelle C. Krueger, "Nursing Administrators' Roles in Research: The WICHE Program," *Nursing Administration Quarterly* 2(4):27–32, 1978.
4. Robert L. Hanson, "Research: A Necessity in Nursing Services," *The Journal of Nursing Administration* 3(3):14, 15+, 1973.
5. Frances Moore, "Research In a Clinical Setting: Promises and Potential," *Supervisor Nurse* 11(6):36–38, 1980.
6. Susan R. Gortner, "Research for a Practice Profession," *Nursing Research* 24(3):193–196, 1975.
7. Margaret L. McClure, "Promoting Practice-Based Research: A Critical Need," *The Journal of Nursing Administration* 11(11):66–70, 1981.
8. Helen C. Chance and Ada Sue Hinshaw, "Strategies for Initiating A Research Program," *The Journal of Nursing Administration* 10(3):32–39, 1980.
9. Avedis Donabedian, "Needed Research in the Assessment and Monitoring of the Quality of Medical Care," Washington D.C., National Center for Health Services Research, DHEW Publications #(PHS) 78–3219, July 1978.
10. William L. Holzemer, "Research and Evaluation: An Overview," *Quality Review Bulletin* 6(3):31–34, 1980.
11. Nancy Jo Davenport, "The Nurse Scientist—Between Two Worlds," *Nursing Outlook* 28(1):28–31, 1980.
12. Ruth B. Fine, "Marketing Nursing Research," *The Journal of Nursing Administration* 10(11):21–23, 1980.
13. Jean Bronstein and Maryann K. Zalar, "Reduce the Incidence of Patient Falls In an Acute Care Setting," Presented at *Nursing Research: Advancing Clinical Practice in the 80s.* Sponsored by Department of Nursing Services, Stanford University Hospital and Symposia Medicus. San Francisco. September 1982.
14. Teresa M. Arsenault, "Slips and Falls: Problem Identification and Resolution By A Primary Nurse," Presented at *Nursing Research: Advancing Clinical Practice in the 80s.* Sponsored by Department of Nursing Services, Stanford University Hospital and Symposia Medicus. San Francisco, September 1982.
15. J.M. Morse, N. Morrow, and G. Federspiel, "Reducing Institutional Iatrogenesis: A Retrospective Analysis of Patient Falls," Presented at *Nursing Research: Advancing Clinical Practice in the 80s.* Sponsored by Department of Nursing Services, Stanford University Hospital and Symposia Medicus. San Francisco, September 1982.
16. Elaine L. Larson, "Research Outside Academia," *Image* 13(3):75–77, 1981.
17. Ada Jacox, "Strategies to Promote Nursing Research," *Nursing Research* 29(4):213–217, 1980.
18. Elaine L. Larson, "The Inquisitive Nurse: Bringing Research to the Bedside," *Nursing Administration Quarterly* 2(4):9–26, 1978.
19. Harriet R. Feldman, "Nursing Research in the 1980s," *Advances in Nursing Science* 3(1):85–92, 1980.
20. Norma G. McHugh and Jean E. Johnson, "Clinical Nursing Research: Beyond the Methods Books," *Nursing Outlook* 28(6):352–356, 1980.
21. J.T. Cuddihy, "Clinical Research: Translation Into Nursing Practice," *International Journal of Nursing Studies* 16(1):65–72, 1979.

UNIT FOUR

FRANCES HOFFMAN

The Cost of Nursing Services

Nursing administrators have traditionally been concerned with the clinical aspects of providing quality patient care. This included assuring that sufficient staff, supplies, and equipment were available to provide that care. In recent years, the nursing administrator has been barraged with additional responsibilities in the financial arena. This emphasis on expenses is a direct outgrowth of the public and governmental concern with escalating health care costs. It is also a reflection of the increasing business orientation of the hospital industry. These changes have several ramifications for nursing as a profession and for nursing administrators in particular.

First, there is an increasing integration of the clinical and fiscal aspects of patient care. When a new technology is developed, not only must an administrator ask "Is this going to benefit our patients?" but also "Can we afford this technology?" Clinical practitioners are becoming more and more involved in answering the financial questions as they develop proposals to include new technologies in their work settings. The nursing administrator must serve as resource and guide to clinicians as they begin this process of integration.

Second, there is the challenge to retain quality in the care provided to patients while increasing the productivity of staff. Nursing administrators will have to be innovative while remaining sensitive to the personal needs of staff. Management reports and accurate data analyses will be vital tools in maintaining an awareness of what kinds of staffing and what scheduling patterns are most effective and efficient.

Finally, there is growing pressure to identify nursing care as a separate cost element—for financial management offices, as entries on patient bills, or both. The need to itemize specific costs to patients has increased tremendously with the advent of the DRG-based prospective payment system. Since nursing personnel are a significant component in the cost of caring for patients, it is important that this component be accurately identified. Many methods are being suggested to achieve an accurate analysis of nursing care costs. The nursing administrator must provide leadership in this area—helping refine those methods that do not include assessment of specific patient care needs as a basis for calculation of nursing costs.

With the increased emphasis on costing out nursing services, nursing as a profession has a singular opportunity. Recognition for the pivotal role of nursing in patient care can be greatly enhanced through the process of cost identification. Cost implies worth. When nursing care is listed as a separate item on a patient's bill, the value of nursing care is clearly communicated. Not only is it communicated to the patient, but also to other departments in the hospital and to administration. Even though the nursing department is not designated as a revenue producer, the implication in costing out nursing services is that nurses contribute greatly to revenues.

It is important that nurses seize this opportunity. Though the "number-crunching" aspects of costing out nursing services may seem grim, the benefits to the nursing profession will more than outweigh the efforts involved.

CHAPTER 20

The Cost of Nursing Care in Hospitals

by Duane D. Walker

How much does nursing care in hospitals really cost? In this article, Mr. Walker explores this issue. He analyzes how the relative cost of nursing care can be determined and how costs of nursing care services can be separated from non-nursing hospital services.

There is a widespread concern about the rapidly escalating costs of hospital care. A national effort has been launched to reduce unnecessary hospitalizations by having physicians perform as many diagnostic and therapeutic procedures as possible on an ambulatory basis. Presumably, more patients are hospitalized because they require continuing nursing care and ready access to physician services.

Acute care hospitals have been under scrutiny and attack for over a decade in regard to their part in the exorbitant and ever-increasing costs of health care. A report of the National Council on Wage and Price Stability recently concluded that during the 1965 to 1975 period, hospital costs and physicians' fees rose more than 50% faster than the overall costs of living[1].

Beginning in 1971 with federal wage and price controls, followed by state rate commissions and voluntary hospital cost-containment efforts, hospitals have been under considerable pressure to control their costs. Nursing service is the hospital's largest department, and therefore has been particularly vulnerable to cost-containment policies.

The nursing service department has been singled out as a major cost in hospital's operating expenditures[2–4]. Yet the actual cost of nursing care is unknown because it is embedded in the daily hospital room charge. The cost of nursing care has been synonymous with the room rate, which is very high by any standard. It is not surprising, therefore, that many assume that the rapidly rising costs of hospital care are due to increased nurses' salaries.

Duane D. Walker, R.N., M.S., F.A.A.N., is Associate Administrator, hospitals and clinics, and Director of Nursing Service at Stanford (CA) University Hospital.

Reprinted with the publisher's permission from *Nursing in the 1980s: Crises, Opportunities, Challenges* (Philadelphia: J.B. Lippincott Company, 1982).

Separating nursing care costs from non-nursing costs

This paper proposes to examine the question, How much does nursing care in hospitals really cost?

To answer the question, we need to probe hidden costs and to find answers to the following interrelated questions:

- How should the relative cost of nursing care be determined?
- Are *all* expenditures in the nursing service operating budget specifically related to direct or indirect nursing care services?

Since these questions, relative to the high costs of nursing care, have been critically analyzed and a preliminary study conducted at a leading university teaching hospital, some background information and initial findings from the study will be presented in order to sort out costs of *nursing care* services from *non-nursing* hospital services.

The setting

Stanford University Hospital (SUH) is a 668-bed private, nonprofit, teaching hospital, owned and operated by Stanford University. Its income is derived primarily from patient revenues (97%). SUH serves as a community hospital for patients from adjacent areas and as a regional medical center for patients with advanced and difficult medical problems.

The primary goals of the Nursing Service Department at SUH are to provide patients with quality nursing care and educational services, and to foster a nursing practice environment that will provide nurses with challenges, satisfaction, and rewards. Some of the programs the department of nursing offers are the following:

- Four-level clinical nursing career ladder
- Department of nursing research
- Continuing education opportunities
- Primary nursing practice
- Distinguished lecture series

• Administrative residency program in nursing management.

The Nursing Service Department is composed of seven major clinical regions, each headed by an assistant director of nursing. Each unit within a clinical region is managed by a clinical nursing coordinator (head nurse). In addition, there is an assistant director of nursing for administrative services and one for educational services; these administrative services provide support to the clinical regions. Overall direction of the department is provided by the associate administrator/director of nursing along with an associate director of nursing. At present, the department employs 1,200 registered nurses, 20 licensed practical nurses, 225 nursing assistants, seven unit managers, and 110 unit clerks.

EXHIBIT 1.
HOSPITAL SERVICES INCLUDED IN THE DAILY ROOM RATE

Direct	Indirect
Direct Nursing	**Indirect Nursing**
Clinical nursing coordinator	Nursing administration
Clinical assistant director of nursing, bedside nursing staff	Nursing orientation
Unit manager, clerks, and equipment technician	Education and development
Direct Medical	**Indirect Medical**
Medical supplies	Medical school contracts
Interns and residents	Anatomic pathology
	Medical staff office
	Utilization review and quality assurance
Other Direct	**Financial Affairs**
Dietary	Financial adjustments
Housekeeping	(Medicare/Medicaid
Laundry and linen	disallowances, bed debts,
Messenger and mail service	discounts and allowances,
Central supply items	provision of Capital)
Minor equipment and	Depreciation (buildings
pharmacy stock	and equipment)
Social services	Patient accounting
Telephone	Finance and data
Admitting	processing
Patient placement	Insurance
Infection control	Interest
Chaplain	Purchasing
	Other Indirect
	General administration
	Maintenance and repairs
	(plant, grounds,
	equipment)
	Personnel
	Utilities
	Medical records
	Office supplies
	Communications
	Facilities protection
	Community relations

The modality of nursing practice consists of primary nursing and team nursing.

Each nursing unit is structured as a separate cost center, and each clinical nursing coordinator, with assistance from a unit manager, prepares the nursing unit's budget. The budgets are based on the projected acuity of illness of the patients to be served. Assistant directors of nursing, assisted by the unit manager, defend their budgets at hospital budget hearings.

It should be noted that the Nursing Service Department at SUH supports the proposition that nursing care is limited only to direct and indirect activities required for the management and delivery of nursing care *per se*. These direct and indirect nursing activities include the following:

Direct nursing care

Those nursing care activities (including the "laying on of hands" in performing nursing functions at the unit level), unit nursing management, and only those recordkeeping, clerical, and management tasks that are required specifically for the provision of nursing care.

Indirect nursing care

Activities performed at the nursing department administrative level, including general administration of the department; nursing supervision (general supervision on evenings, nights, weekends); environmental management; classification of patients; nursing quality assurance programs; nursing staffing and recruitment; nursing educational services (orientation, inservice, and continuing education, patient education programs, other special programs); and nursing research. (See Exhibit 1 for a complete list of direct and indirect nursing activities.)

The method

As a first step, the cost of nursing care must be separated from the plethora of non-nursing tasks and services frequently lumped with nursing under the misleading title "room rate"[5–8]. However, as a prerequisite to this step, the nursing service director needs to take steps to ensure that nursing staff members are indeed performing *nursing* tasks rather than a myriad of other non-nursing tasks. Primary components of nursing care are the direct care requirements of patients and families, which depend upon the acuity of the patient's condition, the necessary related nursing tasks, and the time needed to perform these tasks. These components (acuity, nursing tasks, and nursing time) were identified and quantified at SUH as the basis for a computerized patient classification system that reflects levels of nursing care. This system enables the prediction of staffing needs, and provides a data base for validation of budget requirements and the setting of differential charges for direct nursing care to the patient.

As will be discussed later, this classification system is

similar to others that have been developed, and it has some of the same shortcomings. It has the potential, however, of allowing one to put a more realistic price tag on levels of nursing care throughout the hospital. In order to understand how the patient classification system can be used as a tool to determine the cost of nursing care on a particular unit, the following description of nursing care costs on a adult intensive care unit is presented.

Nursing care costs of intensive care units

On the adult intensive care units (ICUs) at SUH, the patient classification system consists of five levels of direct nursing care that range from the least nursing care required (level I) to the most nursing care required (level V). Each patient's acuity is assessed and classified three times a day by a nurse caring for the patient. The nurse makes this assessment 4 hours before the next shift, which enables adjustments to be made in staffing patterns for that shift. To record each assessment, the nurse completes a form by darkening appropriate squares with a pencil. This form is then read by an optical scanner, and the information goes directly into a computer.

At present, the *pier diem* room charge in the ICUs is based on the five levels of nursing care. Payments for charges are determined on this basis, and were negotiated with third party payers. Although the level of nursing care is identified on the patient's bill, the actual dollar figures for a particular level do not appear on the bill distinct from the room charge.

In the ICUs all *non-nursing* tasks have been reallocated to the appropriate departments through negotiation. Therefore, nurses on these units do *not* perform non-nursing tasks, ensuring that the nursing care charge represents the actual cost of providing nursing care.

Two methods are useful in examining the relative costs of nursing care in hospitals. The first is to examine the components included in daily room charges. To determine the cost of nursing care *versus* the room rate, data were collected for level III nursing care over a 1 month period. The average daily census of patients requiring this care level was 20.

Exhibit 2 illustrates the proportionate daily cost of nursing care *versus* other non-nursing charges included in the average *per diem* rate for level III care. The categories used, other than nursing, were selected to show expenses related to providing services directly to patients ("direct" categories) *versus* overhead costs ("indirect" categories).

The nurse-patient ratio for level III ICU care is 1:1. Patients who are classified as level III have the following nursing care requirements:

- Continuous observation and hourly intervention (nursing activities directed toward evaluating and correcting patient problems or complications).
- Increased number and frequency of vital sign determinations and treatments.

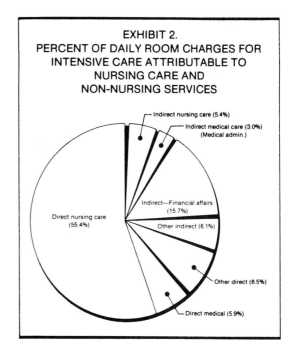

EXHIBIT 2.
PERCENT OF DAILY ROOM CHARGES FOR INTENSIVE CARE ATTRIBUTABLE TO NURSING CARE AND NON-NURSING SERVICES

Indirect nursing care (5.4%)
Indirect medical care (3.0%) (Medical admin.)
Indirect—Financial affairs (15.7%)
Other indirect (6.1%)
Direct nursing care (55.4%)
Other direct (8.5%)
Direct medical (5.9%)

- Vital signs determinations every 15 min. to 30 min.: temperature, pulse, respiration, blood pressure, apical and radial pulses, central venous pressure, electrocardiogram monitoring, and other determinations as indicated.
- Continuous ventilatory support.
- Pulmonary therapy every 30 min. to 60 min.: intermittent positive pressure, breathing treatments, percussion, postural drainage, and other procedures done by registered nurses.
- Continuous drug infusions (vasopressors, vasodilators, and antiarrhythmics).
- Increased monitoring of other parameters with appropriate therapy.
- Blood gases.
- Fluid and electrolyte management.
- Increased monitoring for life-threatening complications.
- Increased care due to total dependency (inability to participate in own care).
- Isolation.

Comparative costs of nursing care versus non-nursing care costs

A second way to examine the relative cost of nursing is to ascertain the share of total hospital charges attributable to nursing. Data were collected and analyzed from a sample of five patients with similar lengths of stay in each of six disease categories ($N = 30$). Since the sample size is small generalizability is limited. However, the data are presented as an exploratory approach in determining and comparing the cost of nursing care with other hospital services.

Charges that make up the average total cost of hospitalization for the sample of 30 patients are presented in Exhibit 3. The total nursing care cost was approximately 50% of the room charge. The percentage may be somewhat high since these patients received intensive care during part of their hospital stay. It should be noted that the table shows mean figures only and does not reflect variations within categories.

Examination of Exhibit 3 reveals that the cost of nursing care accounts for a relatively small proportion of total hospitalization charges (approximately 12% to 20%). In four of the six diagnostic categories, the nursing care cost is similar to the cost of physicians' services. Exhibit 4 represents the proportionate costs of hospitalization when data from Exhibit 3 are combined and the six diagnostic categories are considered as a group. Laboratory charges account for almost the same proportion of the total cost as nursing care.

Although a more comprehensive study is needed to determine the costs of nursing care, the preliminary findings suggest that *actual* nursing care is not as costly as many hospital administrators and physicians would lead us to believe. For example, when 24-hr. one-to-one care is provided by an all-registered nurse staff, as in level III ICU care, the high level of nursing care accounts for approximately 55% of the *per diem* charge. When the cost of professional nursing is compared to that of charges for other hospital services, somewhat less than 20% of the total charges appears to be for nursing care.

Discussion

The general misconception that the cost of hospital nursing care is synonymous with the room rate needs to be corrected. This notion has probably arisen because of the long-standing fiscal practice of combining overhead and other miscellaneous costs with nursing costs, as well as the practice of charging the nursing budget for non-nursing services.

Why has nursing's monetary value and professional identity been buried in this way? Undoubtedly, a large part of the responsibility belongs to nurses themselves. The historical view of nurses as handmaidens has been difficult to change. The subservient attitude that accompanies this view has prompted many nurses to assume responsibility for non-nursing activities that other hospital members have failed to complete.

Nursing administrators need to take more responsibility for fostering the autonomy and decision-making ability of nurses. The nursing budget is a management tool for achieving this end. Not only do nursing directors need to become proficient in budget procedures, but head nurses at the unit level need to increase their knowledge and skills, and play a vital role in fiscal management.

Many nursing directors either do not prepare a budget or do not understand its uses and value[9]. Schmied notes that many directors are remiss in allocating time and energy to fiscal management, even though, as Swansburg points out, "the control of a budget determines who controls nursing service"[10,11]. Furthermore, Stevens proposes that nurs-

EXHIBIT 3.
PERCENT DISTRIBUTION OF CHARGES IN AVERAGE TOTAL COST
OF HOSPITALIZATION BY DIAGNOSIS*

Diagnosis	Room charge (excluding nursing)	Nursing Care	Clinical Professional's Fee†	OR, ER PT OT	Inhalation Therapy	Anesthesia	X-ray and Radiation Therapy	Laboratory	Surgical Supplies	Central Supplies	Drugs	Blood	Total
Coronary artery bypass graft	14.8	14.8	13.9	11.4	2.5	1.3	2.5	19.0	13.2	1.8	4.6	0.1	100.0
Aortic valve repair; mitral valve repair	12.4	12.4	12.6	9.0	2.1	1.0	2.0	13.9	29.5	1.2	4.0	—	100.0
Chronic obstructive pulmonary disease	20.7	20.7	5.7	5.1	9.0	—	6.9	16.8	0.9	5.3	8.7	0.1	100.0
Hodgkins' disease; lymphoma; leukemia	21.0	21.0	5.1	1.6	4.0	0.1	6.6	26.9	0.3	4.5	8.9	—	100.0
Craniotomy	20.5	20.5	22.1	12.4	3.3	1.2	4.1	8.4	1.7	1.5	4.1	0.1	100.0
Thoracotomy; aortic-femoral bypass	17.1	17.1	15.9	14.1	5.8	2.4	6.8	11.5	3.0	1.7	4.5	—	100.0

*Sample of 5 patients in each diagnosis category
†Includes surgeon's fee, where applicable

ing administrators work toward realistic representation on both the expense and revenue sides of the ledger, and recommends that nursing service directors take steps to establish the concept of nursing as a revenue-producing department[8].

To reflect nursing care costs as accurately as possible, levels of care should represent *actual* nursing care, that is, the cost of care when nursing staff are performing only nursing functions. The use of a patient classification system, such as that employed at SUH, is a suitable approach to arriving at a dollar value for various levels of nursing care. This notion has been supported by a number of authors [12–15]. The idea of classifying patients by nursing requirements is not new, and numerous systems have been developed. Although some of the components of the patient classification system are difficult to identify and quantify, soundly developed patient classification systems have proved useful for determining staffing and the nursing budget and setting differential charges for patient care.

Almost a decade ago, Holbrook proposed that nursing care charges be separated from room charges and that they be determined by level of nursing care provided[6]. Recently, a few institutions, such as Massachusetts Eye and Ear Infirmary, and St. Luke's Hospital and Medical Center in Phoenix, Arizona, have initiated charges for nursing care by levels of care, and reflected these charges on the patients' bills[16]. As noted earlier, the actual dollar figures for these charges do not yet appear on the patients' bills at SUH, but it is the appropriate next step in accord with the American Nurses' Association's (ANA) 1977 resolution recommending that "all billing and reimbursement procedures clearly identify both the nature and cost of the nursing care services rendered"[17].

Swansburg recommends that the system of reimbursement for health care costs should not pay for "frills," such as additional food and drinks, daily changes of bed linens, and personal services that patients could perform, provided they are physically and mentally able[3]. Giving patients the option to purchase extra services might be one way of meeting the needs of patients while containing overall costs. Stevens' proposal is similar, and suggests that "it shoud be possible to set price schedules related to both patient needs and standards of care"[8]. This could be accomplished by combining quality control and patient classification systems, and would be useful in nursing and institutional decision making regarding levels of care that could or could not be offered. Either the institution might choose to offer a certain level of care, based on a realistic assessment of its resources, or it might offer a variety of levels and prices, with clients deciding on the price they want to pay.

This concept is analogous to shopping for any item in a free enterprise system. It requires that the seller of the item or service be prepared to deliver that which is purchased. Thus charging for various levels of nursing care requires that the specified level of care will be provided. Nurses may

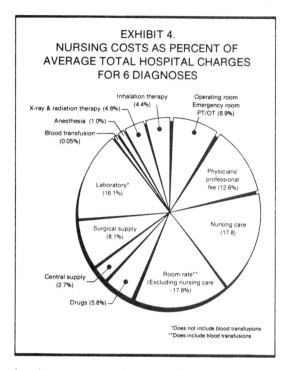

EXHIBIT 4.
NURSING COSTS AS PERCENT OF AVERAGE TOTAL HOSPITAL CHARGES FOR 6 DIAGNOSES

be reluctant to accept the concept that a certain level of nursing care and hospital hotel services will be provided in accordance with choices of the patient. In addition, nurses may have difficulty in accepting the high degree of accountability that goes with identifying and publicizing the monetary value of nursing care. Education of all concerned groups to these changes is essential. Nursing administration needs to work toward changing attitudes of nurses, hospital administrators, other health providers, and perhaps more importantly the consumers.

All groups would benefit from implementation of these fiscal changes. For consumers, benefits will include eliminating the inequitable practice of paying for services not received. Although operating expenditures such as utilities, maintenance, and housekeeping would probably be apportioned equally, a patient who requires and receives minimal nursing care would pay only for minimal care. This patient would not subsidize other patients who receive substantially more hours of nursing care. Consumers would also benefit from the offering of options as to the amount and sources of care or hospital amenities they desire. Such options would not only assist in cost containment, but would also increase the accessibility and scope of services for consumers. An accompanying benefit might be the fostering of self-determination and responsibility, with a lessening of the dependency that hospitals now generally impose on patients and families.

For nurses the anticipated benefits are considerable. Nurses are perceived as an economic drain, rather than as a financial asset. Determining the cost of and charging for nursing care—thereby establishing and validating nurses as income producers—should greatly improve nurses' ability to influence important decisions concerning nursing resources and practice. In addition, the opportunity to demonstrate and establish the relationship between nursing actions and cost-benefits should pave the way for nurses to use their special knowledge and skills more fully.

Finally, the current shortage of nurses may be partly due to frustration brought about through the inability to practice nursing as professional clinicians and teachers, to be valued as important members of the health care team, and to be duly rewarded for the care and comfort they provide their patients. When nurses gain the power and status that goes with recognition of their economic worth, and when their role is more clearly defined through establishment of care levels, they may very well feel more committed to and satisfied with nursing. A satisfied, committed professional nurse is the key to high productivity and quality nursing care.

Conclusion

Despite the central importance of nursing care to hospitalized patients, nursing services have traditionally been included under the hospital's daily room charge instead of as a professional service rendered. As a result, many have come to believe that the cost of nursing care is almost synonymous with daily room charges.

Contrary to popular opinion, nursing care accounts for only about half of the daily room charge for ICUs and may be significantly less in other areas of the hospital. Moreover, for the six diagnostic categories examined here, nursing accounted for only 20% or less of total hospital charges.

Nurses are the largest single group of health professionals employed by hospitals. It is not surprising, therefore, that nursing service budgets have been a target of cost containment programs. Despite a widespread shortage of hospital nurses, there is great reluctance to invest additional resources in nursing. However, if the results of this preliminary analysis are sustained by subsequent studies, it would appear that nursing care is one of the hospital's most economical services. It has also been suggested that the cost-benefit ratio could be significantly improved by breaking the costs of nursing care out of the daily room charge and billing patients for professional services rendered. Nurses would be more accountable for their services, and hospitals would have greater incentives to improve the fiscal management of hotel, maintenance, and other institutional

operating costs.

The question of how to determine nursing care costs will remain without a definitive answer until unsound fiscal practices such as hiding nursing care costs and revenues are abandoned. It is obvious from a preliminary study that nursing care costs need to be separated from non-nursing hospital costs and that the real problem is presenting costs in their room rate disguise. Indeed, the time is long overdue for a more extensive study of the costs of nursing care. One thing appears certain—if nursing in acute care hospitals and other health care facilities is ever to be recognized and reimbursed as an essential professional service, the time for working toward these goals is *now*.

References

1. Council on Wage and Price Stability, Executive Office of the President: The Program of Rising Health Care Costs, p. 3. (Staff Report). Washington, D.C., April 1976.
2. M.K. Mullanne, Foreword. In Donovan H: Nursing Service Administration: Managing the Enterprise, p. 3. St. Louis, C.V. Mosby, 1975.
3. R.C.Swansburg, Cost control in nursing. *Supervisor Nurse* 9, No. 51:3; 12, 1978.
4. T. Porter-O'Grady, Financial planning: Budgeting for nursing, Part I. *Supervisor Nurse* 10, No. 35:3, 1979.
5. N. Baker, Reimbursement for nursing services: Issues and trends. *Nursing Law and Ethics* 1, No. 1:6, 1980.
6. F.K. Holbrook, Charging by level of nursing care. *Hospitals* 46, No. 80:6, 11; 12; 1972.
7. C.P. Jennings, T.F. Jennings, Containing costs through prospective reimbursement. *Am. J. Nurs.* 77, p. 1155: 6, 1977.
8. B.J. Stevens, What is the executive's role in budgeting for her department? *Hospitals* 50, No. 83: 6, 11, 12, 1976.
9. I. Goertzen, Cost effectiveness for nursing: Regulation of hospital rates and its implications for nursing. *Nursing Administration Quarterly* 3, No. 59:11, 1978.
10. E. Schmied, Allocation of resources: Preparation of the nursing department budget. *The Journal of Nursing Administration* 7, No. 31:11, 1977.
11. R.C. Swansburg, The nursing budget. *Supervisor Nurse* 9, No. 40:11, 1978.
12. B. Brown, Editorial. *Nursing Administration Quarterly* 3, No. V:11, 1978.
13. S.K. Evans, R. Laundon and W.G. Yamamato, Projecting staffing requirements for intensive care units. *The Journal of Nursing Administration* 10, No. 34:11, 1980.
14. A. Marriner, Variables affecting staffing. *Supervisor Nurse* 10, No. 62:11, 1979.
15. T. Porter-O'Grady, Financial planning: Budgeting for nursing, Part II. *Supervisor Nurse* 10, No. 25:11, 1979.
16. A Patient Classification System for Staffing and Charging for Nursing Services, p. 12. Phoenix, AZ, St. Luke's Hospital Medical Center.
17. Commission on Economic and General Welfare: Reimbursement for Nursing Services (Position statement), p. 12. Kansas City, MO. American Nurses' Association, 1977.

CHAPTER 21

Variable Billing for Services: New Fiscal Direction for Nursing

by Nancy J. Higgerson and Ann Van Slyck

The authors propose and explain a new fiscal concept for nursing in which patients are billed specifically for nursing services rather than for "routine" services included in the room rate. How is variable billing for various types of nursing service put into effect? What are the purposes, practical benefits, and implications of variable billing? Here the authors answer these questions and describe variable billing systems in effect in two hospitals. The examples will enable nursing administrators to consider adapting variable billing for nursing services in their own institutions.

Nurses are responsible for providing and interpreting clinical care, coordinating a multitude of diagnostic and therapeutic procedures, and facilitating efficient medical practice. The way these responsibilities are carried out determines the standard of care, which in turn determines the hospital's reputation in the community. Although the expenses associated with such nursing care (costs of staffing, supplies, equipment, education, and so forth) are readily identified, the related revenue is often not acknowledged or allocated to nursing units. The nursing profession faces three basic fiscal issues: allocation of revenue to nursing unit cost centers, separation of the room rate into its component parts, and the introduction of variable billing. The first two issues, appropriate allocation of revenue and breakdown of the room rate into its component parts, are objectives that must be dealt with

Nancy J. Higgerson, R.N., M.A., is vice president for Nursing, Abbott-Northwestern Hospital, Minneapolis, Minnesota.

Ann Van Slyck, R.N., M.S.N., is former assistant administrator for Nursing Services, St. Luke's Hospital Medical Center, Phoenix, Arizona. She is currently serving as a nursing consultant.

before the goal of variable billing for nursing services can be reached.

Institutional foundation

What is *variable billing?* It means billing for specific aspects or levels of nursing care, which vary from patient to patient. For variable billing to be successful, the corporation must accept certain assumptions:

- Revenue and expenses are defined and assigned to appropriate cost centers.
- The cost of providing each individual service is identified.
- Patients' bills are based on that cost plus a contribution toward profit.
- Each patient pays only for services received and does not subsidize services received by other patients.

Assumptions specific to nursing should include the following:

- Nursing care is an identifiable entity that can be defined, measured, and costed.
- Nursing care varies with the patient's diagnosis, level of illness, age, and so forth.
- A direct relationship exists between nursing care provided and costs (staff and supplies).

A total commitment to these beliefs is essential if the administrative team is to meet the challenges that occur during the evolution and maintenance of a variable billing system.

Revenue cost centers

Typically, nursing care charges are part of a room rate that includes "routine" nursing services, room, and food. A more logical approach is to establish three cost centers and charge patients separately for (1) nursing services, (2) room (bed and shelter), and (3) food (dietary services). A

EXHIBIT 1.
NURSING CARE RECORDS FOR (A) MEDICAL/SURGICAL
AND (B) BEHAVIORAL HEALTH UNITS AT ST. LUKE'S HOSPITAL

A. Nursing Care Record—Medical/Surgical

St. Luke's Hospital Medical Center ■ Phoenix, Arizona

N = Night Shift; D = Day Shift; E = Evening Shift
B = Breakfast; L = Lunch; D = Dinner

Points	Level		N	D	E
26- 37	1	Sub-Total Acuity 'A'			
38- 55	2	Sub-Total Acuity 'B'			
56- 70	3	Sub-Total Acuity 'C'			
71- 83	4	**Total Points**			
84-103	5	**Acuity Level**			
Date		● ☐ On Pass			
		☐ Private Duty			

DIET	Refused None	B	L	D
NOURISHMENT	Partial			
	Total			

ACUITY 'A'

DIET		N	D	E
	Diet Check	2	2	2
	NPO	2	2	2
	Self	2	2	2
	Assist c̄ Tray	5	5	5
	Sips/Chips	5	5	5
	Intake/Output (Force/Limit)	5	5	5
	Assist Feed	8	8	8
	Total Feed	8	8	8
	Gavage Feed	8	8	8
●	Teaching Feed	8	8	8
●	Complex Total Feed	8	8	8

BATH/LINEN		N	D	E
	Environmental Check	1	1	1
	Tub s̄ Help	1	1	1
	Bath s̄ Help	1	1	1
	Shower s̄ Help	1	1	1
	Self-Help (Bedside)	2	2	2
	H S Care	2	2	2
	Tub c̄ Occasional Check	2	2	2
	Shower c̄ Occasional Check	2	2	2
	Complex H S Care	4	4	4
	Partial Bath	4	4	4
	Complete Bath	4	4	4
●	Complex Bath	5	5	5
●	Teaching Bath/Shower	5	5	5
●	Multiple Baths	5	5	5

MOBILITY		N	D	E
	Sleeping/Resting During Rounds	2	2	2
	Up Ad Lib	2	2	2
	Chair	2	2	2
	BRP	2	2	2
●	Ambulate c̄ Help	5	5	5
●	BRP c̄ Help	5	5	5
●	Chair c̄ Help	5	5	5
	Bedrest c̄ BRP/Commode	5	5	5
	Bedrest	5	5	5
	Restrictive Bedrest	8	8	8
●	Complex Activity	8	8	8
●	Teaching Activity	8	8	8
●	Therapeutic Repositioning	8	8	8
	Total Lift Q _____ H	10	10	10
	Stryker/Circle Bed Turn Q _____ H	10	10	10
●	Soft/Leather Restraints	10	10	10

SUB-TOTAL ACUITY 'A'

	ACUITY 'B'	N	D	E
MEDICATIONS	Medication Kardex Check	5	5	5
	Routine s̄ IV's	8	8	8
	Routine c̄ IV's	15	15	15
	Multiple Meds	15	15	15
	Heparin Lock	15	15	15
●	Teaching Medications	15	15	15
	Routine c̄ Multiple Piggybacks	25	25	25
●	Blood Transfusions/Observation	25	25	25
●	Administrative/Frequent Intervention	25	25	25

		N	D	E
BEHAVIOR	Responsive To Care	5	5	5
●	Dependent Psychologically/New Admit	10	10	10
●	Barriers To Care	10	10	10
●	Confused	10	10	10
●	Disoriented	10	10	10
●	Repetitive Requests	10	10	10
●	Lethargic	10	10	10
●	Comatose	10	10	10
●	Disruptive	15	15	15
●	Hallucinations/Delusions	15	15	15
●	Conflict Of Emotions	15	15	15
●	Threatening Physical Harm	15	15	15

		N	D	E
STATE	Self Reliant	4	4	4
	Routine Admission	7	7	7
●	Short Term Teaching & Counseling	7	7	7
	Assistance c̄ ADL	7	7	7
●	Restrictions	7	7	7
	Pre-Op Preparation	11	11	11
●	Complex Admission/Transfer	11	11	11
	Post-Op/Post-ACU (24 Hours)	11	11	11
●	Physiologically Unstable	11	11	11
●	Discharge Planning/Teaching	11	11	11
●	Communications Barrier	15	15	15
●	Extensive Nursing Care	20	20	20

SUB-TOTAL ACUITY 'B'

ACUITY 'C' (7-14-20) SUB-TOTAL				
TREATMENT/PROCEDURE	ITEMS — FREQUENCY	TIMES		

SIGNATURES								
NIGHT		LPN/NA	Side Rails ↑	**DAY**	LPN/NA	Side Rails ↑	**EVE**	LPN/NA	Side Rails ↑
		RN	Bed ↓		RN	Bed ↓		RN	Bed ↓

● **REQUIRES DOCUMENTATION**

Continued

Exhibit 1. Continued   **B. Nursing Care Record—Behavioral Health**

		N	D	E
	I Milieu 'A' ACTIVITIES			
	'B' BEHAVIOR			
	II Counseling			
	III Somatic			
	Total Points			
	Acuity Level			

Points	Level
15- 37	11
38- 50	12
51- 63	13
64- 79	14
80-100	15

Date

• ☐ On Pass
☐ Private Duty

St. Luke's Hospital Medical Center ■ Phoenix, Arizona

DIET	Refused None Taken	B	L	D	NOURISHMENT

I MILIEU

'A' Activities	N	D	E
Defined treatment plan followed	5	5	5
Free time used constructively without direction	NA	5	5
Dependent on staff for care/participation			
Technically			
• Physical Care: personal hygiene, dietary & fluid needs, orientation to Dx text	10	10	10
Socially			
• Provide for activity attendance/use of program content	NA	15	15
• Arrange for peer socialization	NA	15	15
Dependent on staff for safety			
Precautionary measures:			
• Searching	20	20	20
Phone/visitor restriction	20	20	20
• 2 or more staff for effective care	20	20	20
• Technical preparation for Dx test/Treatment	20	20	20
• 2 or more contacts to achieve test accuracy	20	20	20
• Specific evaluative observation 4 or more times	20	20	20
Special precautionary			
• Restraints/Seclusion	25	25	25
• Suicide	25	25	25
• Seizure	25	25	25
• Smoking	25	25	25
• Elopement	25	25	25
• Isolation	25	25	25
• Oxygen therapy 1 or more sterile procedures	25	25	25
• One to one staff observation q 5-10 min. (critical physical or emotional condition)	30	30	30

II COUNSELING

	N	D	E
• Information interaction (passes leaving/returning)	7	7	7
Group/dyadic interaction			
• Group meetings structured by staff	NA	13	13
• One to one contractual/PRN interaction	13	13	13
Communication barriers			
• Perception & thought distortions (hallucinations, delusions)	19	19	19
• Avoidance of time with staff	19	19	19
• Pt/family goals incompatible with treatment	19	19	19
• Short attention span; poor assimilation	19	19	19
• Physical communication handicap _____	25	25	25
• Cultural _____	25	25	25
• Retardation	25	25	25
• Organically based confusion/disorientation	25	25	25

'B' Behavior	N	D	E
Appropriate to unit activity	5	5	5
Participates in decisions about care	5	5	5
Shares with others own status	5	5	5
Observes and responds to needs of others	5	5	5
Marginal psychological			
• Attends program activities without participating	NA	10	10
• Does activities that do not include interaction	NA	10	10
Marginal physical			
• Remains in room during activity	NA	15	15
• Gives priority to lone or personal activities	NA	15	15
Dependent psychological			
• Unfamiliar with unit and/or program	20	20	20
• Focuses primarily on somatic symptoms	20	20	20
• Lethargic, indecisive	20	20	20
• Verbalizes acceptance of treatment with no follow through	20	20	20
• Refuses to care for self	20	20	20
Dependent physical			
• Unable to care for self (ECT aged toxic)	25	25	25
Locomotion handicap _____	25	25	25
Disruptive (patient/family)			
• Destructive	30	30	30
• Demanding interruptive	30	30	30
• Inappropriate sexual behavior	30	30	30
• Habits offensive to others	30	30	30
• Delusional ideas/prejudices forced on others	30	30	30

III SOMATIC

	N	D	E
Receptive to medication plan	5	5	5
Complex medications			
Four or more times/shift	10	10	10
• Nursing evaluation measures required	10	10	10
• Teaching, information regarding meds, (change, effect, use on pass or after discharge)	10	10	10
Administrative problems			
• Resistive: forcing, tonguing, reminders, dysphagia	15	15	15
Locating due to: _____	15	15	15
• Manipulative for more: repeated requests	15	15	15

NURSE'S SIGNATURES		
Night	**Day**	**Evening**

• **REQUIRES DOCUMENTATION IN NOTES**

cost center is an organizational unit that performs a function and uses specific resources to do so. Cost centers are either revenue- or nonrevenue-producing. *Revenue cost centers* are organizational units that provide identifiable and reimbursable services to the patient. *Nonrevenue cost centers* provide a service or function for which a charge is not generated; thus, revenue is not gained.

A nursing cost center is a logical unit of service such as a nursing unit or a specific nursing service. Each nursing unit and certain nursing service, such as IV therapy, orthopedics, and hemodialysis is a revenue cost center. Nursing administration, staffing, epidemiology, and so forth are nonrevenue cost centers. Some cost centers, such as patient education and nursing education, can be either revenue or nonrevenue depending on the internal financial system and the dictates of external rate-setting groups. Nursing education is usually a nonrevenue cost center, but fees from workshops, seminars, and courses should be credited to the nursing education cost center or to an appropriate component. Whether hospitals can bill patients for patient education continues to be debated between hospitals and third-party payers. Thus, patient education is most often financed by revenues from per diem room charges.

The *room cost center* is also a revenue cost center. The patient is billed a room charge which includes cost of housekeeping, linen, maintenance, equipment repairs, and depreciation. The *dietary cost center* receives revenues gained from charges for patients meals and other nourishment.

With this approach, each of the three functions, room, dietary, and nursing, are accurately identified to the patient. In addition, the revenues and expenses are directly related to providing each function. Identification of nursing service as a revenue producer is the first step toward developing a realistic fiscal system for nursing. This goal must be accomplished before addressing the challenges of variable nursing care charges.

Nursing care charges

Nursing care is difficult to define or classify because of its broad scope, mixture of procedures and processes, and variability with regard to patient mix and nurse interdependence with other health care professionals and services. A viable way to define general services like medical/surgical, behavioral health, and maternity is a patient-classification system. With it, patients' nursing care requirements are defined, and patients are classified according to the level of care they require. For each classification level, the required staffing, in full time equivalents (FTEs) and supplies, serves as the cost basis for the charges. The classification, staffing, and billing system that results reflects actual costs of different levels of care.

St. Luke's Hospital

A model of a classification, staffing, and billing system is found at St. Luke's Hospital Medical Center in Phoenix, Arizona. A classification and charting document called the *Nursing Care Record* serves as the basis for determining both staffing and charges (Exhibit 1). During each shift the nurse (or team member) caring for the patient adds to the Nursing Care Record for that 24-hour period. Numbers in each category of care (diet, bath/linen, and so forth) are circled to describe the nurse's activity or the patient's state or behavior. For example, when a nurse on the day shift in the medical/surgical unit helps the patient to walk, that nurse would then circle 5 in the mobility category, D column, opposite "ambulate c̄ help." The nurses circles all pertinent numbers in each category. Items with dots require narrative charting on the reverse side of the form or on progress notes.

At the end of each shift, the RN responsible for the patient adds up the circled points. Although more than one term may be circled in each category of care, only the one with the highest point value is added into the total. At the end of the 24-hour period, the patient's classification level (acuity level) is determined by referral to the total point range in the upper left-hand corner of the Nursing Care Record. The points and acuity level are recorded on the data processing ticket at the top of the form. At the conclusion of the evening shift the data processing ticket is removed, sent to the staffing office for staffing calculations, and then forwarded to the data processing department for entry into the patient's bill (Exhibit 2).

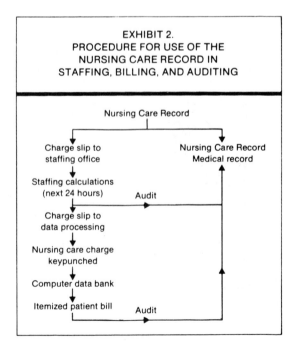

**EXHIBIT 2.
PROCEDURE FOR USE OF THE
NURSING CARE RECORD IN
STAFFING, BILLING, AND AUDITING**

Nursing Care Record

Charge slip to staffing office

Nursing Care Record
Medical record

Staffing calculations (next 24 hours)   Audit

Charge slip to data processing

Nursing care charge keypunched

Computer data bank

Itemized patient bill   Audit

This system of patient classification and reporting has several advantages:

- Key beliefs of the department are included, such as the role of the nurse in educating patients and their families.
- The Nursing Care Record is the official charging document, which combines classification with charting and eliminates a clerical step.
- The Nursing Care Record is designed to make the use of numbers easy; the point system transforms complex qualitative data into simpler quantitative data.
- A single form is used to document nursing care, assess staffing needs, and compute patient's bills.

Staffing

A scheduling matrix, the product of several activity studies, is used to compute staffing needs (Exhibit 3). The matrix defines the number of staff required for X number of patients of Y acuity level. For example, 3.50 FTEs are needed to provide care to 10 class 3 patients in a 24-hour period. Included in the computation for each 24-hour period is a constant factor to account for time spent on fixed and miscellaneous tasks such as shift report, stocking supplies, and attending conferences. St. Luke's has

EXHIBIT 3.
ST. LUKE'S HOSPITAL
SCHEDULING MATRIX FOR TEAM NURSING ON THREE HOSPITAL FLOORS.

Full-Time Equivalents (FTEs) increase with patient number (complete matrix not shown)

Acuity Classification Level

Number of Patients	1 FTE	2 FTE	3 FTE	4 FTE	5 FTE
1	0.23	0.28	0.35	0.47	0.67
2	0.46	0.56	0.70	0.94	1.34
3	0.69	0.84	1.05	1.41	2.01
4	0.92	1.12	1.40	1.88	2.68
5	1.15	1.40	1.75	2.35	3.35
6	1.38	1.68	2.10	2.82	4.02
7	1.61	1.96	2.45	3.29	4.69
8	1.84	2.24	2.80	3.76	5.36
9	2.07	2.52	3.15	4.23	6.03
10	2.30	2.80	3.50	4.70	6.70
11	2.53	3.08	3.85	5.17	7.37
12	2.76	3.36	4.20	5.64	8.04
13	2.99	3.64	4.55	6.11	8.71
14	3.22	3.92	4.90	6.58	9.38
15	3.45	4.20	5.25	7.05	10.05

Note: Matrix shows total care required per patient per day in FTEs for RNs and LPNs (excludes head nurses). Constant FTEs required per day = 0.52.

Daily FTEs required per unit = 0.52 + 0.23 × No. of Level 1 patients + 0.28 × No. of Level 2 patients, and so forth.

EXHIBIT 4.
RELATIVE VALUE UNITS (RVUs) FOR PATIENT ACUITY LEVELS IN THREE AREAS AT ST. LUKE'S HOSPITAL

Acuity Level	Medical/Surgical Unit	Adult Psychiatry Unit
1	1.00	1.00
2	1.25	1.23
3	1.61	1.53
4	2.14	2.00
5	3.04	2.40
	Acute Care Unit	
6	1.00	
7	2.00	

used a fixed constant that is added to the total computation (as noted in Exhibit 3), but as nursing units are converted to all-RN staffing, a different constant factor is built into computations for each acuity level.

Staffing for the medical/surgical and behavioral health (psychiatric) units is computed at 11 P.M. from the evening classification (acuity) levels (recorded on the Nursing Care Record) to project staffing needs for hours starting at 7:00 A.M. If a net change of four or more patients has occurred, calculation is also done at 11:00 A.M. to ensure correct staffing for the evening shift. Owing to changing needs in the acute care units staffing for the following shift is computed 4 hours after the beginning of each shift.

The scheduling matrix reflects the relative values of seven patient acuity levels (Exhibit 4). *Relative-value units* (RVUs) are used to equate procedures or processes that do not require equal amounts of supplies, equipment, and personnel. Relative-value units are established by studying the composition of the procedure or acuity level (time, supplies, and personnel), weighing the various factors according to a preestablished criterion, and computing the relative value of each procedure. The RVUs in Exhibit 4 express the variable amounts of time required to care for patients at different acuity levels. For example, it can be seen that level-1 patients can be cared for in the amount of time it takes to care for one level-5 patient. The RVUs were computed from activity study data and are used in calculating nursing charges for patients at each acuity level.

Charges

The RVUs, daily patient distribution by acuity level, current costs, and patient-day projections were used to establish charges (Exhibit 5). The nursing care charges are summarized on the patient's bill by acuity level, for example, level 2: Medical/Surgical; five days @ $74 = $370. Thus, nursing care is a separate and identifiable charge.

Alternative methods

Other nursing services lend themselves to variable billing. At South Miami Hospital in Miami, Florida, variable charges were created in the emergency, obstetrics, acute hemodialysis, preoperative, and endoscopic departments. Charges at this hospital are based on the costs of performing specific services rather than on a patient-classification system. The method used is to cost one of the following:

- Broadly defined levels of care that are time-based
- Levels of care provided by the hour and half hour
- Specific procedures plus additional time increments per procedure
- Services in addition to those covered by the room rate.

The costing procedure selected depends on the variety and frequency of services rendered, the ease with which a category or level of care can be defined, the availability of the data needed to establish levels and costs, the community's charging practices, and the ease with which the costing procedure can be interpreted and used. The most functional costing procedure is chosen for each situation. In the emergency department, three broadly defined levels of care were established for charging purposes, and a fourth level, with no charge, was defined for wound checks, which had been formerly provided as part of the original visit fee (Exhibit 6). Staffing time and charges for a return visit for purposes of a wound check are incorporated in the level-2 rate. Charges for the three billable levels of care are based on direct and indirect staffing time, as the cost of supplies is negligible; charges for material supplies are itemized on the patient's bill. In the labor room, two levels of care were established based on frequency of observation (intermittent versus constant). For costing purposes, each observation is defined as lasting 5 minutes. Level-1 observation (intermittent) occurs every 30 minutes, and level-2 observation (constant) occurs every 10 minutes. In practice, though, the intermittent contacts are more frequent, and constant observation requires continual attendance to the extent possible. (The charge for the patient's entire stay in the labor room is $45 for level-1 care, $82 for level-2 care.)

The delivery room charge is a fixed fee based on costs determined from a cost study of 25 patients. Due to the local community fee standard, the charge was reduced to $140 to remain competitive. The nursery charge for intensive care provided for infants who are awaiting transport to a level-2 or 3 facility is $100, and the observation charge for infants requiring close observation without monitoring is $40. These charges are in addition to the daily nursery rate and reflect additional nursing time required. The obstetric department does not use a classification system per se for computing staffing time or charges.

The hemodialysis department has two levels of care that are staffing-dependent. In level-1 care, the staff/patient ratio is one nurse to two patients; in level-2 care, it is one nurse to one patient. The supply costs are the same for both levels and are figured into the charges for the first hour. Charges for additional hours include staff time only (Exhibit 7).

In the preoperative suite, in which patients are prepped and medicated for surgery, four levels of variable charges are defined, with the primary cost being staff time (direct time for prepping and medication, indirect time for chart review, transport, and so forth). *Preoperative service* is for patient processing that includes administration of medications but not shaving for scrub prepping. Preoperative service and level 1 prepping fall into the same average time range; thus costs and charges are the same for each, although the two functions are charged separately for statistical purposes. Levels 2 and 3 involve preparation and medication that take different average times to complete (Exhibit 8).

In the endoscopy department, individual procedures are costed with regard to fixed supplies and staff time. All supply costs are incorporated into charges for the base time increment; charges for additional half hours reflect staff time only. Because of the limited number of procedures performed in this department, costing of individual

---

EXHIBIT 5.
NURSING, ROOM, AND FOOD CHARGES AT
ST. LUKE'S HOSPITAL, FISCAL YEAR 1980-1981

Nursing

Acuity Level	Medical/Surgical Unit	Adult Psychiatry Unit
1	$ 59	$ 54
2	74	67
3	95	83
4	127	109
5	180	130
Acute Care Unit (ICU/CCU)		
6	$254	
7	507	

Room

Room Type	Medical/Surgical Unit	Adult Psychiatry Unit
Semiprivate	$ 36	$ 43
Private	72	86
Acute care	72	

Food

Meal		
Breakfast	$ 4.75	$ 4.75
Lunch	6.50	6.50
Dinner	9.75	9.75
Other Nourishment	.00	.50
Food Total	$21.00	$21.50

EXHIBIT 6.
SOUTH MIAMI HOSPITAL
EMERGENCY DEPARTMENT CHARGES FOR
NURSING SERVICES AND ROOM,
FISCAL YEAR 1980-1981

Care Classification Level	Charge
Wound check	$ 0
1	8
2	35
3	80

procedures is a functional approach.

Both St. Luke's and South Miami Hospitals employ variable billing procedures for nursing services in the operating room. Each hospital has defined five levels of nursing services, with cardiac surgery composing the fifth level. Each level includes a number of procedures that require similar staffing, room time, and basic supplies. All procedures are assigned to the most representative level so that like procedures have the same charges (for example, all hysterectomies are included in the same level). Both the time increments and methodology for computing charges for each level vary with the hospital. At St. Luke's, a fixed half-hour charge based on staffing and supply costs is used; at South Miami, costs of staffing and all fixed supplies are added to charges for the first hour and staff time is the cost base for additional half-hour increments. Each system is a product of its hospital's financial system. Exhibit 9 lists operating room rates at each hospital. At St. Luke's, data generated by the variable billing system has been used to justify the addition of staff and facilities.

Auditing

Auditing is as important to the success of variable billing as any component. Efficient auditing, which is crucial to the variable billing system and to the financial outcome, must address (1) accuracy of documentation, (2) case volume/classification-level distribution, (3) staffing, (4) quality of care, and (5) patient billing.

The audit to monitor accuracy of documentation (e.g., Nursing Care Record) should verify:

• Accurate selection of items in each category
• That supporting documentation has been provided when required
• Correct addition of acuity points and level selection
• That the form is technically complete (date, signatures, and so forth).

This complex audit is best performed if each of the preceding points is verified separately.

Monitoring of case volume/classification-level distribution is vital, as revenue is dependent on serving a mix of patients at various acuity levels as well as volume. Check points should be established to alert appropriate personnel when significant shifts in the distribution pattern have occured. It is important that accountability for ongoing review of these data be established.

The audit of staff scheduling (actual versus required) is ongoing. These data need to be shared with the nurses to further their understanding of the relation of patient volume and classification to staffing problems. This audit can also document the need for recruiting efforts if it can be shown that staff numbers routinely fall below those required.

Quality care is monitored by use of outcome and process audits designed by the Joint Commission on Accreditation of Hospitals (JACH). Patient billing is audited by random selection of bills for verification with medical records. Nursing staffs that are involved with this audit can readily see the need for accurate charting.

Education

Groups who need to learn about the variable billing concept include the board of trustees, administration, the financial department, medical staff, third-party payers, patients, and nursing staff. The nursing administrator should provide presentations adapted to the interests and needs of each group on a frequent, regular basis. Nurses,

EXHIBIT 7.
SOUTH MIAMI HOSPITAL
HEMODIALYSIS PROCEDURE CHARGES,
FISCAL YEAR 1980-1981

Care Classification Level	First Hour	Each Additional Hour
1	$270	$15
2	295	30

EXHIBIT 8.
SOUTH MIAMI HOSPITAL
PREOPERATIVE SUITE CHARGES FOR
NURSING SERVICES, FISCAL YEAR 1980-1981

Care Classification Level	Charge
Service	$17
1	17
2	25
3	41

EXHIBIT 9.
OPERATING ROOM RATES AT ST. LUKE'S AND
SOUTH MIAMI HOSPITALS,
FISCAL YEAR 1980-1981

Level	St. Luke's Each Half Hour	South Miami First Hour	South Miami Each Additional Half Hour
1	$ 66.25	$117.00	$ 32
2	91.25	265.00	78
3	111.25	285.00	78
4	142.50	301.00	78
5	226.25	362.00	117

in particular, need assistance with defining professional practices, identifying non-visable tasks and processes, determining "fees for service," and dealing with such ethical issues as occur if actual staffing is below that required.

Summary

The advantages of variable billing for nursing care that

- It identifies revenue nursing cost centers.
- It facilitates systematic control of revenue and ex-

penses, improving budget planning and management.

- It generates a tremendous amount of data that can be used in administrative planning and decision making.
- It is more equitable than past billing practices for the patient, the third-party payer, and the hospital, making it a public relations asset.

The disadvantages of variable billing are that

- Charges at one hospital are not easily compared with those at another.
- The mix of patients at varying classification levels has a significant effect on revenue, thus increasing the possibility of lower revenue.
- More accountability and in some cases more work is required of nursing administrators.

In this article, the practical application of variable billing in acute care settings has been discussed. It is hoped that the information provided here will stimulate nursing administrators to assess the feasibility of implementing variable billing for nursing services as a fiscal practice in their own institutions.

Suggested reading

James Cisarek, Nancy Higgerson, and Ann Van Slyck, "Charging for Nursing Services," (Phoenix: St. Luke's Hospital, Medical Center, 1978.) Available from St. Luke's Hospital Medical Center, 525 N. 18th St., Phoenix, Arizona 85006.

CHAPTER 22

■ Sallie M. Olsen, RN, PhD

The Challenge of Prospective Pricing: Work Smarter

Nursing administrators are faced with the challenge of containing costs under Medicare's prospectively set reimbursement limits. The author suggests that nurses "work smarter" by utilizing the unique aspects of prospective pricing in a program that will maintain professionalism while improving "bottom line" outcomes. A pro-active strategy for administrators within nursing departments, on a hospital-wide basis, and in the entire health care delivery system is described. The author shows how determining nursing costs and revenues by diagnosis can be a way to validate both the cost-effectiveness of an RN staff and a high professional standard of practice. She outlines four elements of a trustworthy, effective change process.

Prospective pricing demands maximum productivity. The federal government estimates its savings on hospital care for Medicare patients will be $3.5 billion in the next 3 years as a result of paying a price prospectively set for the treatment of given diagnosis.[1] Although the greatest savings are expected to be achieved by the reduction of unnecessary stays and the decreased use of ancillary services, the Medicare reimbursement limits will encourage hospitals to weigh each service's contribution to the patients' well-being. Nursing departments will doubtless be asked to cut costs in order to help with the new financial constraints.

Even though prospective pricing is sponsored by the largest single purchaser of health care—the federal government—hospitals with a low Medicare patient population may feel little effect initially. However, because other health insurers will doubtless adopt prospective pricing by Diagnosis Related Groups (DRGs), the Medicare program marks the beginning of a new era in the way health care will be financed and delivered. Making changes now in anticipation of the Medicare constraints can make an important difference in being able to provide cost-effective professional care, both now and in the future.

At first glance, prospective pricing looks like any other "budget tightening" program to which a practical solution is to work harder, doing more work for the same cost or doing the same work at a lower cost. In any hospital, as in any industry or business, some "fat" can be eliminated by fine tuning and emphasizing general productivity measures, i.e., making every minute of work count. Any obvious waste must be trimmed as a first step. In that sense, we will all need to work harder.

Even if it were possible to increase the workload with no cost increase, we would not necessarily cut those costs that Medicare will no longer pay. Prospective pricing defines productivity in a slightly new way: costs of treating a given diagnosis successfully enough so the patient can be discharged. (Productivity under retroactively determined reimbursement rates was the cost of services rendered compared with a standard cost of those services, no matter how effective the service was for the patient.) Therefore, we need to understand nursing productivity in terms of DRGs and to plan strategies that will specifically address the costs and reimbursements from the perspective. While we may have to work harder, we will be more effective if we also work smarter.

Sallie M. Olsen, RN, PhD, is a nursing consultant and a Senior Associate with McManis Associates, a research and management consulting firm in San Francisco, California.

Working Smarter on Three Levels

Because the imperative to reduce health care costs is so clear, all parts of the delivery system will need to develop ways of providing effective care at less cost. Nurse administrators must not only represent nursing's needs but also help develop new cooperative efforts within the health care delivery system that will benefit both the patients and the providers. "Proactive" nursing administrators will be working on three different levels in considering costs and reimbursements under Medicare: (1) the entire health care delivery system, (2) the hospital, and (3) nursing service.

The System-Wide Change Process

Because all parts of the health care delivery system are interconnected, changes in one part affect the rest of the system. Any hospital that wants to position itself specifically to respond to the Medicare constraints should have a strategy team with representatives from all parts of the system—hospital administrators, doctors, nurses, and trustees. This team can assess a variety of competitive options. Such options may include entering new markets with existing programs (*e.g.*, selling a "heart health" program to local businesses) or developing new programs.[2] Nursing can play an important part in helping create and staff new services.

The competitive pressure of prospective pricing is undoubtedly greater on doctors than on any other part of the health care delivery system.[3] Some of the impact on the doctors can ultimately affect nursing. Pressure to shorten hospital stays and serve a greater patient volume may change the kind of nursing service some doctors will need and expect. For example, some doctors will want highly skilled nurses to teach patients self-care, thus hastening discharge. Other doctors may be threatened by nurses who provide out-patient services similar to their own but at a lower cost.

The Hospital-Wide Change Process

Proper adaptation to the new reimbursement system virtually requires the presence of a DRG coordinator.[4] In small- to medium-sized hospitals, the DRG coordinators are often based in the medical records department to coordinate information and guidelines about forms and documentation. In larger hospitals, the DRG coordinator, as an administrator reporting directly to the chief operating officer, will consider all matters related to DRGs both in the hospital and system wide. In the small- to medium-sized hospitals, an administrator will be in charge of planning and implementing the necessary changes that the DRG coordinator would handle in larger hospitals.

The services directly involved with planning and implementing DRGs on a hospital-wide basis are finance, medical records, patient accounts, data processing, utilization review, quality assurance, public relations, admitting, nursing, ancillary services, social service and medical services.[4] The hospital-wide change program will focus mainly on an accurate and timely flow of information. In this regard, nursing will have to make sure that the daily census is reviewed for accuracy and that upon patient discharge, charts are quickly dispatched to medical records. Nurses will have little other DRG paperwork.

It is crucial that nursing not become involved with DRG implementation in a way that will compromise its own position or create problems. For example, with DRGs, doctors must complete charts in a timely manner in order to assure prompt and correct reimbursements. In their recent book on DRGs, Grimaldi and Micheietti repeatedly suggest that nurses remind doctors to close charts.[4] Such urgings will only strain the relationship between the nursing and medical staff. A much better method would be a system of rewarding chart completion rather than burdening nurses with the task of policing doctors.

In close and daily contact with patients, nurses will inevitably be giving information about the Medicare program. Nurses can be instrumental in helping patients understand the need to be preparing for the discharge date established by an initial DRG assignment. Teaching the patient about such constraints and mobilizing all possible resources can make an important difference in the effectiveness of the entire treatment process.

Changes Within Nursing

Prospective pricing calls for only minor changes in documentation. However, the moment a hospital begins to operate under prospective pricing, it should advance a corporate culture emphasizing cost containment with high professional standards. Developing that culture can involve a subtle but far-reaching change process.

If nursing administrators choose to see it as such, prospective pricing can be an opportunity for nursing to increase its accountability, its professionalism, and its control over its practice. Most nursing administrators and nurses have been working toward these goals and need only make some adaptations in order to continue under Medicare constraints.

Determining Nursing Costs and Revenues by Diagnosis

Prospective pricing demands that nurses quantify their work and demonstrate its results. Stated another way, nurses must be able to show what costs they incur and how effective their work is in treating a given diagnosis. This examination of nursing practice by DRGs offers an important opportunity for a nursing staff to determine just what it has to "sell" that is unique and valuable—and whether it generates more revenue than it consumes.

Determining the cost of providing nursing care for each diagnosis is the way to compare productivity within the hospital. It will be obvious, for example, how much was made or lost on hysterectomies as compared with Cesarian sections. By comparing the nursing costs for a given diagnosis treated by the same doctor using similar ancillary services for each patient, the financial effects of nursing care *per se* will be evident. Specific procedures or treatments can then be examined in terms of cost-effectiveness and patient outcome.

In the likely event that several nursing units treat the same DRG, it is also possible to compare costs and results produced by different nursing staffs. Tracking costs by diagnosis provides the opportunity to delineate what nursing does, the result it produces in patients of a given diagnosis, and what it costs to provide that care. By separating nursing costs from basic room rates and hospital expenditures, nursing can compare its cost with the Medicare reimbursement allotment. This is the way to demonstrate what revenue or losses nursing is producing for the hospital.

There are a number of ways to determine nursing costs. Several methods have been developed in large-scale, well-published studies.[4-6] Some hospitals will want to cost out nursing care in these detailed ways. An alternative system, which has the advantage of simplicity, is to code daily nursing intensity for each patient and track the result by diagnosis (Personal Communication, Lou Freund, DRG Systems Associates, Sunnyvale, CA).

All JCAH-accredited hospitals already have a nursing acuity system for determining staffing needs. This system can be used to assess costs by DRGs. A daily acuity for each patient recorded for the entire hospital stay can be converted to the amount of nursing time spent in delivering and documenting direct patient care. Using the hospital's staffing allocation factor, acuity is converted into the number of nursing hours. In one hospital, an acuity level of 1.5 means a med/surg patient will receive 1.5 hours of direct care on the day shift, 1.5 hours on the evening shift, and 45 minutes on the night shift.

The nursing cost includes the salaries and benefits for all the staff on each unit plus a factor for indirect costs. Indirect costs include administrative time, orientation, and education as well as time to plan and coordinate care. Total cost is divided by the total number of patient care hours delivered to get a cost per hour.

Because the Medicare reimbursement rate is based on a group of hospitals in the same geographic area and on costs incurred in a base-rate year, profit or loss will also be a comparison with previous years and other nearby hospitals.

Establishing Cost-Effectiveness of RN Staffing

Pro-active nursing administrators recognize DRGs as a vehicle to demonstrate that a professional standard of practice produces quantifiable results, results with more favorable impact on profits than those produced by LVNs and aides. Such administrators make the costing out of nursing care on a diagnosis basis an opportunity to evaluate staffing patterns and skill mix of the staff. They also see it as a way to increase their accountability and the control over the quality of their care.

"Re-active" administrators, by contrast, see prospective pricing as a demand for cost reduction to which the only possible response is decreasing the number and skill level of the staff. Such a response, particularly if it is one reached without consulting the staff members, can be tremendously damaging to morale. When staffing and skill mix are consistently set at such a level that staff cannot deliver acceptable patient care, it is questionable that there will actually be a cost savings, particularly if staff begin to perform inefficiently or to call in sick frequently as an indication of flagging morale.

Although there is some pressure from non-nursing health care personnel to cut costs by staffing with LVNs and aides, most nurse administrators recognize the cost effectiveness of RN staff. Halloran[7] and Curtin[6] both show that staffing with more RNs can actually cut costs because the time needed per patient is decreased. Halloran's study[8] at Hines VA Hospital showed that an RN staff using nursing diagnoses and assigned by the case method (rather than by tasks) produced better care for lower cost than a staff that included LVNs and aides. If it can also be shown that having RNs deliver care decreases the length of stay, even greater cost savings can be attributed to an all-RN staff.

Other issues must be considered. One administrator pointed out that if she went to an all-RN staff, the union representing them could close down the hospital when it was time to negotiate a contract. She needed to keep a significant number of LVNs (represented by a different union) on the staff in order to keep a balance of power. The availability of skilled nursing personnel is another obvious consideration in determining the most desirable skill mix.

The Need for Control Over Nursing Practice

Although many factors contribute to productivity, a major one is job satisfaction. It stands to reason that an employee who feels satisfied with his or her job will be more productive than one who feels dissatisfied. The single most important factor in nursing job satisfaction is the perception of having control over one's own practice. This means that nurses decide what care is needed and have enough staff to carry out these care plans. How often we have heard nurses with high professional standards complain about not being able to provide adequate nursing care! How very painful it is to see good nurses "burn out" from trying to do more than it is possible for them to do.

There are four factors that can shape the process so that nurses maintain and increase their control over their work while responding to the need for cost containment: (1) information, (2) involvement, (3) building on strengths, and (4) minimizing stress.

Informing the Nursing Staff

A well-informed staff is part of a corporate culture valuing mutual respect and involvement. Nursing staff must understand the history and the rationale of the prospective pricing system. The nurses also need to know what specific information the medical records department will be using to code the correct and most lucrative DRG so they can highlight it in their nursing records. Any changes in charting procedures or information processing must be clearly understood in order to establish and maintain new behaviors.

Since information about prospective pricing has been available in professional publications and in the popular press, it is probable that staff will have preconceived ideas and some misconceptions about "what horrible things will happen to me under prospective pricing." A common worry of many nurses is that prospective pricing may necessitate staff cutbacks or layoffs. There are also legitimate concerns about the wage increase ceilings Medicare accepts despite the outcome of labor negotiations.

Since there are many unknowns about the ultimate impact of prospective pricing, even an aggressive program for keeping staff informed about changes can still leave "holes." If communication between staff and administration is not open and active, nurses can become mistrustful, particularly when they get incorrect or late information about changes that affect their personal financial lives. A sure way to cut productivity is for staff to mistrust their administrator or to fear that the decisions being made about cutbacks will be slow in reaching them.

Involvement of Nursing Staff

Getting the staff members on a unit to examine their productivity and consider methods of improving it is a good way to cut costs. No one knows better how to be more efficient and effective in a job than the person who performs it repeatedly! Productivity improvement groups, or quality circles, are an excellent way to get staff members actively involved in increasing productivity.[9] Quality circles examine problems with a demonstrable cost factor. The task of the quality circle is to research the problem and come up with a way to save money.

Although each circle chooses the problems it will work on, several issues could be appropriate: tailoring staffing patterns to the unit, determining the most cost-effective skill mix, or making nursing care plans more effective. Administration must recognize and implement the proposals for change that come from the circles' research in order to realize the cost savings and to keep staff involved in the process.

Working to reduce the treatment costs of any one diagnosis can involve several hospital departments. Internal reorganization, at least on a temporary basis, will be in order so all personnel involved in the care can problem solve together. Such *ad hoc* groups addressing productivity will need broad-based administrative support to implement their solutions.

Building on Strengths

The best change process is one that utilizes the strengths of the existing situation and makes the fewest adaptations. Every nursing staff has its strengths—in clinical expertise, involvement, or management skills. Administrative acknowledgment and reinforcement of the strengths motivate staff to make changes and try new ideas. Pro-active administrators will utilize the strengths in all three systems (entire health care delivery system, the hospital, and nursing service) to begin and develop changes. An orthopedic unit that has good working relationships with occupational therapy and physical therapy and one involved doctor can be a role model for developing cost-saving measures around "total hip" patients.

The principle of building on strengths applies as well to the nonhuman aspects of the system. Instead of discarding a currently used acuity system because it has some drawbacks and has to be adapted to DRGs anyway, it may be wiser to modify something that is familiar to the staff.

Minimizing Stress on Nursing Staff

Clarifying expectations and providing broad-ranging inservice education and stress reduction classes minimize the negative effects of change. We have already discussed the need for informing the staff. When staff know the specific behavior changes needed and when they have a feeling for the change process itself, they are more likely to make a good and lasting adjustment.

If the movement into prospective pricing means that nursing supervisors increase their involvement in the business and financial aspects of patient care, they may need some educational support. In addition, the supervisors may need help in management skills to help bring out the best in their staff during the change process.

Some inservice education may be needed to teach or remind staff about specific clinical matters. For example, if complete blood tests are no longer going to be done for certain DRGs, staff may need to review the critical signs that indicate when and if an exception should be made. It is also possible that productivity teams will be developing new procedures or protocols that will need to be taught throughout the hospital.

Stress reduction classes that teach how to manage on an unpredictable or diminished income can be useful to staff whose positions are vulnerable to layoffs or cutbacks. Staff who are working when others have been laid off may have guilt feelings that can be addressed in group meetings. Classes to decrease physical and emotional stress that results from change or from increased work can provide an important support to staff.

■ Conclusions

The challenge of prospective pricing will not be met in a single stroke or with a single program, but rather by an evolving process that fosters trust and communication and builds on existing strengths. Understanding the cost and revenues that nursing produces for each diagnosis can lead to increased control over practice and recognition of the benefits of RN staff. Cost containment under Medicare's prospective pricing may well prove to be the ultimate challenge for nursing. By working smarter we can make it the ultimate opportunity to solidify our professionalism.

■ References

1. Grimaldi P. Public Law 97-248. The implication of prospective payment schedules. Nursing Management Feb 1983: 25-7.
2. Nelle S. Market strategy. Hospital Forum. Nov/Dec 1983: 42-5.
3. Sorenson L. Hospitals and doctors compete for patients with rising bitterness. Wall Street Journal. July 19, 1983, 1.
4. Grimaldi P, Micheletti J. Diagnosis Related Groups: a practioners guide. Chicago: Pluribus Press, 1983:3,155,159-61, 166.
5. Horn S, Sharkey P, Bertran D. Measuring severity of illness: homogeneous case mix groups. Medical Care 1983;21(1):14-22.
6. Curtin L. Determining costs of nursing services per DRG. Nursing Management 1983;14(4):16-20.
7. Halloran E. RN staffing: more care—less cost. Nursing Management 1983;14(9):18-20.
8. Halloran E. Staffing assignment: by task or by patient. Nursing Management 1982;13(2):20-6.
9. Thompson P. Quality circles: how to make them work in America. New York: Harper and Row, 1981.

■ Bibliography

Caternnicchio R. A debate: RIMs and the cost of nursing care. Nursing Management 1983;14(5):36-9.
Grimaldi P. DRGs and nursing administration. Nursing Management 1982;13(1):30-4.
Wood C. Relate hospital charges to use of service. Harvard Business Review 1982;Mar/Apr:123-60.

CHAPTER 23

■ Hollie Vanderzee, RN, MSN, and George Glusko, BS

DRGs, Variable Pricing, and Budgeting for Nursing Services

This article focuses on the cost impact of patient acuity on DRGs. The traditional method of routine charges for nursing services is compared with the development of a variable charge structure based on patient classification. Examples of each method are given. The authors also analyze a charge structure based upon patient care requirements and apply the budgeting process to the cost determination of nursing services.

A variable billing system based on patient classification meets three objectives. It establishes a more equitable charge for nursing services provided to the client; nurse managers have more responsibility and accountability in the management of unit finances; and the facility is better able to monitor the cost of each Diagnosis Related Group (DRG).

With the advent of reimbursement by DRG, accurate data are required to enable managers to assess the financial impact each DRG has upon the hospital. Patient classification provides a method for comparing the hospital's actual cost per DRG to its prospective rate. This article compares the traditional method using routine charges for nursing services to a variable charge structure based upon patient classification. Examples of each method are given.

A major portion of the hospital budget, nursing salaries historically have been viewed as a costly expenditure. Through the budgeting process, using a variable charging system, expenses are offset by the

production of revenue. Salary and supply cost can be equitably distributed based on patient utilization.

■ Financial Background

Charge structures vary from hospital to hospital. Before the Tax Equity and Fiscal Responsibility Act of 1982, the majority of hospitals concentrated on maximizing revenues through ancillary services versus the daily accommodation charge. The hospital's daily accommodation charge, or routine care charge, is usually based on a fixed rate per department. Private versus semi-private rate is included in the charge. However, the charge structure does not take into consideration those patients requiring a higher intensity of nursing care, the use of more nonchargeable supplies, or the need for additional services. Depending on the hospital's cost-finding techniques, the daily accommodation charge represents approximately 50% of the patient's cost per day. The accommodation is highly labor-intensive.

■ DRG Cost Accounting

The move to DRG reimbursement was based on the premise that like diagnoses would generate like costs. Traditional cost-finding techniques do not generate an accurate cost per DRG. Cost per DRG

Hollie Vanderzee, RN, MSN, is a private consultant in nursing administration and former Vice-President of Nursing at Glens Falls Hospital, a 440-bed facility in Glens Falls, New York.

George Glusko, BS, is Vice-President of Finance at Polyclinic Medical Center in Harrisburg, Pennsylvania.

calculations are based on accumulated departmental charges by DRG, multiplied by the departmental cost/charge ratio.

Ancillary departments, due to generation of charges based on services rendered or supplies issued, provide an approximate calculation of patient use, but may be distorted due to pricing strategies. Since routine care is typically based on average charge per accommodation, the cost of providing care to higher levels of acuity is never ascertained in the cost-finding techniques.

The following example demonstrates the inaccuracy of traditional cost-finding techniques. Community Hospital wants to determine its cost for the DRG for Laryngectomy. During the year the hospital performed 31 procedures. Table 1 represents a breakdown of the departmental charges accumulated for the 31 procedures using the traditional structure, with an accommodation charge of $100/day.

To convert these charges into cost, the hospital would use statistical cost-finding techniques to allocate direct and indirect costs to the revenue-producing department. Indirect costs include depreciation, interest, heat, light, power, insurance, and administrative expenses. Direct costs are salaries and nonchargeable supplies and expenses. The direct and indirect costs of a given department are added together and divided by the total charges to determine the cost/charge ratio.

With DRG reimbursement, the traditional method of basing charges on accommodations may produce inaccuracies and negatively influence management decisions regarding a particular DRG. Table 2 demonstrates the DRG cost for Community Hospital.

After the cost per DRG is computed, it is compared with the prospective rates paid by Medicare. In the Community Hospital example, the charge was based on accommodation charge versus a charge for services rendered.

Table 1. Departmental Charges for 31 Laryngectomies Using the Traditional Routine Services Charge Structure

Department	Charge ($)
Operating room	9000
Recovery room	3000
Cardiology	2000
Physical therapy	1000
Pharmacy	7000
Medical supplies	5000
Room and board	25,000
Total charges	52,000
Number of DRG cases	31
Total patient days	250
Average length of stay	8.1
Average charge per case	1677

Table 2. Departmental Charges for 31 Laryngectomies Comparing the Traditional Routine Services Charge Structure with the DRG Cost

Department	Charge ($)	Ratio	DRG ($)
Operating room	9000	0.75	6750
Recovery room	3000	0.65	1950
Cardiology	2000	0.70	1400
Physical therapy	1000	0.55	550
Pharmacy	7000	0.50	3500
Medical supplies	5000	0.80	4000
Room and board	25,000	1.10	27,500
Total	52,000		45,650
Total cases	31		31
Average charge/case	1677	0.89	1473

Improving Cost-Finding Techniques

More accurate cost accounting is accomplished through the development of a variable charge structure for nursing services based on patient acuity and nursing administration's assessment of labor and nonchargeable supply costs per acuity level. This charge replaces the accommodation charge. Required gross departmental charges are generated using historical data based on average patient acuity levels per nursing unit.

Table 3 reviews the unit's historical patient days by acuity level with required patient revenues at breakeven to offset the unit's direct and indirect costs. In this methodology, indirect costs are items such as interest, depreciation, heat, light, power, insurance, and administrative expenses. Direct costs are comprised of salaries and nonchargeable supplies and expenses.

To develop a cost to charge ratio, the direct and indirect costs are added together and divided by the total charges. This represents an alternative to the $100 per patient day charge.

Determining Salary Cost Per Classification Level

Since the restructured daily charge per classification level has been based upon the nurse administrator's assessment of labor and supply costs, and labor represents the major portion of the cost, the methodology for establishing the staffing cost per classification level must be sound. Many patient classifica-

Table 3. Restructured Nursing Unit Revenue						
Classification	Percent per Category	Patient Days		Daily Charge ($)		Gross Revenue ($)
Level 4	20	2400	×	170	=	$408,000
Level 3	30	3600	×	124	=	446,400
Level 2	35	4200	×	70	=	294,000
Level 1	15	1800	×	30	=	54,000
		12,000				1,202,400

tion and staffing systems have established the number of nursing hours required per patient per shift at each level of acuity. To determine the cost of nursing services the nurse administrator must take this process one step further and establish the mix of personnel required at each level.

A variety of factors is considered in determining mix and forecasting labor requirements per level. The classification system considers items such as admission and discharge patterns, changes in occupancy, number of transfers, changes in acuity, and routine daily activities. Additional factors to be included in the planning portion of the budgeting process are: the short- and long-term goals of the nursing department; new policies and procedures impacting staffing; the addition of new services; changes in role expectations; or the nursing model being used.

Nursing care is given in a continually changing environment. Therefore, the nursing administrator must be alert to those changes that impact patient care, staffing, and/or supply needs. Since each nursing unit is a revenue-producing department in the variable charge structure, the nurse manager of the unit should be an integral part of the planning and decision-making process. As the manager closest to patient care and unit activities, the head nurse plays an important role in determining need and monitoring expense.

Based on historical acuity data and forecasted projections for the coming year, the nurse administrator determines the number of patient days expected in each classification level and the number of nursing hours per patient per day required by each level. In Table 4, the nursing hours per patient per day have been identified and multiplied by the patient days for each acuity level. This calculation determines the hours per year per classification level.

Determination of staff mix per level of acuity is the next step in the cost-finding process. A variety of factors beyond the scope of this article influences the nurse administrator's decisions concerning mix. Table 5 provides one example of staff mix per level of acuity. The percentage of registered nurses, practical nurses, and nurse aides have been multiplied by the total nursing hours required per year for each level. The result is the required hours per year for registered nurses, practical nurses, and nurse aides in each level.

The total number of productive hours per year is found by adding Levels 1 to 4 together for each category of employee. This is the basis for determining the direct labor cost in the variable charge structure. Productive costs are found by multiplying the total hours required in each category by the average hourly wage for that group of employees.

The data in Table 5 are also used to determine the number of FTE required for each category of personnel. One FTE is equal to 2080 hours. Using 32,040 hours, the total number of registered nurse hours

Table 4. Patient Days per Acuity Level					
Classification	Percent per Category	Nursing Hours per Patient Day	Patient Days	Hours per Year	Percent of Hours
Level 4	20	8	2400	19,200	31
Level 3	30	6	3600	21,600	35
Level 2	35	4	4200	16,800	28
Level 1	15	2	1800	3600	6
	100		12,000	61,200	100

		Percent per Level			Hours per Level		
Classification	Hours per Year	RN	PN	NA	RN	PN	NA
Level 4	19,200	80	20	—	15,360	3840	—
Level 3	21,600	60	40	—	12,960	8640	—
Level 2	16,800	20	50	30	3360	8400	5040
Level 1	3600	10	40	50	360	1440	1800
	61,200				32,040	22,320	6840

Table 5. Determination of Mix

required, and dividing it by the number of hours for one FTE, results in the need for 15.4 FTE. The same process is used to determine the number of practical nurses and nurse aides. The master staffing plan for the unit is developed from the FTE requirement. The nurse manager assesses patient acuity data and unit activity indicators to assign staff to shift.

Productive hours have been determined by classification level in this article. Prior to completing the budgeting process, nonproductive hours, fringe benefits, nursing administration, and staff development must be calculated. Additional items for inclusion vary from facility to facility, *i.e.*, overtime hours, meeting times for Quality Circles, call pay, educational days, holiday and weekend differential.

Nonchargeable supply costs vary from facility to facility. The number of nonchargeable items charged to a nursing unit should either have a routine charge established, or be part of the acuity system. The same process used for staffing could be applied to supplies to determine the cost per level of acuity. This article has focused upon staffing since labor represents 90 percent of the cost.

Conclusion

Arriving at a variable daily charge for nursing services has been based upon the labor and supply cost per acuity level, as determined by the nurse

administrator and historical patient acuity data. In Table 3, the required budgeted gross patient revenue of $1.2 million was generated by the restructured accommodation charge. The variable charge structure has considered distribution of patient days per acuity level, staffing requirements, and supply needs in the budgeting process. The traditional average charge of $100 per patient per day has been changed to reflect acuity. Additional charge items could be generated for extraordinary cost items such as isolation, special dietary consultation, patient education, etc.

The need to develop a nursing variable charge structure is essential with DRG reimbursement. Due to the nature of DRG groupings, acuity distributions will vary by DRG. Therefore, it becomes important to evaluate the hospital's profitability per DRG. This article offers one approach to the development of a charge structure that can be accepted by both finance and nursing departments. Financial accounting for intensity, using patient classification data, is useful in screening potential DRG outliers, since outliers are based on excessive average length of stay and/or excessive costs incurred. Patients requiring additional nursing care generate excessive costs.

Nurse administrators and financial officers considering this method should remember that there are validity and reliability problems inherent in many patient classification systems. This does not represent an overwhelming obstacle, rather a factor to be considered and evaluated.

UNIT FIVE

CAROL D. SPENGLER

Nurse – Physician Relations

Throughout its history, Nursing has struggled for recognition of the significant contributions it has made to patient care. This struggle has continued in all settings where nurses are found to work regardless of their roles. The significant role that nursing plays in health care has not been well understood by other health care providers, administrators, or the public. Ironically, the group that nurses have worked most closely with, namely physicians, has been the most resistant to understanding, acknowledging, and supporting the contributions made by nurses to produce effective patient care. A common complaint of nurses is that there is a lack of acknowledgment from physician co-workers regarding their clinical knowledge and skills in the provision of patient care. When a patient progresses and does well, it is often the physician alone who is credited with this success. Nurses also report that in many settings they are restricted from fully using the knowledge, skills, and capabilities that they have due to physicians' resistance to change.

Although changes in the nurse–physician relationship appear to be occurring at a remedial pace, they have, however, been evolving in a mostly positive direction. Early in their professional history, nurses cared for patients without knowing what specific medications, ointments, herbs, and so forth the physician had taken from his "little black bag" and administered to the patient. Over time, the physician not only shared this information with the nurse but eventually delegated responsibilities to the nurse. Now, only rarely, does the physician carry out some of these responsibilities. Many enlightened physicians now recognize and acknowledge that nursing and medicine must operate as a partnership if effective patient care is the desired outcome.

In this section, a contemporary view of the nurse–physician relationship is provided. Johnston describes a formula for success for fostering improvement in this relationship. She points out that hospitals, in an attempt to provide a more positive and rewarding work environment for nurses who were in short supply, began to focus on the often troubled nurse–physician relationship. Malpractice issues related to poor nurse–physician communication also served as an important impetus to address this concern. Scarce resources (nurses) and economic constraints also increased the desire of some hospitals to get maximum productivity from their nurses by allowing them to more appropriately use their skills and knowledge. Johnston describes major changes made by one community hospital to enhance the way that nurses and physicians work together in an integrated practice approach. She defines this as a collaborative practice program. The outcome of such a program is improved patient care and greater job satisfaction for nurses.

"Associated Practice" is the model described by Elpern and associates that provides for professional collaboration between the nurse and physician. This group of nurses and physicians point out that planning, patience, and risk taking are essential in establishing a successful associated practice. The authors point out that the "traditional relationship between physicians and nurses in which physicians personally prescribed, supervised, and directed nursing activities is today both unnecessary and unrealistically restrictive." A desire on the part of both physicians and nurses to address patient care needs in a more comprehensive and satisfying way is the driving force that leads to establishing an associated practice.

Major changes in health care financing and competition for the health care market are driving organizational changes in some hospitals that could bring about new areas of conflict between the nurse and physician according to Sheedy. In many hospital settings, the position of vice-president of medical affairs (or medical director) is being added to the hospital management team. Depending on the placement of the vice-president for medical affairs in the organization and the reporting relationship of the vice-president for nursing, this new role could be hazardous to the practice of nursing.

The evolving relationship between nurses and physicians is not yet viewed as "consistently progressive and positive" in nature. In a time of turbulence, great change, and dwindling resources, physicians and nurses are presented with strategy choices that will have an impact on their continued professional viability. If either or both elect a defensive turf-protecting stance, they may miss the opportunity to evaluate the system, join forces, and collaborate to maximize the capabilities of each professional group. The health care system will now demand that hard choices be made. The survival of some health care institutions will depend on the nature of these choices. When complementary practice between nurses and physicians is encouraged and supported, effective patient care and a viable institution will result.

CHAPTER 24

Improving the
Nurse-Physician Relationship

by Phillippa Ferguson Johnston

Health care professionals are calling for more collaboration between physicians and nurses, recognizing the influences of these relationships on patient care and job satisfaction of nursing professionals. This article presents one hospital's successful formula for fostering effective nurse-physician relationships.

Improving the working relationship between physicians and nurses has become one of the top priorities on management's agenda in many hospitals. The need to provide a more rewarding work environment to recruit and retain RNs is one reason hospitals give for seeking better nurse-doctor rapport. Another is the desire to reduce the chances of patient injury and malpractice claims that can result from poor nurse-physician communication. Still other managers assert that in a time of economic constraints, the hospital must get maximum productivity from its nursing staff— and that means allowing nurses to use *all* the skills and training they have.

Whatever the motive, hospitals are attempting to fashion major changes in the way physicians and nurses work together. Some institutions have limited goals: for example, to improve nursing morale or to encourage physicians to treat nurses with more respect. Other hospitals have more grandiose objectives involving collaborative practice. Opposition to these changes does not reside exclusively with the medical staff; in various hospitals, resistance also has come from management, from the governing board, and from within the ranks of the nursing staff itself. Primarily, however, the most serious obstacle to expanding the nurse's role in patient care comes from physicians.

At Greater Southeast Community Hospital in Washington, D.C., we have made major changes in the way our nurses and physicians work together. Nursing is no longer

Phillippa Ferguson Johnston, R.N., M.S., is Assistant Administrator, Patient Care Services, Greater Southeast Community Hospital, Washington, D.C.

task-oriented; head nurses are accountable for every patient on their units, and our nurses apply skills of problem solving, observation, diagnosis, and treatment through increasingly integrated practice with physicians. As a result, RN recruitment and retention is no longer an acute problem, and nursing morale is measurably up. Physician complaints about nursing are down sharply, and physician praise for nursing care occurs regularly. A collaborative practice program is working on more than half our units, with the rest expected on-line within a year.

We made all of these changes without open rebellion by our medical staff—no small accomplishment. Had we told our physicians three years ago that we wanted to expand nurses' roles and increase nurses' salaries, the response would have been less than overwhelming support. The way we went about making changes may be helpful for other hospitals that seek to maintain and build medical staff support for improving the nurse-physician relationship.

1. *Avoid "charged" words.* When physicians hear about "assertiveness training," "joint practice," "professional nurses," and other common, but loaded terms, a whole host of pejorative meanings springs to their minds. If battles must be fought, fight over substance, not semantics. We talked to physicians in terms of "improving care of the patient" and "solving the problems physicians had with nursing" and found we struck responsive chords.

2. *Build nurses' clinical competence and clinical credibility.* Physicians honestly question whether nurses can assume the diagnostic and treatment responsibilities they seek. It is management's job to be sure that the nursing staff has the clinical preparation necessary to meet new standards of performance. Giving nurses more responsibility without adequate training is like throwing fat onto the fire. We built clinical competence in various ways: writing specific performance standards, aggressive in-service education, and utilization of highly trained clinical nurse specialists to serve as role models and perform on-the-job education. Building clinical competence leads to clinical credibility. Too often, nursing seeks the reverse: It asks for deference from physi-

151

cians before demonstrating its own competence.

3. *Create a problem-solving structure.* Physicians and nurses will have communication problems as long as there are patients. All professionals working together encounter such problems. In hospitals, these problems often are allowed to fester without resolution, leading to an undercurrent of hostility that poisons nurse-physician communication and hampers effective patient care. It is management's responsibility to create a problem-solving structure that seeks to resolve problems as close to the bedside as possible and on behalf of the patient. When a nurse has a problem—a physician is nonresponsive or abusive, for example—the accountability structure for resolving problems should be clearly defined and promptly implemented. The same applies to physicians. Communication problems arising in daily care should be resolved on behalf of the patient at the lowest level possible—they don't belong on the desk of the director of nursing or the medical director or at the quality assurance committee meeting.

4. *Support the nurses.* If nurses are clinically competent and they assert their competence within their roles, management must support them. When individual nurses at Greater Southeast question a physician's order or a failure to respond to certain signs or test results, they do so with a strong clinical background, And so, when nurses raise questions—on behalf of the patient and through the accountability structure—we support them to the wall.

5. *Create a prospective problem-solving structure.* A forum is needed where physicians and nurses can work out recurrent problems. At Greater Southeast, we have created collaborative practice committees on a unit-by-unit basis. The committees are initiated and staffed by nurses, but physicians participate, bringing and helping resolve problems. The bywords for involving physicians on committees are "be results-oriented" and always make the central question "What is best for the patients?"

6. *Stop blaming the doctors—and start listening.* If we are going to reverse the "us versus them" mentality, we need to focus on problem solving. We found that physicians had a number of justified complaints about nurses, just as nurses had legitimate problems with physicians. Only by opening a dialogue and working through the accountability structure and the collaborative practice committees did we begin to move toward problem resolution and a better working relationship.

These ideas are not magical or remarkable. But formulating them and keeping them in mind has helped us make very significant changes in nursing practice and nurse-physician relationships.

CHAPTER 25

Associated Practice: A Case for Professional Collaboration

by Ellen H. Elpern, Mary F. Rodts,
Ronald L. DeWald, and James W. West

*The establishment of a successful nurse-physician asso-
ciated practice requires planning, patience, and a willingness to take calculated risks. The nurse executive can lend
credibility and support to the nurse in associated practice by
understanding the concept, providing a climate for acceptance of such practices, and by clarifying the role of the
nurse associate in relation to other professionals in the
organization. In this article the authors describe models for
associated practice, as well as the measures necessary to
ensure peer and patient acceptance and effective health care
delivery.*

Substantial changes are occuring in the delivery of patient
care. The primary providers, nurses and physicians, have
been increasingly motivated to seek professional arrangements that will ensure the highest quality care for their
patients and provide satisfaction for themselves. A particular professional arrangement for nurses and physicians,
here termed associated practice, is gaining attention and
credibility.

In its simplest terms, associated practice means that a
physician and a nurse jointly assume responsibility and
accountability for delivering care to patients. It is synonymous with joint or collaborative practice. As it will be used
in this paper, the term "associated practice" refers to a

Ellen H. Elpern, R.N., M.S.N., is Assistant Professor, Department of
Medical Nursing, Rush University College of Nursing.

Mary F. Rodts, R.N., M.S., is Assistant Professor, Department of
Surgical Nursing, Rush University College of Nursing.

Ronald L. DeWald, M.D., is Professor, Department of Orthopedic
Surgery, Rush Medical College.

James W. West, M.D., is Assistant Professor, Department of Medicine,
Rush Medical College.

 *Associated Practice, Pulmonary Diseases
**Associated Practice, Spinal Surgery

situation in which a physician and nurse, through voluntary
negotiation, mutually share responsibility for care of a specific population of patients. It is important to emphasize
that the associated practice arrangement is one that is
voluntary, negotiated, and collegial. Each professional person brings to the practice a perspective and expertise which
help both participants manage the broad spectrum of problems and concern that patients have.

The climate

Numerous factors have contributed to a shift of emphasis in
nurse physician relationships from hierarchical to collaborative. The many advances in science have left us with complex and highly technical diagnostic and therapeutic capabilities. People are living longer, many with chronic diseases. Medical and nursing care has become increasingly
specialized. This progress in care managment has led to
increasing demands on and options for physicians and
nurses.

Patients, too, have become more sophisticated in their
expectations of health care providers. The traditional relationship between physicians and nurses in which physicians
personally prescribed, supervised and directed nursing
activities is today both unnecessary and unrealistically restrictive. Today's nurses are aware of the valuable contributions they can make to patient care. They seek opportunities
to demonstrate their clinical competencies and to favorably
affect the care patients receive. When opportunities are
blocked that are within the capabilities of nurses, frustration
and dissatisfaction are inevitable results.

Associated practice is one response to the desire of both
nurses and physicians to better address patient care needs in
a responsive, comprehensive and satisfying way. At Rush-
Presbyterian-St. Luke's Medical Center (RPSL) in Chicago, Illinois there has been growing interest and activity in
the area of associated practice. Nurse-physician practice
teams have been established in several of the clinical areas.

Models for associated practice

Three models for associated practice have been developed at RPSL that provide a logical division for the various ways in which a practice may be established. These models are: (1) the associated practice in which the nurse practices in the outpatient clinical setting; (2) the associated practice in which the nurse practices within the outpatient and inpatient clinical settings; and (3) the associated practice in which the nurse practices entirely within the inpatient clinical setting.

Similarities exist in each model. The nurse associate must have at least a masters level preparation and expertise in a specific area of clinical practice. The associate works in conjunction with a physician or group of physicians in the management of a specific patient population. In all models the nurse is responsible for nursing care and management of the particular population of patients. This is a basic motif. Exactly what distinguishes nursing management from physician management is not always easily categorized. Nonetheless, the criteria for nursing practice in each model should be established in an effort to identify guidelines which indicate the scope of nursing practice. These criteria change as nurse competencies increase.

The nurse associate whose practice is based in the outpatient setting is responsible for patient assessment, follow-up care, education of the patient on health maintenance, and identification of health problems. Nurses in this setting conduct triage and refer patient problems beyond their scope of competence to the physician associate for continued assessment.

The responsibilities of nurse associates in the outpatient setting vary from practice to practice depending on the backup they have. The practitioner in a small rural community with a patient who has a complex medical problem will need to assess the patient, relay this assessment to the physician associate, implement treatment with his/her input, and make plans for further care. The nurse associate in a large medical center has the benefit of easy access to a physician or emergency department.

The nurse associate who has inpatient and outpatient responsibilities incorporates the same responsibilities as stated in the first model, but also is concerned with the inpatient population. The nurse oversees the care each patient receives, identifies future needs of the patient, discusses these needs with the physician associate and primary nurse, establishes goals for the patient and is a consultant to the primary nursing staff. By providing data acquired in the outpatient setting, continuity of care is enhanced.

This type of practice is feasible if the location of the outpatient setting is geographically near the inpatient setting, if the nurse associate is free of other office duties such as making appointments or answering the phone, and if the hospital or medical center has established guidelines to allow associated practice nurses to function. This is the most

common type of associated practice at RPSL. Associated practices currently exist in the departments of medicine and surgery. Each associated specialty practice offers different role content to the nurse, depending on the needs of the patient population and the individuals available to address them. The associated practice which includes both the outpatient and inpatient settings offers nurses the opportunity to fully utilize their assessment skills, knowledge base and decision-making capabilities, it also provides a hospital-based clinical setting which many nurse associates find extremely rewarding.

The model of associated practice in which nursing practice is confined to the inpatient setting is being investigated for possible implementation at RPSL. This model would be most useful in the inpatient setting where there is no resident physician coverage. In most instances patient management decisions would be specified by the physician or found in protocols developed for commonly occurring health problems.

These three models of associated practice exist in various forms throughout the country. Associated nursing practice, however, varies because of: (1) the type of medical practice; (2) the size and location of the patient population; (3) the patient population's acceptance of associated practice; and (4) the resources available to the practitioners.

Establishing an associated practice

The physician and nurse enter into an associated practice after each has had the opportunity to review his or her professional qualifications, philosophical goals for patient care, and the competence each would bring to the practice. In most cases the nurse and physician have had the opportunity in the clinical setting to obtain some information as to how they would work together as colleagues. At the very earliest stage of establishing an associated practice, several important aspects of that practice need to be discussed. These would include the nurse-physician colleagial relationship, division of responsibilities, time commitment, financial reimbursement, and future professional goals for each person.

The ability of the nurse and physician to relate to each other in a colleagial manner is most important. Colleagues must be able to accept and respect each other for the expertise and other qualities they bring to patient care. The nurse and physician must understand that questioning a colleague's aproach to patient care is not an accusation of poor patient management; rather, it is a stimulus to growth of competence and better patient care. The colleagial climate must be nourished to enable discussion of all aspects of patient management and to identify the necessary steps that will lead to the desired outcome for each patient.

This very special colleagial relationship should also be evident to the patient population. The patients' acceptance of the joint approach to patient care will be enhanced if they are assured that the associates work well together. A simple introduction such as "This is my associate" is very reassuring to the patient, and also helps establish identity, credibility and respect.

The division of responsibilities in the nurse-physician relationship needs to be outlined when the associated practice is first formed. The nurse and physician will continue to develop their supplemental and complemental roles; for this reason, responsibiltities may need to be reviewed and altered at a later date. In general, the physician deals with medical management of each patient while the nurse handles the nursing care.

The nurse in an associated practice is not there simply to make the life of the physician easier. This is not the primary goal, although in many instances this certainly is the case. The nurse is there to help provide more complete health care services to the patient population. Prior to the associated practice, these services may not have been offered to the patient or they may have been handled hurriedly and incompletely by the physician or secretarial staff under his/her direction.

The physician and nurse need to look at the time commitment each will need to make if the practice is to evolve successfully. An associated practice will require at least one year of concerted effort before the benefits to all will be seen. A commitment to education and discussion during that first year is necessary so that each associate will learn the other's strengths and ideologies. An associated practice should not be established without thought and a commitment to a long-term association.

The specific structure of the association between the nurse and physician may take any of several forms. The nurse and physician may work together on a full time or part-time basis. The nurse may be a partner in the practice or an employee of the practice corporation. In other instances, the nurse may be an employee of the hospital or medical center. In this situation, the practice corporation usually assumes responsibility for reimbursement to the institution for all or part of the nurse associate's salary and benefits.

Most nurses and physicians feel uncomfortable dealing with the income for a nurse in associated practice. The nurse and physician need to negotiate the income of the nurse on the basis of relative worth and input. There should be no limitations set on the earning ability of the nurse.

It is also important for the nurse to make sure that, aside from income, other benefits such as health insurance, disability, vacation, time to attend professional meetings, and profit and pension have been provided. The nurse also must make sure that malpractice insurance is sufficient to cover nursing practice.

Future professional goals for each person need to be reviewed when the associated practice is developed. Certain goals may require time away from the practice. For instance a nurse may return to school for further education or the physician may take a sabbatical. This time away from the

practice should be seen as a way to improve the practice. Both persons need to make adjustments in order that the practice continue to operate in an efficient manner during an associate's absence.

Organizational supports

As the models previously discussed demonstrate, associated practice may include both the inpatient and outpatient settings. Private outpatient practice occurs outside the confines of an institutional setting and is not subject to institutional controls. Establishment of the nature and scope of each practitioner's outpatient role is, with few exceptions, at the discretion of the physician and nurse as long as they remain within the dictates of the state nursing and medical practice acts. This is not the case in the hospital setting.

The relationship between hospital organization and the staff physician typically is such that physicians report directly to the board of trustees through a medical staff organization. Physicians usually are not employees of the hospital and are outside the general bureaucratic lines of authority. As professionals, the scope of physicians' clinical activities within the hospital are delineated and approved by the physician's peers.

The relation of the nurse associate to the hospital organization is less easily defined. Most nurses who practice in hospitals are employees of the institution. They are staff members of the department of nursing and are subject to clear departmental and institutional lines of authority. This may also be true of the nurse associate. In other instances, the nurse associate may not be part of the hospital bureaucracy and, therefore, must apply for practice privileges. In either circumstance, certain characteristics of the hospital organization can influence whether the nurse in associated practice is openly opposed, merely tolerated, or effectively integrated into the health care team.

The type of hospital setting in which the nurse and physician in associated practice are most easily integrated is, simply, one in which physicians and nurses are accustomed to communicating with one another. As basic as that concept seems, many hospital organizations are structured in ways that are not conducive to professional communication and collaboration. Whatever the rhetoric may be, it is not difficult to spot institutions that place low value on professional nursing practice. In such institutions, it is not unusual to find the nursing operation organized under hospital administration with departmental status and reporting relationships much like other services such as housekeeping, laboratories and central supply. The director of nursing is not part of the mainstream of communication, relying on the administrator to whom she reports to represent the nursing enterprise when decisions are made. Rather than participating in joint decision making with physicians and administrators, nurses at all levels in the organization may be charged with the time-consuming responsibility for the provision of support services such as clerical assistance, dietary services and transport. At the unit level, nursing may be organized and accountable more for functions, tasks, teams and shift-based routines than individual patient needs. In such an environment, physicians and nurses would have little opportunity for or inclination toward the joint decision making that collaborative practice implies.

The concept of collaboration is more viable and credible one in institutions where physicians and nurses interact at all levels. Collaboration requires a structure that provides for interaction among physicians, nurses and administrators. The nursing division that incorporates the principles of decentralized decision making and primary nursing are most conducive to professional practice. Nurses will be more practiced and skilled in negotiation, calculated risk-taking and nurse-to-nurse consultation on practice issues and problems. Physicians are more predisposed to appreciate the benefits they and patients realize when nurses are able to contribute to and better coordinate plans for patient management.

These structural elements may provide an environment that fosters associated practice, but they do not preclude the necessity for careful role negotiation between the nurse associate and the chief nurse executive of the institution. It is our belief that nurse associate credentialling for inpatient activities should be through the nursing division rather than through the medical staff organization. Representatives of nursing administration are best qualified to review the credentials of nurses who wish to practice within the institution. Logically, the nurse associate should bear accountability to the nursing division for nursing activities performed in the hospital or medical center. Once approval for clinical privileges is granted, the nurse executive may desire to inform representatives of medicine and hospital administration.

Establishing institutional relationships

As nurses become increasingly professional in their practices and as expanded roles for nurses continue to proliferate, the nurse executive at some time will encounter the question of clinical privileges for non-hospital based nurses. Whether this situation have yet arisen, it seems prudent that the nurse executive have a well deliberated approach ready. This planned anticipatory approach will ensure an orderly process without the chaotic, prolonged and sometimes impassioned struggle that ensues when important groundwork has not been laid.

Preliminary work on addressing the question of clinical privileges for the nurse associate must begin with the knowledge of the local nurse practice act and pertinent rules and regulations. Contacting the state nurses association may also provide information on local position statements or guidelines for granting clinical privileges to nurse practitioners. The experiences of nurisng divisions in other insti-

> ## "The philosophies of the institution and the nursing division should be reviewed in order to determine if these statements will support the concept of associated practice."

tutions may be helpful sources of information.

Next, institutional attitudes toward the concept of the nurse-physician practice team should be assessed. The philosophies of the institution and the nursing division should be reviewed with particular care in order to determine if these statements will support the concept of associated practice. The attitudes and reactions of key physicians, administrators, and nurses should be evaluated. The understanding and support of these individuals are absolutely crucial.

Once such support has been ascertained, a mechanism for the petitioning and granting of practice privileges should be established. In organizations where a nurse staff organization is operative, such a mechanism should already exist. If this is not the case, an appropriate body will need to be defined. Questions to be addressed will include:

- What qualifications must a nurse associate possess to practice in the particular institution?
- How shall credentials be submitted and reviewed?
- What are the conditions and duration of appointments?
- How shall evaluation and continuation of privileges be managed?
- What functions will the nurse associate assume within the hospital?
- What will be the relationship of the nurse associate to the nursing staff? resident staff? attending physicians?

At RPSL, nurse associates hold graduate degrees in nursing. They are licensed by the Illinois State Board of Nursing and possess advanced knowledge and skills in a particular area of clinical practice. They are practice associates of a physician or physicians who have staff privileges at Presbyterian-St. Luke's Hospital. Application for clinical appointments are handled through one of the seven clinical nursing departments. Consistent with the nursing philosophy at RPSL, all nurse associates hold, in addition to clinical appointment, a faculty appointment at the Rush University College of Nursing. The nature and scope of responsibilities in the College are negotiated directly with the chairperson of the nursing department. The College of Nursing compensates the nurse associate for the percentage of time devoted to faculty activities. The remainder of the nurse's income is negotiated with the physician. Clinical appointments are made for a one-year term and are reviewed annually. The duration of the faculty appointment varies according to academic rank.

Most nurse associates at RPSL have contact with both inpatients and outpatients. Depending on patient needs and office resources, the nurse associate may see outpatients for specific, limited activities or may become the predominant care provider. In the inpatient setting, all communications regarding nursing care are channeled through each patient's primary nurse. This arrangement focuses accountability on the primary nurse for the nursing care provided during hospitalization, and ensures that coordination between the outpatient and inpatient departments is maintained. There is resident staff coverage on almost all units; all medical orders are coordinated by these physicians. On units where resident physicians are not in attendance, the nurse associate may write orders, which are countersigned by the physician associate within 24 hours. Because RPSL uses an integrated hospital record, the nurse associate charts on the patient progress notes, along with all others involved in the patient's care.

If nurse associates are to function effectively within the hospital, they must be prepared to address the concerns of their co-workers. In our experience, physicians, particularly house officers, will question where the nurse associate fits in the schema of inpatient management. Some will test the competence of the nurse associate and may be initially skeptical about accepting consultation from a nurse. Staff nurses also may have questions about how the nurse associate fits into the nursing care structure. They must be assured that during a patient's hospitalization, the nurse associate assumes a consultant role to the nursing staff. Responsibility and accountability for nursing management during hospitalization must lie with the primary nurse.

Summary

Successful associated practices usually do not occur seren-dipitously. The physician and nurse form an association after much thought and discussion, and usually on the strength of a previous professional relationship. An asso-ciated practice represents a long-term commitment between professionals whose main impetus for this association is more complete patient care management.

When physician and nurse have established a collabora-tive relationship, they must "sell" their associated practice to patients they serve, to other professionals, and to those who administer the institutions where they will practice. There is no one best way to ensure acceptance. Issues of competence, credibility, competition and control are likely to arise des-pite careful planning. These issues are best dealt with in a straightforward manner if the association is to thrive.

Associated practices may become more commonplace as physicians and nurses realize that collaboration will en-hance patient care and the patient population will view this change in their health care routine as a bonus. The admin-istrator will find associated practice an innovative and excit-ing way for optimal patient management. After all, the key to all health care provision is a more satisfied and better cared for patient population.

CHAPTER 26

■ Susan G. Sheedy, BSN, MPH

Vice-President of Medicine/ Vice-President of Nursing:
Collaboration or Conflict?

In the current environment of Diagnosis Related Groups and competition for the health care market share, there is a significant increase of vice-president of medical affairs or medical director positions on the hospital management team. This partnership is seen as vital for the survival of private practice physicians and hospitals. What does the addition of this role mean to the nursing administrator? What is the likelihood of a confusion of responsibilities between the vice-president of nursing and the vice-president of medical affairs or medical director? What involvement should the vice-president of nursing have in the vice-president of medical affairs or medical director's job description? These are some of the questions discussed in this article.

Many nursing administrators are familiar with the president of the medical staff as a voluntary or paid elected physician who conducts the monthly medical staff meeting and attends management meetings when his or her private practice permits; or the part-time voluntary or paid medical director of a specific service who approves or revises patient care policies for that service and conducts a part-time private medical practice. However, as the physician glut becomes a reality and competition for patients yields partially filled appointment books in the physician's private practice, part- or full-time salaried positions will be far more attractive to the private practitioner. In addition, with the advent of preferred provider organizations, business coalitions, and reimbursement based on Diagnosis Related Groups, a strong partnership will need to evolve between hospitals and physicians unlike any we have seen in the past. Thus many organizations are reviewing their structure and the role for physician leadership whether it be titled vice-president of medical affairs or medical director.* In most instances, it will be a paid position. The physi-

cian may or may not be in private practice. The position may have line responsibilities and will be more involved in the operations and policy making of the organization.

■ Broader Issues

What are some of the broader issues the board, medical staff, and administration will have to address as this stronger partnership evolves? A particularly difficult issue will be whether these positions should be filled by a physician who will remain in private practice. This discussion inevitably leads to two schools of thought: (1) the only way for a physician salaried by the hospital to maintain credibility with the private attending staff is to be in private practice, or (2) the physician salaried by the hospital must not be in private practice since he or she will be in a conflict of interest position. The conflict will be that the salaried vice-president of medical affairs will be competing with other members of his or her service/ hospital when in private practice, yet will be expected to represent their interests when acting as the vice-president of medical affairs. The proponents of the latter view state that at hospital policy meetings the physician in private practice should vote with the following priorities in mind and thus lessen the conflict of interest situation. (1) Will this decision/policy

Susan G. Sheedy, BSN, MPH, is Vice-President, Nursing, Baptist Medical Center Princeton, Birmingham, Alabama. At the time this article was written, the author was Vice-President, Nursing, Methodist Hospital of Indianapolis, Indiana.

*To be referred to hereafter as vice-president of medical affairs.

affect my practice or my chief referral sources? (2) Will this decision/policy handicap another private practice group who are my competition? (3) Will this decision/policy support a strong internal and external hospital operation? Obviously, the last priority needs to be first or the future viability of the institution is tenuous. This is the central issue discussed by medical staffs, boards, and administration as they consider the position of vice-president of medical affairs.

Another concern on the part of physicians is the issue of the corporate practice of medicine by a hospital. Projects discussed at hospital administrative meetings, such as emergicenters, geriatric centers, and sports medicine centers, represent, from the physician's viewpoint, examples of the hospital overstepping its boundaries. This split loyalty to profession and hospital places the physician in the dilemma of voting to protect the interests of private medical practice or voting to ensure the survival of his or her institution in a competitive health care market. Clearly, physicians and hospitals may be pursuing the same markets in order to survive.

Assessment of Need for Vice-President of Medical Affairs

As the discussion of this need continues, nursing administrators should be familiarizing themselves with the issues and be requesting to be a part of the deliberations. How does one prepare for such a discussion? To begin to understand how this position of vice-president of medical affairs might affect the institution and the nursing department, one needs to ask some questions: Will this affect the role of the nurse administrator? If so, How? What expectations of the role does the nurse administrator have? What are some functions that need physician leadership? Depending on the organization and proposal for the position's structure, a myriad of questions could develop.

Regardless of the proposed structure, given the addition of a vice-president of medical affairs, the nurse administrator's role will change. How it will affect the nurse administrator will depend on the proposal. With hope, the process will include the nurse administrator as the structure is being reviewed. The most useful input the nurse administrator can have is to pose the question: What medical affairs/issues are unaddressed or lack continuity due to rotation of service chiefs or medical staff officers? Some of these unaddressed functions in medical affairs could be the following:

1. Develop a physician recruitment plan to be reviewed by the medical staff and administration.
2. Coordinate the search process for physician recruitment.
3. Orientation of new physicians joining staff.
4. Chair a utilization review committee for his or her specialty.
5. Develop and chair overseer physician committees to monitor patient care, examples: intensive care committee, newborn intensive care committee, oncology committee, etc.
6. Responsible for medical staff compliance with JCAH, State Board of Health, and other regulatory agencies.
7. Advise and recommend the addition or exclusion of major new medical or technology programs and expenses in line with corporate objectives.
8. Meet and counsel physicians who are not in compliance with the service's patient care policies.

If there are any affiliations with medical schools by the hospital, several other functions could be added, such act as liaison with the university medical school, recruit private attending physicians as faculty for medical education, develop policies for private attending physicians who are faculty. The position needs to satisfy institution-specific functions.

Depending on the size of the hospital, the vice-president of medical affairs could perform these functions for the whole hospital with input from the medical staff, or in a large hospital each service chief could perform these functions for his or her service.

Vice-President of Medical Affairs Organizational Structures

It is clear that physician leadership is needed to complement the administrative team. The placement of the vice-president of medical affairs in the organization is significant. The two most common structures are (1) vice-president of medical affairs as an equal with other vice-presidents or assistant administrators including the vice-president of nursing (Fig. 1) or (2) as an equal with other vice-presidents or assistant administrators but, with the vice-president of nursing/director of nursing reporting to the vice-president of medical affairs (Fig. 2). When reviewing Figure 2, the question must be asked: What is the purpose of the director of nursing reporting to the vice-president of medical affairs? If there are not enough functions for a position of vice-president of medical affairs, then the position is not needed or is only needed part time. For the additional

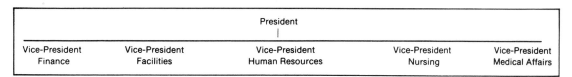

Figure 1. Administrative team structure with vice-president of medical affairs as an equal to other vice-presidents.

salary expense of a new position, the institution should be gaining some function that no one else other than a physician could do. Thus the position should be capitalizing on "physician-only knowledge" rather than trying to make the physician an operations manager. Indeed, Figure 2 underemphasizes the need for *medical* leadership and dilutes the expertise a physician could bring to such a position. The physician's major contributions should be an understanding of his or her medical colleagues and medical politics in the institution, awareness of national and local issues in health care and their effect on the medical profession, the interface of the medical profession and other health care professions, and an awareness of the quality of medical practice in the institution. The physician then acts as an educator and interpreter of medical profession/staff issues with the board and administration and as an educator and interpreter of administrative issues to the medical staff. To add nursing as an additional responsibility to the vice-president of medical affairs is to underestimate the expertise nursing administration demands and the need of the institution to have medicine *and* nursing at the top level of decision making. In addition, the nursing administrator's only loyalty is to the institution as in Figure 1. In Figure 2, the nurse administrator's loyalty is to the physician who hires, evaluates, and terminates. The physician's split loyalty to his or her medical profession and his or her colleagues, partners, and referral sources can compromise the nursing administrator's strong support of the institution.

Over the last several years, the literature has abounded with studies of nursing as a reaction to the nursing shortage. Such reports as the National Commission on Nursing recommend "nursing should be recognized as a clinical practice discipline that needs to have authority over its management process."[1] The same study goes on to urge trustees and health care administrators to "promote and support complementary practice between nurses and physicians" and that they (board and health care administrators) "examine organizational structure to ensure that nurse administrators are part of the policy making bodies of the institution and have authority to collaborate on an equal footing with the medical leaders in the institution."[1] From the American Association of Critical Care Nurses and the Council of the Society of Critical Care Medicine comes a collaborative practice statement that further enhances the need for nursing and medicine to be equals in the organizational structure: (1) responsibility and accountability for effective functioning of a critical care unit must be vested in physician and nurse directors who are on an equal decision making level; (2) the organizational structure of a critical care unit must ensure that physicians are autonomous when dealing with issues that affect medical practice; and (3) the organizational structure of a critical care unit must ensure that nurses are autonomous when dealing with issues that affect nursing practice.[2]

Thus the model that would seem most in keeping with the recommendations made by these two groups after in-depth analysis of the nursing profession would be a collaborative one between the vice-president of medical affairs and vice-president of nursing, as shown in Figure 1. It would be a model wherein the vice-president of medical affairs and vice-president of nursing would be equal in authority and decision making for their respective responsibilities with equal input to corporate level policies and decision making. With a collaborative model there is

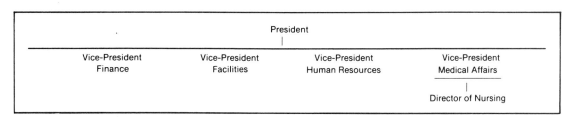

Figure 2. Administrative team structure with vice-president of medical affairs as an equal with other vice-presidents, but with the director of nursing reporting to him or her.

a comprehensive understanding lent to all patient care activities. The most noted statements or studies are the National Commission on Nursing and the collaborative statement of the American Association of Critical Care Nurses and the Council of the Society of Critical Care Medicine. Memberships represented leaders in medicine, nursing, and other fields. They do not support one profession governing another. Thus nurses and physicians in these two national groups, via their knowledge and findings, affirm that nurses should control nursing practice and physicians should control medical practice.

References

1. National Commission on Nursing Initial Report and Preliminary Recommendations. Chicago, 1981:2,9,62.
2. The Organization of Human Resources in Critical Care Units. Focus on critical care. February 1983:43-4.

UNIT SIX

JANE A. FANNING

Computers

Recently, I had a discussion with a friend regarding the entrance of her $2\frac{1}{2}$-year-old child into nursery school. She informed me that one reason why she had chosen the school was because it offered computer basics as part of the curriculum. The $2\frac{1}{2}$-year-old was soon on his way to learning computer skills and becoming a computer literate adult in the twenty-first century.

By contrast, and take no offense, most nurses practicing today are computer illiterate. In addition many nurses have computer phobia or, at best, an avoidance behavior evidenced by little desire to learn to use a computer. Many nurses take false comfort in ill-founded advice that it is unnecessary to know about computers. The vocabulary of MIS, hardware, modem, software, user-friendly, CRTs, "on-line," and real-time remains unknown to them.

Whether one practices in acute care or in an ambulatory setting, whether one focuses on clinical direct patient care, management, education, or research, nursing has a new imperative. The imperative is knowledge and a level of comfort with computer technology. This does not mean that one needs to obtain a doctoral degree in computer science to practice nursing now or in the future. It does mean, however, that at least a general knowledge of basic computer sciences, terminology, and some specific uses or applications of the computer is needed to replace confusion, fear, and ignorance. Survival into nursing's twenty-first century at least partly depends on how well nurses currently learn and adapt to computer technology and automated information systems.

What are the nursing applications of computers? What automated systems could be developed to meet present needs? How can nurses plan effectively for the acquisition of automated information systems and then effectively implement them? The reprinted articles selected for this section provide answers to these and other important questions.

Catherine Carpenter's article *Computer Use in Nursing Management* reviews the status of automatic data processing in health care and notes the lack of involvement of nurses in the computer revolution in hospitals. As computer potential is realized nursing administration depends increasingly on computers to organize data to augment budget preparation; to gather patient classification and acuity data; to develop recommended staffing, scheduling, and statistical reports; to update current employee information files; and to assess the quality of care monitoring: These are just some vital computer uses. Further, with the advent of DRGs, it is to the nurse administrator's advantage to measure workload and staffing by way of daily patient acuities and translate this into accurate costs for nursing care. Large amounts of data, including administrative, fiscal, and clinical information, are organized efficiently and effectively through automatic data processing. Carpenter asserts that the nursing administrator should take an active role in computer-acquisition decisions to meet the daily operation needs of the department and also to help in middle- and long-range decision making. She also elaborates on ways to avoid problems in the complex process of system planning and discusses the importance of integrating nursing systems with hospital systems.

Rita D. Zielstorff advances answers to "Why Aren't There More Significant Automated Nursing Information Systems?" A lack of any of the five factors she lists may decrease the chances for success. The necessary ingredients include: (a) a strong trained leader, (b) a good idea, (c) a data base amenable to computer manipulation, (d) adequate financial and administrative support, and (e) a successful implementation of the system. In addition she relates reasons for nursing's lack of research grant requests involving computerized information systems in the clinical setting. She concludes her article with optimism about nursing's ability to incorporate good ideas into well-designed information systems to assist with clinical decision making and ultimately to contribute meaningful data for research. Nurses have demonstrated strengths that are needed in the successful process of system installation.

The final article in this section by Erica L. Drazen focuses on the practical elements involved in planning and implementing an automated hospital information system. She details a planning framework to assist successful decision making in the complex process of acquiring an automated system. In order to avoid costly disasters in the selection of automated systems, she concentrates on the importance of evaluating cost impacts of computerization and details the process of cost benefit analysis. Cost benefit analysis as a planning tool is complex, and the author believes that direct cost savings may not be the major benefit of implementing an automated system. Her review of an erroneous cost analysis helps the buyer beware and more critically evaluate a purchase. Her planning framework starts with important questions: (1) Do I need a system? (2) What system will best meet my needs? and (3) Will the system work as planned? Answers to these questions are basic whether the nurse shops at a local mall for a home computer or investigates through vendors a system for a work setting.

The articles in this section review where we are today and suggests some of the future directions for nursing in the computer revolution. Computers have brought space-age technology down to earth and they have put enormous new power in the hands of the courageous and willing learner. An acceptance of the challenge to become computer literate exposes important future frontiers to nurse leaders.

CHAPTER 27

■ Rita D. Zielstorff, RN, MS

Why Aren't There More Significant Automated Nursing Information Systems?

This article answers the question posed in the title. The author maintains the following factors must exist if a significant computerized nursing information system is to prove successful in clinical settings: a) a strong leader whose training includes research and computer sciences; b) a "good idea" that is practical, researchable, and will attract support; c) a data base amenable to computer manipulation; d) adequate resources, including administrative support, money, hardware, personnel, and authority; and e) successful implementation of the system.

At the 1982 Symposium on Computer Applications in Medical Care held in Washington, DC, the Plenary Session saw a panel of five physicians address the topic of how computerized information systems contribute to the quality of medical care. Four of them presented specific examples of how the systems they had developed were assisting in day-to-day medical decision making.[1]

I wondered when the day would come that one or more nurses would be invited to be on such a panel. I learned during the meeting that the session chairman had asked for nursing representation, but no one could name an automated nursing information system that was significantly influencing nurses' clinical decision making on a day-to-day basis.

A similar topic was brought up at a recent meeting sponsored by the National Center for Health Services Research (NCHSR) and the University Hospitals of Cleveland. The purpose of that meeting was to explore the status of automated nursing information management systems, with the intent of providing direction for research and development. It was pointed out that the vast majority of grant requests to the NCHSR over the past 2 decades for research in

using computers in health care came from physicians. Very few requests came from nurses; of those few, less than half a dozen had been approved or funded. Why have so few good proposals come from nurses?

Dr. Harriet Werley, now Associate Dean for Research at the University of Missouri School of Nursing, has been asking this question for many years. She and Dr. Margaret Grier of the University of Illinois convened a Research Conference on Nursing Information Systems in Chicago in June 1977. The meeting gathered together "individuals knowledgeable about and interested in identifying and computerizing data bases relevant to nursing care"[2] in the hope of identifying and catalyzing further research in that area. At that time, it was apparent that those persons who were deeply involved in research related to identifying the nursing data base were totally separate from those who were intimately involved in specifying and implementing computerized information systems. The meeting served a valuable purpose in bringing together these two groups, but the basic question remained unanswered: "Why is it that nurses do not design research and development proposals to identify a basic set of nursing data pertinent to any area of practice, test the data in settings receptive to computerization, and see to it that appropriate portions are incorporated into compu-

Rita D. Zielstorff, RN, MS, is Assistant Director, Laboratory of Computer Science, at Massachusetts General Hospital in Boston.

terized health are information systems?"[2]

If one examines the conditions that have promoted the successful development of significant medical systems, it becomes apparent that there is no single answer to this question. Just as plants require a variety of elements in appropriate sequence and balance in order to thrive, it appears that a certain mixture of elements in proper sequence and balance is necessary to nourish the development of significant medical information systems. And when one looks at the many opportunities that have existed in the past (and that exist at present) for the development of similar systems in nursing, it is possible to point to the absence of one or another of these elements to explain why no significant system has evolved.

This is not to say that there are no successful computer-based nursing information systems. In fact, there are many. But even the staunchest supporters of these systems would admit that, for the most part, they do not involve automated decision making (or even automated decision support) for day-to-day clinical care; and they do not contribute to data bases that are easily manipulated for clinical research purposes. To my mind, these are two essential characteristics of a significant automated information system. Without these characteristics, a computerized system is simply a tool that facilitates the many tasks related to transcribing, transferring, recording, and billing patient-related data.

Five elements are essential to the development of information systems that support clinical decision making and research: a) a strong leader, b) a good idea, c) data amenable to computer manipulation, d) adequate resources, and e) successful implementation. Examining each element in detail provides some clues as to why medicine has succeeded where nursing has not.

systems (AAMRS) in the United States, Kuhn and Weiderhold observed the following:

> A high level of motivation and strong leadership appeared to be a key to success or potential success. A strong individual was involved with development and implementation of every major AAMRS. In most cases the person was a physician turned computer specialist. It appeared that if the leadership was not there, or would leave the project, that the likelihood of success would be significantly impaired.[3]

What are the characteristics of these leaders and are there comparable individuals in nursing? There is no question that these leaders possess creativity, ability, expertise, commitment, and charisma. And certainly no one would disagree that nursing possesses its fair share of charismatic and able leaders. It is in expertise and commitment that we falter. There is at present a large cadre of physicians who possess dual degrees in engineering and medicine or in computer science and medicine; and who by virtue of their advanced education are well versed in research methodology. In nursing, this combination and level of expertise are extremely rare. Without a solid foundation in research and computer sciences, it is impossible for nurses to provide leadership in developing significant nursing systems.

Many physicians gained their knowledge of computers informally, through their own initiative and by long-term exposure to experts. Their commitment and experience made up for their lack of formal education. At the same time, much of their wisdom and judgment are the direct result of years of experience in the field, including some rather spectacular failures. Many nurses who might be in a position to learn this way simply do not stay in the field long enough to gain either the expertise or the wisdom.

▌A Strong Leader

Those who are knowledgeable in medical informatics can quickly name a handful of computer-based medical systems that are generally agreed to be significant or important. Each of these systems is associated with the name of a particular physician who has exerted strong leadership over the years. Everyone recognizes that these systems are really the fruit of the labors of many capable individuals; yet without the creative force engendered by their leaders, it is likely that these systems would never have come into being.

In a report summarizing the characteristics of successful automated ambulatory medical record

▌A "Good Idea"

A leader without a goal is like a car without a motor: neither will ever get anywhere. The best medical systems have been founded on a good idea—one that is worthy of research, has useful applications, and attracts support in the form of resources. Nursing is at no disadvantage here. There are just as many good ideas for the application of computers to nursing problems as there are in medicine. Perhaps even more, since nursing has so much further to go!

Good ideas, however, don't always sell themselves. The commitment, forcefulness, and resourcefulness of the leader play a crucial part in gathering resources and bringing the idea to realization.

Data Amendable to Computer Manipulation

Without exception, significant medical information systems deal with data that are machine readable. That is, patient-related data are stored in a coded format that allows the computer to differentiate between a diagnosis and a medication; to evaluate results of laboratory tests; and to recognize combinations of events and values that should be brought to the provider's attention. This is not the result of computer magic, but of painstaking effort to develop (or to find and utilize already developed) coding schemes, accepted normal value ranges, and valid clinical rules for practice.

Medicine is at a distinct advantage here, because the science of medicine is far more advanced than the science of nursing. Those who work in the design and development of nursing information systems constantly bemoan the fact that there are so few clinical problems in nursing for which the etiology, symptoms, treatment, and expected outcomes are known. There are no known probability estimates for prevalence or incidence of common nursing problems; or for relating symptoms to diagnosis, or treatment to outcome. Indeed, there is neither a standard terminology nor a widely accepted format for data gathering. It is impossible to derive hard and fast rules for computer assistance in decision making with such an ill-defined data base.

Adequate Resources for Implementing the Good Idea

"Resources" is an umbrella term for many things. First of all, the leader must have legitimate authority to decide which ideas will be implemented, and he or she must have support at higher administrative levels. There must be adequate financial support for carrying out the project. Finally, the leader must have at his or her command the hardware resources and the personnel capable of carrying out the good idea.

Here again, the imagination and commitment of the leader are crucial factors. The resources cited do not come as a gift-wrapped package. In many cases, today's leaders in medical computing are also experts in grantsmanship. Often they sought and obtained joint university/hospital appointments; the monies they brought in have entitled them to administrative responsibility over the personnel and hardware needed to carry out their projects. With legitimate authority over these resources, they have been able to expand and carry out their ideas. Today, as federal grants become scarce, they are resourceful enough to seek other sources of funding.

If one examines the field of computer science in nursing, it becomes apparent that the combination of high level administrative support, authority over personnel and resources, and initiative in finding financial support for independent nursing research projects, simply have not existed in a clinical care setting in this country. There are currently many nurses who serve important, even critical, posts in the administration and coordination of large computer systems. But almost none of them has the authority or the resources to carry out research ideas independently.

Successful Implementation

There are innumerable instances of bright and able leaders who conceived a wonderful idea for appropriately using a computer, and who gathered the resources needed to develop the system that would have carried out the idea, only to see the system fail in daily use. This is usually due to problems with one or more of the following: system design, user environment, or installation methods.

Among the many potential design problems are systems that are too expensive or too cumbersome to use; or systems that are so insensitive to users' needs that they threaten the very people they were supposed to assist.

Since every system influences and is influenced by the environment in which it is used, a certain symbiosis must occur in order for a significant system to thrive. This is not to say that today's important systems thrive in *every* environment in which they are placed, only that there must be *some* environment in which they contribute meaningfully to patient care. Of course, the more transferrable a system is, the greater the impact it can make on daily care and on research efforts.

When a system based on a good idea fails to thrive, it is sometimes difficult to determine whether the system itself was designed badly, or whether the environment was simply unsuitable; or, to confuse matters even further, whether the method of implementing it was the major problem. In a revealing portrait of an important medical computer system that was ultimately withdrawn, Lundsgaarde et al. declare:

 . . . Many of the human and organizational problems associated with the demonstration of the PROMIS system could have been avoided, or at least neutralized, if the developers had paid more attention to contextual social variables affecting system users rather than to the ideological or technological goals of the system developers.[4]

There is a growing body of literature concerned with why systems fail, a topic much too complex to be covered in this paper. Suffice it to say that the implementors of today's significant automated medical systems have managed, by virtue of ability, training, acquired wisdom, or good luck, to see that their good ideas were implemented with well designed systems. Furthermore, they successfully placed these systems into the environments for which the systems were designed, somehow circumventing or expertly managing the human problems associated with installing computer systems in health care settings.

Are nurses capable of doing this? Most certainly! Many of us are still weak in design skills because of our inexperience in system design, but consider our sensitivity to human needs, our skills in management, our ability to communicate with the entire spectrum of health care workers, and above all, our experience in implementing change. These combine to give us extraordinary strengths in the most delicate phase of system implementation: installation of the system. There is hardly a single major automated system in this country that has not had a nurse employed in this capacity. Given that all other elements are present for the development of significant nursing information systems (and that is a *very* large "given"), then certainly we can use our innate strengths to foster the installation of these systems.

When nursing can provide an environment where all of these elements exist, then perhaps we will see the development of automated nursing information systems that assist with day-to-day clinical decision making and contribute meaningful data for research.

References

1. Blum BI, ed. Proceedings of the sixth annual symposium on computer applications in medical care. New York: IEEE Computer Society Press, 1982.
2. Werley H, Grier MR. Nursing information systems. New York: Springer Publishing Company, 1981:ix, 321.
3. Kuhn IM, Wiederhold G. The evolution of ambulatory medical record systems in the U.S. In: Heffernan HG, ed. Proceedings of the fifth annual symposium on computer applications in medical care. New York: IEEE Computer Society Press, 1981:82.
4. Lundsgaarde HP, Fischer PJ, Steele DJ. Human problems in computerized medicine. Lawrence, Kansas: University of Kansas, 1981:2.

CHAPTER 28

Computer Use
in Nursing Management

by Catherine R. Carpenter

Nursing interest in computer use is on the increase; to date, however, its focus has been on clinical applications. Manually processing the volume of information needed to effectively and efficiently manage a modern nursing department becomes more difficult daily. This paper investigates published nursing management computer applications. It points to the need to look beyond the simple administrative to true management information systems, and outlines a role for the nurse administrator in preparing and implementing automatic data processing (ADP) plans.

Hospitals and information processing

While information is an essential management resource in any enterprise, hospitals are more dependent on this resource than most. This reflects the nature of health care. Davis stated that an organization's need for information increases with the uncertainty of the task, the number of elements relevant for decision making, and the interdependence of organizational units[1]. The modern hospital requires that a large number of departments cooperate to restore clients to health. This is a task which is nothing if not uncertain, given the complexity of the human organism and varying perceptions of what health is. To these must be added the information required of hospitals by regulatory bodies and third party payers.

It is estimated that between 7 and 10 billion dollars a year are spent by hospitals in the acquisition and communication of information—a figure representing 25 to 33 percent of the hospital budget[2]. Information is an expensive necessity, and can be made more so by managers who either don't

Catherine R. Carpenter, R.N., M.S. is a Major in the Army Nurse Corps stationed at Tripler Army Medical Center, Honolulu, Hawaii.

The author wishes to acknowledge the unstinting support of Gary B. Carpenter, M.D. in the preparation of this paper.

The opinions or assertions contained herein are the private views of the author and are not to be construed as official or as reflecting the views of the Department of the Army or the Department of Defense.

know what information they need, or confuse it with data. Data becomes information only when it "has been processed into a form that is meaningful to the recipient and is of real or perceived value in current or prospective decisions"[3]. This problem has become more acute as automatic data processing systems make their way into hospitals.

A computer is a complex and expensive machine which performs a simple operation: it takes data, organizes it, and communicates it faster and more accurately than a human being[4, 5]. The prime purpose of a computer is to provide accurate and relevant information with which to make clinical or managerial decisions. The benefits of computerization, whether cost saving or quality care, are dependent upon what the manager does with that information.

Hospitals have lagged behind industry in implementation of ADP systems and show considerably less sophistication in their use. This reflects the complexity of computer applications required in health care, as well as management timidity and ignorance. Computer use in hospitals began in the sixties with fiscal applications expanding to materials management and personnel administration in the seventies. Interest then developed in designing medical information systems to collect and process clinical data. Finally, the need for greater efficiency suggested that not only should direct communication between all these systems be developed, but also that data collected by both systems be stored in a data base separate from the programs and accessible to both. Few hospitals have adopted such "fully integrated hospital information systems." Austin maintains that, although substantial progress has been made in clinical and administrative uses of computers, even integrated systems are oriented towards support of day to day operations rather than towards management planning and control. Systems to support long range management decision making are still in a primitive stage[6].

The proliferation of administrative and clinical ADP systems in hospitals has not been without criticism. Herzlinger feels that hospital information systems are more oriented towards providing for the information needs of external agencies—which may not be information needed by the hospital. Conversely, where the information is appropriate, managers don't know how to use it[7, 8]. Veazie thinks that hospitals have more information than they can use, a problem complicated by their inability to measure its worth[9]. LaViolette states unequivocally that hospitals have more computer technology than they can handle, acquired faster than the experience or managerial controls can be developed to operate them effectively[10].

"Notwithstanding the key role of nurses in health care, they have been little involved in the hospital computer revolution."

Despite the problems surrounding the implementation of computer technology in health care, not a single author advocates a retreat to manual information processing. They agree that a system as complex as the hospital makes ADP a necessity, for "without adequate information processing, the parts of the system cannot integrate their efforts"[11]. Their proposals vary in minor details, but all argue that hospital management must become more involved in planning for, phasing in, and managing what may very well be the biggest single capital expenditure a hospital will make.

Nurses and information processing

Notwithstanding the key role of nurses in health care, they have been little involved in the hospital computer revolution. There are a number of reasons for this. Tomasovic blames the data processing experts for threatening and alienating medical and nursing staffs[12]. Zielstorff feels that the problem is one of education; that nurses are lacking the basics of the technology, with little oportunity to learn from more knowledgeable persons[13]. Werley and Grier state that nurses are so involved with the immediate care of patients and families that they become "myopic when it (comes) to influencing the system of which they are critical components"[14]. The possibility of nurse involvement has been virtually ignored (with the notable exception of Austin's excellent book) in the major nonnursing literature devoted to hospital computer applications[15–17].

Nurses are becoming more aware of the potential computers have for enhancing the care they give. This is evident by an increase in the number of published articles, plus the appearance in 1980 and 1981 of the first two books on nursing and computers. Yet the majority of articles in nursing journals, even administration journals, are concerned with clinical applications of computer technology and their planning and management. The clinical emphasis is easily explained: nursing's primary focus is on patient care, where most of the interest lies; and the primary concern of nursing management is patient care[18]. Despite all published evidence of interest, clinical ADP systems are less common than administrative systems because of their cost, complexity, massive staff education requirements, and resistance of potential users[19–21].

Nursing management applications

Very little has been written by or for nurses on nursing service administrative applications, with the exception of a number of articles on nurse scheduling programs. Furthermore, there is nothing on a true management information system for nurse administrators, nor on nursing's potential contribution to an overall hospital management information system. This may reflect Stevens' contention that nursing is one of the last divisions to participate in a computerized system[22]. The nurse administrator is not thereby relieved of seriously considering her information needs and what ADP might do for her. Broad areas of concern must be two: nursing administrative information necessary to manage the daily operations of the department; and nursing management planning and control information to assist middle and long range decision making.

Administrative information systems

Administrative ADP uses are many. Staffing requirements can be determined, generally as a function of patient acuity data[23–25]. There is even an experimental hospital information system in Great Britain which determines staffing needs directly from the care plans entered into the computer[26]. Scheduling, the assignment of specific individuals to shifts, has also been implemented; with the exception of one article, however, these reports have never been published in nursing journals. The ADP applications mentioned above need a close man-machine interaction and are based on an overall cyclical rotation pattern[27, 28]. Computer programmers have attempted to program individual scheduling preferences[29, 30]. There have been efforts to use computers to store staff inservice education records. These programs allow supervisors to use accurate information for evaluation, allow employees to keep track of CEUs for licensing, maintain a record for accrediting agencies, and are a source of data for planning and research[31, 32]. A quality assurance program generates large amounts of data, but to date there has been only one published attempt to use a computer to process such data[33]. Nurse managers also make extensive use of budgetary feedback generated outside the nursing department. To date, there have been no published attempts to integrate this data with nursing generated data.

Management information systems

It is difficult to deal with an administrative system in

isolation—it invariably overlaps with the least developed yet potentially most useful computer application: a management information system. According to Alter the conventional ADP system only permits users to obtain specific sets of data in the form of standard reports at set intervals. A true decision support system would generate standard reports, plus generate data in response to a specific user request[34]. A management information system should be able to: rapidly retrieve isolated data items, such as total hours worked by part time LPNs; retrieve and compare sets of data in differing ways; estimate the consequences of decisions through modeling or simulations; and propose decisions to the manager. In short, the nurse manager should expect more of a computer than automatically generated reports.

Austin lists five management information needs of the modern hospital[35]:

1. Information to assist in setting objectives and in long range planning
2. Information to assist in short term demand forecasting and work planning
3. Information to assist in resource allocation and cost control
4. Information to assist in performance and quality control
5. Information to assist in overall program evaluation

It is obvious that nursing department information must contribute to an overall hospital management information system. Furthermore, such a system should be programmed to fulfill the needs of nurse administrators as well as hospital administrators. There are a few rudimentary systems available: Hospital Administrative Services (HAS), Professional Activity Study (PAS), and CASH. They cannot, however, be tailored to individual hospital needs; each provides information with a different focus, and there is considerable lag time between data input and information output[36]. There have been isolated modeling attempts by hospital administrators and a very primitive simulation attempt by nurses[37, 38].

It is important for the nurse administrator to understand that a management information system will not spring full grown from an existing administrative information system —it must be programmed separately. It is hard to justify, for it is as hard to quantify the effects of improved decision making as it is the effects of quality care. Yet the question "What information do I need to make appropriate management decisions.?" needs to be asked even if the system itself must wait for implementation. According to Alter, "The process of defining the system is every bit as valuable as the system produced"[39].

The nurse administrator's role

The abysmal lack of nurse input in hospital administrative and clinical ADP development cannot continue. Otherwise we will end up attempting to cope with our problems using a tool designed by others according to their perspective of our situation. Nurse involvement must be active, and must start with the nurse executive educating herself about data processing. She may have a nurse expert in computers on the hospital data processing committee, but the nurse executive must have sufficient knowledge to direct and evaluate that expert's work.

Knowledge will also be necessary to enable the nurse executive to contribute to final ADP decisions. For example: what type of system should be chosen—preprogrammed or one programmed to specifications? Should clinical or administrative systems be begun first? In which departments? How can these changes be accomplished most smoothly? Somers is insistent that these decisions must remain the responsibility of a management team consisting of the chief executive officer and the hospital department heads. This team will be able to view the needs of the organization as a whole, laying aside territorialism. The department heads must be as responsible for the success of the system as they are for that of their own departments[40]. ADP knowledge will assist the nursing director in determining what can and can't be done with a computer, and what may be possible but not justifiable fiscally. The wise director will also attempt to both educate her supervisors and tap their perceptions regarding information they need to manage.

Somers also outlines the role of the nurse executive in the planning process:

1. She must know where her department is: the current philosophy, goals, structure and functions as they really are.
2. She must know where it should be going: she should have well developed ADP objectives which coordinate with hospital-wide and interdepartmental objectives.
3. She must know what resources are available to assist her in getting there: what dollars are allocated, what her personnel's capabilities and attitudes are, does the hospital already have a computer—what can it do?
4. She must actively assist in the process of designing and evaluating alternative ways of meeting her objectives.

The nurse executive's role in the implementation of the ADP plan involves allocating resources intelligently: choosing the right people for the project; providing space, supplies, and administrative support (including an active personal interest); and working towards acceptance of the plan by her supervisors.

Evaluation of the ADP project is the most frequently neglected part of ADP implementation. Wooldridge and London give several reasons for this: fear of having to redo all the work if it isn't right; fear of the personal and career consequences of a negative evaluation; too much involvement in other projects; and, worst of all, not being able to evaluate the project because there were no formal, reasoned, quantified objectives against which the ADP system could be measured[42]. An evaluation is also a very expensive, frequently underbudgeted business. But while parts of an evaluation require the expertise of the data processing department or an outside consultant, Zielstorff maintains that the nurse executive, indeed any user, must judge each aspect of the system on two levels[43]:

1. Does it do all that it is supposed to do? (For this you need those quantifiable objectives!) and
2. Does it help, make no difference to, or hinder the user?

"The key to a successful ADP plan involves allocating resources intelligently."

Caveats

Not a single author suggests that managers do without ADP; they do vary in their enthusiasm and the problems they perceive. Wooldridge and London list what they consider good reasons for not having a computer[44]. By considering these carefully, the nurse executive may come to realize when a proposed system should be delayed, or may be able to devise ways to avoid problems.

1. A computer system cannot improve or replace bad management—it will only make it worse. Lesson: get your own house in order first.
2. A computer (or the computer experts) may alienate your staff. Lesson: start brushing up on the change process.
3. Reprogramming is difficult if not impossible for multiple reasons. Programming is in itself difficult. Hospitals rarely have their own programmers and any change requires rehiring one at additional expense. It involves the time and frustration of another "debugging" period for the new program. A change in a nursing portion of a hospital information system may well impact on the programs of other departments, thus requiring both negotiation with them and a far more extensive reprogramming than might have been initially envisioned. Lesson: know exactly what you want when you start, or at least before programming begins.
4. Confidential information is at risk.
5. The high technology costs spiral; everything costs more and takes longer. Lesson: hospitals typically underfund their information systems activities[45]. You may have to remind others on the management team of this.
6. Mistakes are magnified. There may be no more errors than in the old system, but they happen faster and take longer to find and correct.

7. Finally, there are some things that people do better.

After digesting the reasons for not having a computer, it also helps to consider the most common mistakes that can be made in their development[46]. Forewarned is forearmed.

1. Attempting a system that must be all things to all people at once. Lesson: Modular implementation is best. Do one or two functions at a time. Don't start with the worst problem you have.
2. No nurse on the project team.
3. No provision for interdepartmental systems communication from the outset. Lesson: Isolated systems mean double sets of data and increased vulnerability to error.
4. Demanding that the system produce every conceivable report. Lesson: Ask yourself "Why do I need it?"
5. Insufficient managerial support. Lesson: Show interest and support the effort. If you don't, who will? This also means using it once you have it!
6. Design by committee. Lesson: Keep the team small.
7. Technical marvels fail if not user-oriented. Lesson: Get your supervisors involved in management system planning.
8. Loose project control. Lesson: The project manager may know computers and systems inside out, but if she can't manage you might as well forget it!

The key to a successful ADP system is the same as that to a successful nursing department—good management. Managers who are involved in the project from design through evaluation. Managers aware of the pitfalls and armed with plans to avoid them. There is no way to manage a department without coordinating large amounts of administrative, fiscal, and clinical information. The nurse-manager must determine how the computer might assist her, and become involved in systems development as soon as possible.

References

1. Gordon B. Davis, *Management Information Systems: Conceptual Foundations, Structure and Development* (New York: McGraw-Hill Book Company, 1974), p. 123.
2. June B. Somers, "Information Systems: The Process of Development," *The Journal of Nursing Administration* 9(1):53, 1979.
3. Gordon B. Davis, *Management Information Systems: Conceptual Foundations, Structure and Development* p. 32.
4. Robert L. Rees, "Understanding Computers," *The Journal of Nursing Administration* 8(2):4–7, 1978.
5. Robert A. Piankian, "Computer Hardware: Operation, Applications, and Problems," *The Journal of Nursing Administration* 8(2):10–15, 1978.
6. Charles J. Austin, *Information Systems for Hospital Administration* (Ann Arbor, Mich.: Health Administration Press, 1979), pp. 220–238.
7. Regina Herzlinger, "Management Non-information Systems in Health Care Organizations," *Health Care Management Review* 1:71–76, 1976.
8. Regina Herzlinger, "Why Data Systems in Nonprofit Organizations Fail," *Harvard Business Review* 55:81–86, 1977.

9. Stephen M. Veazie, "Management of Computerized Systems Noted," *Hospitals* 54(7):97–102, 1980.

10. Suzanne LaViolette, "Too Much Technology, Not Enough Control," *Modern Healthcare* 11(5):102 & 104, 1981.

11. Stephen M. Veazie, "Management of Computerized Systems Noted," p. 97.

12. Elizabeth R. Tomasovic, "'Turning Nurses On' to Automation," *Hospitals* 46(9)80–86, 1972.

13. Rita D. Zielstorff, ed. *Computers in Nursing* (Wakefield, Mass.: Nursing Resources, 1980), p. x.

14. Harriet H. Werley and Margaret R. Grier, eds *Nursing Information Systems* (New York: Springer Publishing Company, 1981) p. ix.

15. George A. Bekey and Morton D. Swartz, eds. *Hospital Information Systems* (New York: Marcel Dekker Inc., 1972).

16. Morris F. Collen, ed. *Hospital Computer Systems* (New York: John Wiley and Sons, 1974).

17. Roger H. Shannon, ed. *Hospital Information Systems* (New York: North-Holland Publishing Company, 1979).

18. Barbara J. Stevens, *The Nurse as Executive* (Wakefield, Mass.: Nursing Resources, 1980), p. xiv.

19. Charles J. Austin, *Information Systems for Hospital Administration,* p. 164.

20. Gary L. Hammon, "The Future of Hospital Information Systems," *Hospital Information Systems,* ed. Roger H. Shannon. (New York: North-Holland Publishing Company, 1979), p. 351.

21. Alan F. Dowling, "Do Hospital Staff Interfere with Computer Implementation?," *Health Care Management Review* 5(4):23–32, 1980.

22. Barbara J. Stevens, *The Nurse as Executive,* p. 352.

23. James A. Bahr, et al. "Innovative Methodology Enhances Nurse Deployment, Cuts Costs," *Hospitals* 51(8): 104–109, 1977.

24. Ronald Norby, et al. "A Nurse Staffing System Based Upon Assignment Difficulty," *The Journal of Nursing Administration* 7(9):2–24, 1977.

25. Chris E. Brouhard, et al. "A Management Information System to Monitor Nursing Care Hours," *Management Information Systems: A Collection of Case Studies* (Chicago, Ill.: American Hospital Association, 1978), pp. 41–59.

26. Christina R. Henney and Richard N. Bosworth, "A Computer Based System for the Automatic Production of Nursing Workload Data," *Nursing Times* 76: 1212–1217, 1980.

27. Hira Ahuja and Robert Sheppard, "Computerized Nurse Scheduling," *Industrial Engineering* 7:24–29, 1975.

28. Donna J. Ballantyne, "A Computerized Scheduling System with Centralized Staffing," *The Journal of Nursing Administration* 9(3): 38–45, 1979.

29. Michael D. Warner, "Scheduling Nursing Personnel According to Nursing Preference: A Mathematical Programming Approach," *Operations Research* 24 (5):842–856, 1976.

30. L. Douglas Smith, et al., "A Computerized System to Schedule Nurses that Recognizes Staff Preferences," *Hospital and Health Services Administration* 24 (4):19–33, 1979.

31. John M. Dixon, et al. "A Computerized Education and Training Record," *Computers in Nursing,* ed. Rita D. Zielstorff, pp. 59–62.

32. David L. Moon, "Data Processing in Staff Development," *Nursing Management* 13:23–25, 1982.

33. Marsha Barney, "Measuring Quality of Patient Care: A Computerized Approach," *Supervisory Nurse* 12: 40–44, 1981.

34. Stephen L. Alter, "How Effective Managers Use Information Systems," *Harvard Business Review* 54:97–104, 1976.

35. Charles J. Austin, *Information Systems for Hospital Administration,* p. 221.

36. Charles J. Austin, *Information Systems for Hospital Administration,* p. 224–225.

37. Mark Chase, et al., "Modeling a Hospital Entrance System," *Dimension Health Services* 57(1):16–20, 1980.

38. N. Duraiswamy, et al., "Using Computer Simulations to Predict ICU Staffing Needs," *The Journal of Nursing Administration* 11(2):39–44, 1981.

39. Stephen L. Alter, "How Effective Managers Use Information Systems," p. 104.

40. June B. Somers, "Information Systems: the Process of Development," p. 54

41. June B. Somers, "Information Systems: the Process of Development," p. 55–56.

42. Susan Wooldridge and Keith London, *The Computer Survival Handbook* (Boston: Gambit, 1973), p. 140.

43. Rita D. Zielstorff, "The Planning and Evaluation of Automated Systems: A Nurse's Point of View," *The Journal of Nursing Administration* 5(6):22–25, 1975.

44. Susan Wooldridge and Keith London, *The Computer Survival Handbook,* p. 32–39.

45. Regina Herzlinger, "Why Data Systems in Nonprofit Organizations Fail," p. 82.

46. A.S. Walker, "The 10 Most Common Mistakes in Developing Computer Based Personnel Systems," *Personnel Administration* 25 (7):39–42, 1980.

CHAPTER 29

Planning for Purchase and Implementation of an Automated Hospital Information System: A Nursing Perspective

by Erica L. Drazen

Planning for purchase, implementation, and use of an automated hospital information system is critical to its success. The planning process involves assessing needs, evaluating alternatives, selecting a system, and implementation support. Although an evaluation of costs and benefits of alternative systems is useful in planning for and selecting a system, the assessment can be very complex, and the assumptions used in the analysis are critical. Most benefits of automated systems are the result of improved timeliness, accuracy, and access to information, and these are difficult to value in dollars.

Why you should be interested

Your hospital currently is purchasing or will in the near future purchase automated information systems which may have profound impacts on the way care is delivered within your institution. These systems may provide better information for nursing care, greatly aid in the record keeping process, and may come to be viewed as invaluable by your nursing staff. They may also be a costly disaster. Proper planning is essential in making the decision to automate, selecting the right system, and receiving benefits from the automated system you purchase.

One thing is certainly true: If you are not involved in planning for future automated systems in your hospital, you should be. Therefore, when I was asked to write an article for *The Journal of Nursing Administration* on evaluating costs of automated information systems, I enthusiastically accepted.

The editors stated that the purpose of the article was to help nursing administrators be more informed participants in the evaluation of automated systems. I was asked to write an article about methodologies used to evaluate the cost impacts of automated information systems, which would focus on methods for predicting labor savings. After writing a 10-page introduction, which I thought did not touch on all of the important issues, I gave up.

Problems with cost-benefit analysis as a planning tool

The reasons for my problems in writing the article were twofold:

- *Evaluating cost impacts of Automated Hospital Information Systems is a very complex process, and developing methodologies for such studies is probably best undertaken by evaluation researchers.* There are, in my opinion, no validated, practical methodologies within the public domain which can be used as a guide in conducting a study. Many of the methodologies used in the past have been later shown to be based on faulty assumptions. A review of evaluation methodologies, which analyzes 10 methodologies used in past studies (in 192 pages), is available as a resource to any nursing administrator who wants to pursue this complex subject[1].

- *I do not feel that direct cost savings, especially labor reductions, are the major benefit of implementing an automated information system.* The *major benefits* of any of these automated systems are the increased timeliness, accuracy, completeness, and accessibility of information used in patient care delivery and management of the delivery process. I think evaluation of cost savings (and particularly of labor savings) should be only one component of an evaluation of automated systems.

You may be asked or required to prepare a cost-benefit analysis when you are deciding to purchase a system, or a cost-benefit analysis may be prepared by an outside consult-

Erica L. Drazen is Manager of the Health Care Technology Unit at Arthur D. Little, Inc., Cambridge, Massachusetts. She received a B.S. in Mechanical Engineering from Tufts University and an M.S. in Mechanical Engineering from the Massachusetts Institute of Technology. She is currently a doctoral candidate in Health Policy and Management, Harvard University School of Public Health.

ant or a system vendor. I urge you to be very careful to review such an analysis for its reasonableness, especially if you will be required to deliver all the cost savings promised. I will next illustrate some of the problems with an erroneous cost-benefit analysis of an automated laboratory information system. I will consider only those benefits most relevant to nursing—those accruing to users outside the laboratory itself.

With this automated laboratory system, laboratory test orders can be entered at a terminal at the nursing station, automatically checked for conflict with diet and medications, and transmitted in seconds to the laboratory without risk of their being misplaced, or having missing patient identification. The results also can be checked against normal ranges, compared with past results to identify outliers and possible errors, and can be available in the nursing station seconds after they are complete. The status of the test can be checked at any time. In addition, test results can be displayed to show trends over time, correlations with treatment, etc.

There are several benefits of such an automated system to nursing:

1. Test orders and results will not be lost (or delayed and assumed lost), nor will tests be invalid because of conflict with diet and medications. Therefore, fewer tests will have to be reordered. The elimination of unnecessary repeat tests—which may account for 5 percent of all test orders—is one benefit of the system.
2. Since test results will be available sooner, therapy may be initiated sooner, and patient stays reduced—another benefit of the system.
3. There will be fewer telephone calls to and from the laboratory to check on the status of tests and to obtain results of STAT tests. This will save the nursing staff time.
4. Quality information needed for patient care will improve. Information will be available sooner; more information, for example, on trends, will be readily available for use in decision making; and there will be more checks on information to ensure its accuracy.
5. The information on tests conducted for each patient will be automatically transferred to the accounting system, so billing will be more complete and accurate.

Moreover, the (erroneous) cost-benefit analysis shows a cost savings of $650,000 per year associated with the benefits cited above (see Exhibit 1).

I agree that the five benefits listed above may be major potential benefits of a laboratory information system (from a nursing perspective), and they might be reasons for purchasing a system. However, none of these benefits will result in cost reduction to the hospital which would offset the cost of the system's purchase.

I would like to review these "savings" to illustrate some of the potential pitfalls in a cost-benefit analysis.

EXHIBIT 1.
(ERRONEOUS) COST ANALYSIS*

5 percent decrease $5.50 supply savings/patient day x 200 patients x 365 days	= $ 20,000
2 percent decrease 8 days x $200/day x 9,000 admissions	= $290,000
¼ hr./patient day x 200 patients x $13.50 x 365 days	= $250,000
5 percent increase in charge capture x 9,000 admissions x $200 laboratory costs/admission	= $ 90,000
	$650,000

*Assumes 200 patient average census, 9,000 admissions per year, 8-day length of stay.

---

1. A change in the number of unnecessary repeat tests (due to lost results, conflicts with medications, etc.) will result in a decreased cost of the patient's treatment. The patient's bill will be less, and ultimately the savings will be reflected in lower health insurance costs. However, only if the hospital is being reimbursed a fixed cost by diagnosis will this result in increased income for the hospital.
2. A change in hospital stay benefits the patient and community, but does not save money for the hospital (except as above).
3. Assume that nurses spend an average of 5 minutes per shift per patient in telephoning for test results, and this was totally eliminated with the automated system. With an average occupancy of 200 patients, the total daily savings would be 50 hours of nursing time per day. However, does this mean that you now need nine less nurses and can save the hospital $250,000 per year in personnel expense? Most surely not, because the time savings cannot be aggregated across shifts and wards. The benefit will be in more satisfied nursing staff, not direct cost reductions.
4. The quality of care benefit is probably the most important system benefit, and it cannot be quantified or expressed in dollar terms.
5. The improved charge capture is unrelated to *costs* of service. The cost of a laboratory test is incurred when the test is performed, and exists irrespective of billing. Therefore, improved billing does not result in a decrease in cost of care to the patient or society; it *may* result in increased revenue to the hospital for a small group of patients, but not for the majority of patients who are covered by cost-reimbursement set rates.

Although faster turnaround, reduced need to call for laboratory results, more timely initiation of therapy, and improved accuracy of data all may be important benefits of automated laboratory services, they probably will not reduce nursing staff needs or the hospital budget. A decision based on cost savings might be the right decision, but would be made for the wrong reasons. Making the right decision for the right reasons requires different planning tools.

A planning framework

There are three essential attributes for the successful implementation of an automated hospital information system:

1. You should have a need for the system,
2. The system should meet that need, and
3. The system must work.

Therefore, the three essential elements of the planning process are:

1. Determining need for a system,
2. Selecting the best system, and
3. Assuring that the system will function as planned.

Needs assessment

Needs assessment is the most critical and most neglected step in the process. A proper needs assessment will help ensure that if you buy a system it will represent a solution for your problems, not just the most advanced, the most complex, or the most costly possible system.

Needs assessment starts with a list of information problems or needs in each department. You must identify the unmet needs of the laboratory, the pharmacy, and the nursing stations. It is important not to exclude needs that seem unrelated to an information system—for example, word processing for the radiology department or scheduling assignments in nursing. After a list of needs is developed these must be ordered on the basis of priority; essential requirements must be identified. The second step in the needs assessment process is to obtain consensus among departments and administration on the priorities of the hospital—these will form the basis for making decisions about the purchase of automated systems.

After you have defined a list of requirements you then have to specify what information is needed, how much data should be available, how accessible the data should be, and how data should be displayed. For instance, you may want to keep *all* inpatient information in active storage within the system, but only keep outpatient data for 7 days. Or, you may want to integrate laboratory data with a display of the patient's medications. Where you are unsure of your requirements, decisions can be postponed until future planning resolves them.

Evaluation of costs and benefits

At this stage you have defined what your system would do; now you need to decide whether to buy one.

Although I have outlined the potential pitfalls in relying on a cost analysis as the only planning tool, in order to compare alternative systems it is important to analyze the costs of automating and to quantify, where possible, the benefits you expect from each system.

Net costs of automating can be estimated by:

Initial system cost (obtained from vendors or other sources)
+ Operating cost (maintenance, personnel)
- Cost of any automated systems being displaced
- Cost of any personnel being displaced (the system may automate whole jobs in some departments—for instance, in admitting, registration, or billing—and permit staff reductions).

"You need to consider whether the vendor . . . will be able to . . . upgrade the system to meet future needs."

Many noncost benefits of automation can be quantified. This usually requires a study of the existing operating process to determine:

How long it takes for late results to get back?
How many results are lost?
How many tests are reordered because results are not found?
What is the rate of discrepancy between ordered and administered medications, etc.?
How many test results are filed in the wrong chart?
How many outpatients are seen without medical records?

It is then quite simple to estimate the possible changes in this information which might be effected by automation and to estimate the net benefits of automation. When costs have been totaled and benefits estimated, the question to be answered is: Is it worth "X" dollars (the expected net costs) to effect these changes (the expected net benefits)?

This analysis can be performed for single applications, for example, for automation of the laboratory or pharmacy, or for an integrated system.

If you make a decision to purchase a system, the next part of the process is selecting the system.

System selection

You want to select a system that meets your needs and will deliver the benefits you have predicted. That means it must contain the correct hardware design and software applications.

Selecting the hardware is relatively easy since it changes less frequently than software. Usually, what you see is what you get. It is important to determine whether there will be enough terminals available to access and retrieve data, and whether the terminals can be used easily by the required staff: for example, Is the system designed so that *nurses* are required to *type* requests into the system? Will the terminals fit in the space you have available?

Although an initial screening of hardware can be made by visiting shows, receiving literature, or visiting the vendor, in order to evaluate the equipment it is essential that you view it in actual operation; therefore, site visits to hospitals already using the equipment must be part of the evaluation process.

Evaluation of whether software will meet your requirements is more complex. Every vendor offers software which has some unique features, which may or may not be of benefit to you.

You need to decide what capabilities you want and also how much data are needed, what type of displays you need, etc. Again, discussion with current users, whose patient care requirements are similar to yours, is very helpful in evaluating different options. You need to be very cautious of the assurance that the software you need, although not currently standard, will be "no problem" to develop. It may or may not be a "problem." However, asking the vendor to put a priority on developing a unique feature just for your installation, with the likelihood that it will work on the first try, will most likely lead to problems.

You also need to consider whether the vendor you select will be able to continue to upgrade the system to meet future needs. You must ask yourself: is the vendor investing in research and development; do they have a commitment to the industry; do they have the next generation of products in mind; will these products be compatible with your system, etc.?

Successful implementation

The third critical planning step is to be sure that the system works well when it arrives—both technically and operationally. Of course, you must write performance specifications into the system contract. The American Hospital Association has developed guidelines which can be used in writing technical specifications for your system[2]. Despite the best planning and selection efforts, you will probably want to change some aspects of the system after it has been installed. Therefore, it is important to plan flexibility into the contract.

System reliability is also essential. Obtaining a "proven" system, one which has worked well in prior installations, is some assurance of reliability. If you decide to be the first purchaser of any system features, it is important to verify that they have been well tested within an operating environment, and that they are not critical to the operation of other system applications.

Another way to ensure initial system reliability is to pretest the system in your own environment. The safest way to do this is to run automated and manual systems in parallel during a test period. However, this often results in an increase in the workload which is not acceptable.

A useful strategy is to put the system into use gradually—for example, automate one section of the laboratory, or one ward. The "bugs" of the system can be worked out during the initial trial, where they will have only a limited impact on hospital operations.

Another key to successful system implementation is training. Usually, the vendor offers initial "classroom-style" training of the staff. This is not enough. Hands-on experience with the system is also necessary. You should arrange to have access to a system (usually one located on the vendor's site, to which you have access over telephone lines). This system can be made available to your staff for leisurely practice and familiarization, or can be integrated into the formal training program. Whenever this system is available for training, a knowledgeable person must be available to answer questions.

During the initial implementation of your own system, it is also essential that a knowledgeable person be available to conduct training sessions, and perform troubleshooting whenever the system is in use. (This may mean that knowledgeable help must be available 24 hours a day, 7 days a week.) Anything less may result in the development of negative feelings toward the system, which will take a long time to overcome. It is also important to keep a log of technical and operational problems with the system, for use in planning future systems. A log of training questions and issues (based on calls for assistance) will be useful in designing future training materials and programs. Plans also need to be made for ongoing training to orient new employees or introduce new system features.

Finally, it is important to make evaluation of the system an ongoing process. You should monitor the system in use to see if expected benefits are being realized, and to identify changes in the system or operations that would result in enhanced system benefits or reduced costs.

References

1. Arthur D. Little, Inc., *Methods for Evaluating Costs of Automated Hospital Information Systems,* 1980. *Summary* available free from NCHSR Publications and Information Branch, Room 7-44, 3700 East-West Highway, Hyattsville, MD 20782. Complete Report available from NTIS, Springfield, VA 22161. Reference No. PB 80 178593, cost $17.50, or from Erica Drazen, Arthur D. Little, Inc., Acorn Park, 20A/257, Cambridge, MA 02140, cost $17.00.
2. American Hospital Association, *Hospital Computer Systems Planning: Preparation of Request for Proposal.* (840 North Lake Shore Drive, Chicago, IL 60611 : AHA Catalog No. 1445, August 1980).

UNIT SEVEN

CYNTHIA M. FREUND

Trends and Issues

It is much easier to identify trends and issues today than to predict trends and critical issues for the future. For example, in 1983 federal legislation mandated a new financing mechanism for the medicare program — a prospective payment system (PPS) based on diagnostic related groups (DRGs). This new payment system signalled a new trend, one that would result in radical changes in the methods of financing all health care services and programs. The signal was deafening and the entire health care industry was preoccupied with it. DRGs drew everyone's attention: they were discussed in the corridors and board rooms of health institutions; they were the central topic of national, regional, and local conferences; and they dotted the literature and mass media. Thus, it was not difficult to predict the new fiscal order and related trends and issues.

In contrast, other trends and issues emerge in a more subtle fashion. They are not made apparent by some radical change and they may not draw a lot of attention initially. Rather, they evolve gradually and become identifiable as a trend mid-course or *post facto*. Such evolving trends, however, often turn out to be as significant as more overt ones. The articles collected in this section are representative of the more subtle but significant trends evolving in nursing administration.

In the past, the chief nursing officer was commonly known as the director of nursing; today, this person is viewed as an "executive" with all the prerogatives, privileges, and responsibilities accorded other executives. The nurse executive is not only responsible for the daily operations of the nursing organization; as an executive, he or she has a responsibility to lead the nursing organization, with a clear vision of the future. One way to establish a clear vision and future direction is through strategic planning, as described by Fox and Fox in *Strategic Planning for Nursing*. Fox and Fox identify many advantages associated with strategic planning, but say that, "The development of a keen sense of direction for nursing is first among the benefits of the formal planning process."

Nursing executives' concerns can not be limited to the internal environment of the nursing organization. Fox and Fox recommend basing plans and strategies not only on nursing's internal environment but also on its external environment. This notion is reinforced in Sheridan's article, *The Health Care Industry in the Marketplace: Implications for Nursing*. Sheridan describes free market systems and economic theory and examines the effect of recent economic trends on the health industry and nursing. She too suggests that nurse executives be cognizant of the external environment: "For nursing to survive, nurse administrators must develop strategies based on economic theories and realities." Likewise, O'Toole and O'Toole take the nurse executive away from their internal environment into the realm of interorganizational cooperation and coordination. In *Negotiating Cooperative Agreements Between Health Organizations*, they point out that ". . . the solutions to health care problems cannot be found in a single organization." Many solutions require cooperation and coordination of several institutions. The growth of multi-institutional systems will increase the demands on nurse executives for cooperation and coordination; negotiating skills will be crucial for success in these new forms of interorganizational relationships. Furthermore, the nurse executive's increasing sphere of influence within his or her own institution also requires a keen sense of the negotiation process. Thus, O'Toole and O'Toole's exploration of negotiation has relevance for the nurse executive both within and outside of his or her own organization.

While moving from an operational role to an executive role, nurse executives are also creating a new environment and a new relationship between themselves and professional nursing staff. McClelland notes that "Management and nurses are mutually dependent on one another. Their relationship is characterized by symbiosis, not domination and submission." Although McClelland, in *Professionalism and Collective Bargaining: A New Reality for Nurses and Management*, uses a highly charged issue to make her point, she believes that ". . . health care professionals must play complementary roles rather than competing roles. . . ." Warren, in *Accountability and Nursing Diagnosis*, makes a similar point. She suggests that a taxonomy of nursing diagnoses not only provides a scientific base for nursing, but also serves as a link for managerial and professional conjoint accountability. Hunt and associates, in *Networking: A Managerial Strategy for Research Development in a Service Setting*, emphasize the nursing executive's responsibility for encouraging professionalism by ". . . creating a climate conducive to research." They describe a network that was developed between three hospitals for the purpose of promoting research. Although McClelland, Warren, and Hunt and associates use different frameworks, they all reinforce the notion of interdependence between the nursing administration and the professional staff.

In the six articles in this section, two major themes or trends run throughout. One is the changing focus of the nurse administrator's role, which is evolving from an operational to an executive role. The second is the nurse executive's responsibility to nurture and support the professionalism of nursing. If nursing is to survive and be effective in a highly complex and rapidly changing environment, nursing must have a clear vision for itself, professional practice must thrive, and all nurses must be united and cohesive in their efforts.

CHAPTER 30

The Health Care Industry in the Marketplace: Implications for Nursing

by Donna Richards Sheridan

Recent economic changes have had a substantial impact on health care. For nursing to survive, nurse administrators must develop strategies based on economic theories and realities. Reaganomics is based on many of Milton Friedman's theories and frameworks. This article explores these theories as they apply to future nursing opportunities. As a nurse administrator you feel the economic crunch—now it's time to base your strategies on these realities.

Traditional health care delivery systems currently face a variety of economic challenges resulting from shifts in supply and demand for health care and pricing changes within the health care industry. Health care costs are escalating rapidly and taxpayers demand financial accountability from health care providers. Since the '60s consumers have become more knowledgeable about health care and now seek more information to make their own choices regarding health care. Increased types and numbers of providers create a new competitive environment in the supply side of the market. General economic policy shifts such as supply side economics (encouraging people to work and invest by cutting taxes), reduction in the size and scope of government, and the new federalism (the return of many federal government functions to the state level) are forcing a response by the professions.

The nursing profession stands to lose or gain much during this period of change. Understanding current trends and their probable effects on general economics and the future direction of the health care industry is essential for professional survival and, if appropriate strategies are designed to deal with these effects, advancement of the profession.

This article uses Milton Friedman's economic framework[1] to explore the economic situation as it applies to nursing. Friedman's explanation of free market essentially

is based on the economic classic *Wealth of Nations* by Adam Smith[2], the father of modern economics. Friedman's support of a strong marketplace is reflected in the core of Reaganomics—a current reality for each of us. The concepts underlying Reaganomics contrast with the opposing views of John Galbraith[3], a Keynesian advocate of extensive governmental programs and budgeting to maintain a high level of employment while accepting increased taxes to support these programs.

The free market

The power of the free market

The market transmits accurate information as sellers (suppliers) meet buyers (demanders) and goods or services are exchanged willingly between the two for a price. The relationship of quantity supplied to quantity demanded determines the price for which the good is sold. Prices perform three functions: the transmission of information; an incentive to use the least costly methodology for production; and a determinant of who gets how much of the product. The price system transmits information to those who need it, without clogging the "in baskets" of those who don't. This mechanism is efficient because the people who are in a position to use the information, both suppliers and demanders, seek each other out.

Two current threats to the market

Two recent serious threats to this free market system exist in many industries, including health care. These threats, monopoly and inflation, have had serious untoward effects on industry and on the economy. Through executive and legislative changes, however, both threats are being attacked. And, this war on monopoly and inflation has grave consequences for health care providers.

Supply side economics attacks inflation by fostering decreased government size and spending and increasing

Donna Richards Sheridan, R.N., M.S., is Management Development Coordinator at Stanford University Hospital, Palo Alto, California and an MBA candidate at Pepperdine University, Malibu, California.

value spending (i.e., getting more value for your money). Therefore patients will do more "shopping around" for their care. Attacks on monopolies and antitrust interventions change territorial norms of the health care providers. Therefore, health care providers will begin to "sell" their services to maintain or increase their territory. These issues lead to increased supplier competition in health care.

Other interferences in the health care market

Too much government. Thomas Jefferson, like Adam Smith, saw concentrated government power as a threat to the ordinary man. Jefferson viewed government as an umpire: "a wise and frugal government, which shall restrain men from injuring one another, which shall leave them otherwise free to regulate their own pursuits of industry and improvement"[4]. Friedman points out that now "one government policy after another has been set up to 'regulate' our 'pursuits of industry and improvement,' standing Jefferson's dictum on its head"[5]. This extensive government expansion has skyrocketed the national debt to a record 90 billion dollars. Financial accountability and cutbacks are essential to avoid the collapse of an overinflated economy.

Friedman states, "Extra government spending has been paralleled by a rapid growth in private health insurance"[6]. Between 1965 and 1977, total medical care spending doubled its fraction of the national income. The inevitable result has been steep increases in health care prices.

Third party payers. Consumers (demanders) usually do not buy directly from sellers (health care providers). Direct consumer outlays account for only 32.4 percent of the health care dollar. Private insurance pays for 26.6 percent and government picks up the largest part of the tab—39.7 percent[7].

Friedman explores this problem with the non-direct payment system in the following table:

You are the spender

Whose money	On whom spent	
	You	Someone Else
Yours	I	II
Someone Else's	III	IV

In category one, you are spending your own money on yourself—an incentive to get value for your dollar. In category two, you are spending your money on someone else—the same incentive exists. In category three, you are spending someone else's money on yourself—your incentive to save is decreased (e.g., expense account eating). In category four, you are spending someone else's money on still another person—very little incentive to save [8].

Government and private insurance companies act within the latter two categories, which provide little incentive to get value for *our* dollar. Furthermore, their program administration costs and their profits also are deducted from our money.

Medical monopoly. Monopoly, control over a particular commodity by one producer or a cartel of producers, distorts the price system of the market by preventing prices from freely reflecting conditions of supply and demand[9]. Medicine comprises a monopoly because, by definition, pure or absolute monopoly exists[10] when a single firm (in this case the American Medical Association) is the sole producer of a product for which there is no close substitute.

"Two recent serious threats exist to this free market system..."

The absence of competitors is explainable primarily through barriers to entry. Newhouse believes entry into medicine is restricted because one must have a license to practice[11]. That license is attainable only after completing medical school where barriers to entry exist through rationed number of entries or the inconvenience and expense of medical education abroad.

Friedman believes that a monopoly seldom can be established in a country without overt and covert government assistance in the form of a tariff or some other mechanism[12]. The United States government does support medical schools with tax money. In addition, the American Medical Association maintains physician territorial rights by extensive congressional lobbying and securing key positions on third party provider boards.

Government and economic trends

Decreased government

Galbraith[13], renowned economist of the Kennedy era, espouses a large government philosophy. During the 1975 economic crisis in New York City, Galbraith advised that there is no problem that cannot be solved by spending more money. The cost of this strategy has ended in a current national debt of 90 billion dollars.

Friedman, by contrast, believes you can't solve problems by throwing money at them. He goes even further saying, great government spending, excessive government interference, and paternalistic government programs affect the very fabric of our society by

- Weakening the family
- Reducing incentive to work, save, innovate
- Reducing accumulation of capital and
- Limiting our freedom [14].

Reagan's election has been interpreted as a voter demand for new economic policies and less government spending[15]. Several national polls indicated that Reagan's supply side economics was expected to lead the way to an improved economy[16, 17]. Based on Friedman's theories, however, supply side economics emphasizes "the negative effects of higher tax rates on peoples' willingness to work, save, and invest...and limits money supply to contain inflationary pressures"[18].

The intent of Reagan's policies is to increase private sector production by decreasing government involvement. Before Reagan took office, says De Witt, the health care industry had little hopes of seeing the end to onerous regulations[19]. Now, according to McCann, counsel for the American Hospital Association's Division of Legislation and Regulation, "The Reagan Administration clearly is more interested in looking at programs to determine whether they are needed, what their objectives are, and whether the regulations meet those objectives[20].

Increased competition

In the mid-1970s, the Supreme Court ruled that the "learned professions" are subject to antitrust law[21]. The American Medical Association has been sued for its ban on advertising. Lower courts upheld a Federal Trade Commission ruling that such restraint is anticompetitive[22]. Other such challenges to antitrust law include a fee schedule for member-doctor services set by a county foundation in Arizona, which violates the Sherman Antitrust Act[23]. Refusal to reimburse clinical psychologists unless billed through an MD is the basis of a suit in Virginia against Blue Shield[24]. The Federal Trade Commission is questioning if doctor-controlled prepaid medical insurance plans restrict competition[25]. In Ohio seven antitrust suits have been filed since 1975, one of which charges an illegal boycott forced the closure of a Health Maintenance Organization[26]. Removal of restraints will increase competition and provide impetus for innovations in health care delivery.

Physician competition also will increase as the predicted oversupply of U.S. physicians becomes a reality. Although expected to occur in 1990, some observers believe physician oversupply already has begun[27]. Emily Friedman[28] predicts the realities of competition among physicians will include:

- Physician income will fall—the average net income of MDs already fell between 1970 and 1980[29].
- Board-certified physicians will move to small towns—a trend which has begun[30].
- Specialists will provide some of the care previously given by generalists—another trend which has begun [31].
- Doctors will initiate a visit from a patient[32].
- California's attempts to decrease the influx of physicians into the state include writing a tough new licensing examination[33].
- Nurse practitioners will be at risk—"The major effect will be on nurse practitioners, who have done the most to take

over health assessment, physical assessment, and counseling"[34].
- MDs are trying to regain what was once considered less desired health care territory and now is provided by nurse practitioners and physicians' assistants—using such methods as limiting scope of practice or, as is the case in eleven states, threats of arrest for practicing medicine without a license[35].

"Removal of restraints will increase competition and provide impetus for innovations in health care delivery."

- Competition, among specialists, for parts of the body is expected to intensify[36].
- Foreign medical school graduates will be excluded[37].
- Women physicians who often prefer group practice will face increased competition from male physicians who will accept the group practice alternative given less private practice career choices[38].
- Salaried positions for hospital physicians are expected to become more common[39].
- Physician-controlled emergency centers will pull profits away from such hospital services as laboratory, surgery, and radiology[40].
- Fad medical treatments for such conditions as obesity, behavioral problems and sports injuries will increase [41].
- Physicians may spend more time with individual patients, explain treatments, provide emotional support, provide more convenient office hours, walk-in serv-and free consultations[42].
- More care may be provided to patients now neglected in prisons, mental institutions and long-term facilities as well as the chronically ill and the elderly confined to their homes[43].
- The house call may make a comeback.
- Territorial battles are predicted between physicians and hospitals, physicians and nurses, and physicians with each other.

Other health care professionals have already begun competitive activities. Spurred on by an oversupply in their field, professionals often use legislative lobbying to open up creative opportunities and to try to block entry into their territory by competing fields.

Dentistry is one such example of a health care profession glutted with practitioners. New dentists have difficulty starting a practice. Even many established dentists promote their services through advertising. Group practices offer such incentives as a free first visit, and weekend or evening services. Even so, bankruptcies are no longer rare among young dentists[44].

Pharmacists are another group experiencing competition. Increasingly, pharmacists no longer own their stores, and are employed within bureaucracies. With the advent of advertising and generic naming of products, competitive pricing for medications is commonplace—a practice once considered unethical and illegal.

Hospitals also compete among themselves, Health Maintenance Organizations, and some privately-owned individual services such as laboratories. Expensive equipment, often quickly outmoded, is purchased to lure physicians to bring patients to their facility.

With too many hospitals opening after passage of the post-World War II Burton-Hill Act, many began to face bankruptcy in the seventies. Since then, some hospitals have incorporated, a popular business strategy, allowing diversification of assets during changing economic times[45].

Strategies for the nursing profession

The effects of the changing economy will not leave the nursing profession untouched. Nursing must be ready to meet the inevitable challenges of increased competition and the free market system. Strategies must be devised to meet competition and increase the profession's foothold in current territory. Goals toward which the profession should move include:

Legislative. Nursing practice needs to be clearly defined in the Nurse Practice Act to reflect the realities of current practice. Rather than lagging behind practice, the law should be at the forefront of our newly assumed responsibilities.

Also, nursing must use collective power. The effect of combining our two professional organizations, the American Nurses' Association and the National League for Nursing would be synergistic, increasing our power considerably. Rather than diffusing our power by hanging out our dirty laundry for the world to see, let us join together and air our conflicts within one organization.

Instead of working on separate goals, we must unite to achieve our common goals of quality health care and increased professional status. With one strong representative organization, paid lobbyist positions should increase. Lobbyists not only need seek government money, of which there will be little, but also develop a sphere of influence and power as has the American Medical Association. This power can be used to advance the rights of consumers in health care choices and support direct payment by third party payers to nurses and other non-physician health care providers.

Competition. Nurses must learn to compete in the marketplace, and raising our image is a priority in this

effort. We need to protest television shows and literature which detracts from our image. We must inform patients, families, and friends what today's nurses do.

As traditional patient advocates, nurses must continue to teach health care and become more visable and available directly to the consumer. Innovative methods to reach the public must be explored.

"Because of less available government funding, nurses must be assertive in seeking private foundation money..."

We must write and speak not only to our professional colleagues but also to consumers. The body of knowledge essential to professional status demands recording in the literature. Health care knowledge needs to be shared with the public through consumer journals; books; childrens' television programs, books, and comics; videocassettes, large print books, and senior center programs for the elderly; and recordings for the blind. Preventive medicine *is* nursing—treating people, not body parts. Educating for prevention and best level of wellness is traditionally a nursing role—let's mark this territory and compete here.

Also, nurses need to stake out newer found territories in addition to such old standbys as gerontology, alcoholism counseling, midwifery, stress counseling, and critical care nursing.

Nurses must sit on third-party payers' boards and boards of other community organizations to help frame policies. In addition, we need to contribute to development of precedents in health care institutions through policies, grievance procedures, and bargaining on practice issues.

Research. Moreover, nurses must become more involved in research as the basis and foundation of practice. Because of less available government funding, nurses must be assertive in seeking private foundation money to advance nursing research and patient care goals.

The value of nursing care must be clearly defined and separated out from room charges. Patient care provided by nurses should be clearly identified on hospital and other health care bills; and patients should be charged by the level of nursing care received.

Studies analyzing nursing care cost-benefits are timely and essential. Insufficient data exists to justify our gut feeling that many aspects of health care are provided more efficiently and effectively by nurses than other health care professionals. Quality, efficiency, and cost-containment must be linked through research.

Education for management. Nursing must continue to

develop professional leaders and seek new techniques to prepare nurses for these challenging roles. Management development courses must be offered to new nurse managers. Graduate degrees in nursing administration need to include economics, finance, and marketing courses to prepare nurse executives for today's demanding management roles.

Nursing education. Educators need to explore and teach the latest nursing roles along with more traditional roles. Use of nursing research as a basis for practice needs to be integrated into all practice courses, rather than included only in pure research courses. Education and service must recognize their interrelated dependencies and support each other—decreasing adversary roles is not enough.

Conclusion

Although there will always be shoddy products, quacks and con artists, on the whole the consumer is best protected by market competition, says Friedman[46]. And market competition is affecting the health care field.

"No one has clearly articulated the limits of competition or the impact of competition on various types of providers and actual delivery of health services," says Colloton[47]. But, as McNerny adds, "For every force there will be a countervailing force. Progress will be evolutionary, through competition, voluntary efforts, and regulation"[48]. It is essential that the nursing profession prepare for and be flexible during this challenging period.

References

1. Milton Friedman and Rose Friedman, *Free to Choose* (New York, N.Y.: Avon, 1979).
2. Milton Friedman, *Free to Choose*, p. 303.
3. John Galbraith, *The New Industrial State* (New York, N.Y.: Houghton, Mifflin, 1978).
4. Thomas Jefferson, Inaugural Address, 1801.
5. Milton Friedman, *Free to Choose*, p.xix.
6. Milton Friedman, *Free to Choose*, p. 103.
7. Ibid.
8. Milton Friedman, *Free to Choose*, p. 107.
9. Milton Friedman, *Free to Choose*, p. 221.
10. Ibid.
11. John P. Newhouse and Vincent Taylor, "How Shall We Pay for Hospital Care?," *The Public Interest* 23: Spring 1971, pp.78–92.
12. Milton Friedman and Rose Friedman, Ibid.
13. John Galbraith, Ibid.
14. Milton Friedman, *Free to Choose*, p. xviii.
15. Bradley R. Schiller, "Reagan-Economics," *An Update to the Economy Today* (New York, N.Y.: Random House, 1981), ch. 15.5.
16. CBS-*New York Times* poll, Sept. 16, 1980, as reported in *An Update to the Economy Today,* Ibid.
17. "Gallup Poll," *U.S. News and World Report*, Jan. 26, 1981, p. 23.
18. Bradley R. Schiller, " Reagan-Economics," ch. 15.5, p. 6.
19. Cynthia DeWitt, "Can Reagan Really Reform Regulations," *Hospitals*, July 16, 1980, p. 87.
20. Ibid.
21. "The Spiraling Costs of Health Care," *Business Week*, no. 2725, February 8, 1982, p. 61
22. Ibid.
23. Ibid.
24. Ibid.
25. Ibid.
26. Ibid.
27. Emily Friedman, "Doctor, the Patient Will See You Now," *Hospitals,* September 16, 1981, p. 117.
28. Ibid.
29. G. Grandon and J. Werner, "Physicians' Practice Experience During the Decade of the 1970s," *Journal of the American Medical Association,* 244: December 5, 1980, p. 2514.
30. W. Schwartz et al, "The Changing Geographic Distribution of Board Certified Physicians," *New England Journal of Medicine* 303: October 30, 1980, p. 1032.
31. L. Aiken et al, "The Contribution of Specialists to the Delivery of Primary Care," *New England Journal of Medicine* 300: June 14, 1979, p. 1363.
32. G. Wilensky and L. Rossita, "The Magnitude and Determinants of Physician Initiated Visits in the United States," World Congress on Health Economics, Lindey University, the Netherlands, September 1980.
33. "G.M.E. in California Again Under Scrutiny," *New Physician* 29: October 1980, p. 15.
34. Emily Friedman, "Doctor, the Patient Will See You Now," p. 121.
35. "Physician Interrelationships with Allied Health Personnel" *Illinois Medical Journal* 158: August 1980, p. 72.
36. R. Welbur, "Physician Surplus: The Role of Specialists," *Internists* 21: March 1980, p. 15.
37. Graduate Medical Education National Advisory Committee, "Summary Report to the Secretary," Department of Health and Human Services, Vol. 1 (Washington, D.C.: Health Resources Administration, September 30, 1980).
38. L. Freshnock and L. Jensen, "The Changing Structure of Medical Group Practice in the United States, 1969–1980," *Journal of the American Medical Association* 245: June 5, 1981, p. 2173.
39. M. White and R. Culbertson, "The Oversupply of Physicians: Implications for Hospital Planning," *Hospital Progress* 62: February 1981, p. 28.
40. P. Ellwood and L. Ellwein, "Physician Glut Will Force Hospitals to Look Outward," *Hospitals* 55: January 16, 1981, p. 81.
41. Emily Friedman, "Doctor, The Patient Will See You Now," p. 127.
42. Ibid.
43. Ibid.
44. P. Froiland, "Filling Time,"*TWA Ambassador* 14: April 1981, p. 57.
45. Cynthia DeWitt, "Getting Down to Business," *Hospitals*, October 1981, p. 76.
46. Emily Friedman, "Competition and the Changing Face of Health Care,"*Hospitals*, July 16, 1980, p. 64.
47. J.W. Colloton, oral testimony on S. 1968, the Health Incentives Reform Act, by the Association of American Medical Colleges, to the Subcommittee on Health, Committee on Finance, U.S. Senate, March 19, 1980.
48. Walter McNerny, Testimony on S. 1968, the Health Incentives Reform Act, to the Subcommittee on Health, Committee on Finance, U.S. Senate, March 19, 1980.

CHAPTER 31

Strategic Planning for Nursing

by Dorothy H. Fox and Richard T. Fox

Strategic planning is a systematic approach to decision making. Nurse administrators who rely on formal planning and measurement of outcomes are more likely to assure consistent high performance from their departments than those who rely on intuition. Planning can serve as motivation for nursing personnel if they are allowed to have some input into it. Not only is nursing practice advanced by strategic planning, as this article shows, but scarce resources can be conserved.

Overall department performance improves when a formal, systematic planning method is substituted for habitual reliance on intuitive or "gut feeling" approaches to decision making[1–3]. Any management group that does not plan ahead is risking a series of crises in its operations[4].

These observations are particularly applicable to departments of nursing, which have tended in the past to neglect formal planning because of (1) heavy demands for immediate solutions to daily crises, (2) the consequent relegation even of thinking about future events to last on the list of priorities, and (3) the lack of knowledge and experience in creating a formal planning program and then integrating it into the overall management of the nursing department. The best interest of nursing will be served if those responsible for its direction become more aware and knowledgeable about the benefits to be derived from strategic planning and about the process itself. The following five principles are basic to the strategic planning process[5]:

1. Critical thinking about past, present, and future states of affairs aids in the development, implementation, and evaluation of a well-formulated plan.
2. Sensitivity to the needs of the institution and its personnel, as well as to the clientele it serves, is fundamental to

strategic planning.
3. A structured plan is flexible, readily adaptable to environmental changes.
4. Accuracy is increased when outcomes related to goals or objectives can be measured quantitatively and not just described qualitatively.
5. Advanced planning is positively related to the making of sound decisions in the present.

Strategic planning defined

Planning is broadly defined as the art of formulating beforehand a detailed scheme for accomplishing one or more goals. Strategic planning uses techniques designed to conserve scarce resources while working toward goals[6]. Drucker provides a more detailed definition:

> Strategic planning is a continuous, systematic process of making risk-taking decisions today with the greatest possible knowledge of their effects on the future; organizing efforts necessary to carry out these decisions; and evaluating results of these decisions against expected outcome through reliable feedback mechanisms[7].

In short, the formal planning approach specifies desired outcomes, maps out actions to be taken, and then measures the degree of success in achieving the desired goal.

The nursing administrator who undertakes strategic planning is forced to think critically about the organization's mission and the department's philosophy. Reflection must occur before setting into motion the logistics for developing, implementing, and evaluating a blueprint of the department to deal with events proactively, rather than reactively. A strategic plan for nursing is a systematic way of giving direction to decision making in the present for the future well-being of the department, its patient clientele, and the institution.

Steiner explains what strategic planning is not. It is not

> an attempt to blueprint the future in a static, rigid manner . . . strategic plans are subject to periodic revision based on technological advances and other environmental changes.

Dorothy H. Fox, Ph.D., R.N., is a Nursing Management Consultant in St. Louis, Missouri.

Richard T. Fox, Ph.D., is a Professor in the Department of Hospital and Health Care Administration at Saint Louis University in St. Louis.

[Nor does strategic planning] prepare massive, detailed, and interrelated sets of plans . . . strategic planning methodology can range from very simple to highly complex, depending upon needs of the department and of the organization as a whole[8].

Participants in planning

The main participants in the formal planning process are those in nursing administration who are responsible and accountable for directing and coordinating the department —the chief nurse (regardless of title) and associate or assistant directors. Choice of primary figures in planning depends on size and complexity of the department, along with its philosophy toward centralized versus decentralized decision making. The planning committee that represents a cross section of nursing management is an example of the decentralized end of the continuum. Centralized decision making membership is restricted to top nursing administration.

Individually and together, planners utilize a number of valuable resources internal and external to the department and to the institution in order to be well informed about issues subject to planning. Concerns voiced internally by lower level management and nursing staff alike are important cues that often stimulate various phases of the planning process. Incorporating nursing personnel's input into the planning program promotes a sense of professional satisfaction throughout the department[9,10]. Even indirect participation motivates workers to achieve goals and thus is an important element in establishing a successful strategic planning program for nursing[11,12].

Benefits of strategic planning

An array of benefits resulting from the application of strategic planning principles are described in the literature[13–19]. This type of planning for future activity is particularly beneficial to the department because it provides a sense of direction to the organization over time; it functions as a control mechanism by setting limits and monitoring variance from the intended course; it helps to conserve both capital and human resources; it deals concretely with complex projects or programs in multistage time sequences; and it is a source of professional satisfaction for the planning group[20].

The development of a keen sense of direction for nursing is first among the benefits of the formal planning process. Planners in different facilities may choose varied courses of action for a number of reasons. Some may work toward maintaining a status quo; others may progress rapidly toward newly identified goals; and still others may strive to be somewhere between the two extremes. Regardless of which path is followed, active involvement in a strategic planning program coordinates and guides present and future department activities.

Control mechanisms operationalized through formal planning indicate whether a department is proceeding on course as anticipated or is off course to a significant degree. Although planning helps deter nursing management from making decisions contrary to a selected course of action, some deviations are bound to occur. No guarantee can be given that all decisions made initially by the planning group will fit perfectly to situations as they develop. When significant deviations evolve, however, planners representing nursing administration are alerted to the need to investigate and judge how best to cope with the unplanned variances. Because the strategic planning process is both flexible and adaptive, it allows planners to accommodate themselves with relative ease to unforeseen contingencies and to apply corrective actions necessary to rectify a problem or redirect a planned course.

The conservation of scarce resources is an additional advantage resulting from the planning process. It is given that any degree of activity on the part of the organization absorbs scarce resources. If a department of nursing's management group persists in making gut-feeling or short-sighted decisions with no well-defined objectives in mind, the result is misdirected activity that more often than not inappropriately absorbs costly resources. On the other hand, if management chooses to think critically about where the department is going, why, and by what means, then the outcome is deliberate, directed activity that decreases the chances of wasting these same resources. Both material and human resources are conserved by using a formal strategic planning model.

Strategic planning is especially helpful when undertaking a complicated, multiple-stage project or program. Its worth depends upon the complexity of the project or program. Formal planning is most valuable when a new project must be developed in several stages over time, with each stage directly dependent upon the successful completion of a former stage. In order to address these interrelated tasks creatively, effectively, and economically, specifications are necessary to show how complex parts of the system fit together over time.

Finally, results obtained from strategic planning involvement can be both personally and professionally rewarding in terms of satisfaction perceived as planners work together in developing, implementing, and evaluating a comprehensive planning program.

Strategic planning as a process

Although the exact number of steps in strategic planning is rather arbitrary, the process itself is made up of five principal phases of action: (1) identification of institutional values and mission; (2) data collection and processing; (3) determination of goals and objectives; (4) implementation of operations; and (5) evaluation of and reaction to results

(Exhibit 1). Given the dynamics of interactions among these five phases, which usually occur within an uncertain environment, a general systems conceptual framework helps to place the complex planning process in perspective[21,22]. A systems viewpoint is advocated here because it is "a way of thinking about a problem and structuring an analysis in terms of the major issues, the critical variables, and the linkage among variables and subsystems"[23].

From values and mission to goals and objectives

Values are fundamental to the process of health planning. Values, according to Blum, "make up the steering mechanism which guides impetus for change"[24]. A value system is a composite of multiple, basic beliefs and ideas held by an individual and society. The value systems of individuals in policy-making positions—members of the governing board —strongly influence the direction of the institution. The board assumes responsibility for examining and determining its basic purpose or mission. The mission openly acknowledges in very general terms the ultimate end being pursued by the organization. Gaining a good understanding of the philosophy and intent of the institution's policy-making body is a necessary starting point in strategic planning for the department of nursing.

The terms *goal* and *objective* are commonly interchanged, but they are distinct. A goal is a general description of an aspiration or a desired state of affairs. Etzioni explains that goals are important because they set general guidelines for organizational activity; constitute a source of

legitimacy justifying activity; and serve as criteria for evaluating accomplishment[25]. Goals are more tangible than the mission; nevertheless, they must be broken down into more concrete elements called objectives. Multiple objectives are generally linked to a single goal. Objectives are defined as specific end points or targets, achievement of which brings about the reality of the goal. Each of the objectives must be stated in clear, concise, and measurable terms. Precision in operationalizing objectives requires prime consideration because they direct the concentration of resources. Objectives also serve as standards for evaluation.

Finally the progressive linkage—values to mission to goals to objectives—is directly related to the hierarchy of the organizational structure. The mission statement initiated by the policy-making group functions as a general directive to top administration, who use it when compiling official goals for the institution. Institutional goals are next transformed into more explicit goals and objectives at the department level to be operationalized at still lower levels in the hierarchial arrangement. Although values implied in the mission statement may appear to lie dormant, these values become actualized as the department of nursing's goals and objectives openly address the dynamic state of nursing practice.

Data collection and processing

Before deciding upon goals and objectives for nursing, planners must first gather baseline information about the

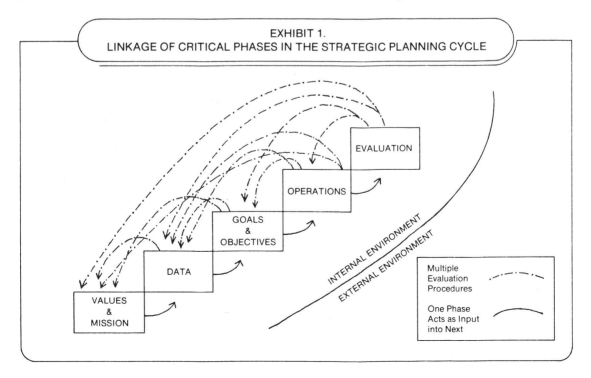

EXHIBIT 1.
LINKAGE OF CRITICAL PHASES IN THE STRATEGIC PLANNING CYCLE

EVALUATION

OPERATIONS

GOALS & OBJECTIVES

DATA

VALUES & MISSION

INTERNAL ENVIRONMENT

EXTERNAL ENVIRONMENT

Multiple Evaluation Procedures

One Phase Acts as Input into Next

present state of nursing affairs and then identify key factors and trends that ultimately affect the department and its patient clientele. For example, utilization rates and case-mix data of various nursing divisions over the past year or two need to be systematically gathered and carefully analyzed.

Either formal or informal data collection and processing may be used by planners. The formality depends upon the type of information sought, its availability, its intended use, the degree of accuracy needed, the depth and rigor of analysis projected, and, of course, associated cost. One would make the assumption a priori that detail and precision of data are positively correlated with cost. Ancillary departments, such as institutional planning, personnel, and financial management, usually have on hand a substantial amount of data that are directly relevant to strategic planning for nursing. Data sources external to the institution should not be overlooked. Although more informal and less quantitative, other primary sources include professional associates and literature reviews. Regardless of source, a critical study of (1) selected information concerning nursing productivity and technological advances, (2) marketing capabilities and innovations, (3) physical and social work environments of personnel, and (4) political issues and legal requirements is done to acquire the necessary insight. A clear understanding—both qualitative and quantitative—of the nursing department's internal and external environment is strongly recommended.

Steiner stresses that the more systematically the changing environmental factors and key trends are assessed, the greater is the accuracy in gauging the impact of change[26]. For example, forecasting is an assessment technique used by many institutional planners for the purpose of systematically choosing issues to be given priority in planning. Forecasting is an attempt to find the most probable course of events or range of possibilities. Forecasts used by the department of nursing may be generated by institutional planners or by others in the hospital who have statistical expertise. Should nurse planners decide to produce their own forecasts, basic business statistics textbooks, plus others devoted exclusively to forecasting, can be consulted[27,28]. Forecasts should be better than best-guess estimates of the future state of events. At the same time, relatively simple constructed trend lines can be very helpful to nurse planners. Steiner warns that forecasting is simply a projection of the future based on present and past information; it is incapable of dictating the future[29]. Blum supports the use of forecasting, explaining that when historical parameters are examined and a forecast made to show where these are going, a description of the future environment begins to emerge.

Deciding among alternatives

Choosing among goals and searching for the best means for reaching them is the next major task to be undertaken by the planning group. Decisions associated with this task can be made by employing one of several decision-making methods, ranging from a simple group consensus to a complex, quantitative decision matrix using probability measures based on conditions of certainty, risk, and uncertainty[31–33]. Certainty means that full knowledge of consequences of an action is at hand; risk refers to partial knowledge and the probability of consequences; and uncertainty means that little or no knowledge of outcome is immediate and the probability of possible results is unknown.

Using information gathered earlier, planners must first evaluate and then decide among alternative goals and their objectives. Reaching a group decision is ordinarily preceded by serious, in-depth discussions centering on such things as perceived versus real needs, professional capabilities within the department, availability of other resources and their associated costs, ideas concerning various operational aspects, and probable consequences if different actions were to be actualized.

The *nominal group process,* which is akin to the Delphi technique, is a relatively simple method for identifying and then prioritizing goals and objectives for the nursing department's strategic plan. The primary objective of the nominal group approach is to reach a general agreement by rank-ordering pertinent data while participants work within a creative, nonthreatening environment[34]. The approach assumes that there is no difference in authority status among participants, thus establishing a sense of equality that helps to reduce individual inhibitions and premature evaluations.

Initially the nominal group is noninteractive; each planner has the same opportunity to express preferences independently about department goals in the presence of peers but via individual written listings. Research has demonstrated that noninteracting groups are significantly superior to interacting groups in generating information, with the latter spending long periods of time on a single train of thought and constraining the opportunity for creative thinking[35–37]. Next, in round robin fashion, data are collected for group notation. Each item expressed is then discussed in greater detail for the purpose of clarification and evaluation. Last, individual ratings of the importance of suggested goals are summed mathematically, indicating the group's rank-order preference. The final result is a constructive resolution of differences in terms of suggested best of alternative goals to be formally submitted to the chief nurse for approval as a working document for the department. Objectives are then substituted for goals, and the nominal group process is repeated until the task of drafting goals and specific objectives thought necessary to reach the desired states is complete. Additional time and effort are directed now toward refining statements to meet operational qualifications, meaning that each objective must be defined by a set of quantitatively measureable characteristics (Exhibit 2). Although planners also examine qualitative characteristics, quantitative measurements are likely to be more accurate for comparing what was wanted with what was obtained. It is evident that the nominal group approach creates a controlled environment where each planner is strongly motivated to accomplish the assigned task of choosing among goals and objectives[38]. The procedure is productive as well as relatively quick and easy.

Implementation of operations

Operations is the action phase of the strategic planning process, where a number of the department's personnel now become actively involved. The conversion of plans into policy and practice is the main reason for the planning process. It is important to note that this phase is directly linked to all other management functions, such as organizing, directing, and controlling.

The strategic plan for nursing now progresses beyond definitions of objectives into the reality of setting into motion mechanisms designed to support a successful operational phase. Expanding upon department objective 2—to decrease nurse turnover to 20 percent maximum—a career ladder advancement program might be activated. This is one method used to retain nurses currently employed, thus reducing the rate and cost of turnover (Exhibit 2). Activating such a program calls for a sequence of steps to be performed to integrate it into the department's and institution's personnel policies and practices. Rationale and logistics for change in criteria for hire and promotion must be determined and clearly communicated to those affected by the change, regardless of position or status within the organization. Acceptance of such a policy change is enhanced when sincere efforts are made to (in)directly involve both management and staff in its development, implementation, and evaluation. Similar measures discussed here in operationalizing a new advancement program would also apply to department objective 3—to substitute 10 percent of licensed practical nurses with the same percentage of experienced registered nurses (via attrition) for the purpose of increasing quality of nursing care.

The development of a monitoring system for the periodic review of concrete data specific to department objectives is an important component of the operational phase. It should be designed to track the overall turnover activity among nursing personnel plus other critical factors. Needed are monthly figures showing the number of nurses who resign from the various nursing divisions along with the corresponding number of hours used for orientation of their replacements. Likewise, the number of substitutions of registered nurses in place of licensed practical nurses is needed, as are separate breakdowns for each category of personnel in terms of nursing care hours utilized per patient day, based on patient acuity measurements, and salary expenditures. Finally, the development of quality measurements for monitoring nursing services provided by each category of personnel is crucial.

Evaluation of results

Evaluation is often thought of as the final action signifying closure of a sequence of related events. In planning, however, evaluation or the comparison of actual outcomes against desired outcomes occurs not only at the end of the process, but also at each of its preceding critical phases (Exhibit 1). Evaluation is divided by Poister into two general categories: formative evaluation, done periodically while the planned program or project is underway, and summative evaluation, carried out at its completion[39].

For example, formative evaluation takes place before a program is put into operation; economic feasibility is often the main issue examined. Depending upon feedback received, revision or updating may substantially modify the original plan's goals and objectives. Formative evaluation can reveal flaws in the structured plan, allowing them to be

---

EXHIBIT 2.
NOMINAL GROUP GOAL AND
OBJECTIVE SELECTION

(hypothetical)

Mission Statement

The aim of this institution is to promote the physical and psychological well-being of the community which we serve.

Institution Goal

To employ a proper balance of professional and nonprofessional personnel who will deliver high-quality patient care services in a cost effective manner.

Department Goal

1. According to our recent, validated patient classification measurements, to maintain a mean standard of 3.4 direct nursing care hours per patient day for an 85 percent rate of occupancy of this 100-bed, general medical-surgical facility. Allocate 105,485 hours (total) to direct nursing care to be given by 50.5 full-time-equivalent (FTE) nurses.

2. Decrease our nurse turnover (total) to 20 percent maximum. Allocate 2424 hours to the orientation of 10.1 FTE replacement personnel; that is, up to 240 hours or 6 weeks per FTE replacement using a competency-based type of orientation program.

3. Through attrition, substitute 10 percent of licensed practical nurses with the same percentage of experienced registered nurses.

Note: Standards are quantified for the purpose of periodic and final comparisons; that is, desired verses actual outcomes. Second, this exhibit illustrates only a portion of a total strategic plan, noting linkage of interrelated department objectives to the mission statement. Finally, this example is limited to direct nursing care hours and orientation hours for FTE replacements in this 100-bed acute care facility.

corrected in advance of completion of the program, thereby saving valuable resources. For instance, criteria developed to classify professional nursing personnel into three clinical groups for career advancement may need to be made less stringent if expectations prove unrealistic when measured against academic preparation and demonstrated competency in nursing. Formative evaluation may also signal the need for planners to revert to the data-gathering phase for the purpose of adjusting the goals and objectives appropriate to changing environmental conditions. Responsible institution of timely changes while developing or implementing the strategic plan can help assure its successful fulfillment.

Summative evaluation is generally more comprehensive than the formative evaluations that precede it. Its purpose is to identify and measure final outcomes of a new program or project against the desired objectives. Quantitative comparisons are recommended because of the greater degree of objectivity involved with their interpretation. An agenda for a final evaluation usually concerns resources; progress reports are made on operations, output, and impact. Analyses are conducted regarding the utilization of manpower and materials; the transformation of resources into products and services; the outputs in terms of volumes of activity, such as units of service produced; and the impacts or changes in, say, patient care delivery or the health status of clients. Note the difference between the terms *output* and *impact*. Output measures units of service produced over time, whereas impact measures changes in characteristics of the target population due to services consumed[40].

In summative evaluation measurements can be made by using rather simple mathematical manipulations of numbers—subtracting either absolute value or percentage achieved from absolute value or percentage intended (Exhibit 3). Such calculations can give a good indication of how close to the target the completed program or project falls. Examination of the nurse turnover summary data in Exhibit 3 indicates in general that the rate of turnover among nurses over a 12-month period was reduced to 17 percent, or 3 percent less than the standard 20 percent. However, a closer look at division breakdown shows that Surgical A had twice the rate than was intended, while Surgical B maintained its 5 percent maximum. Both of the medical divisions demonstrate an even greater reduction in turnover than was expected; that is, 1 percent each as compared to 5 percent anticipated. Although it can be said that objective 3 presented in Exhibit 2 has been reached for the department as a whole, a possible problem area, Surgical A, is discovered, requiring further investigation as to patterns and reasons for turnover.

Planners may prefer to use more sophisticated statistical methods (parametric or nonparametric) which, of course, provide increased accuracy in findings—significant or no significant difference between actual and intended. Finally, after selected analytical techniques have been applied to

EXHIBIT 3. ANNUAL REPORT: NURSE TURNOVER SUMMARY

Division	Beds	FTE Personnel	Intended %	Actual %	Difference
Medical A	25	12.6	5	1	4% under
Medical B	25	12.6	5	1	4% under
Surgical A	25	12.6	5	10	5% over
Surgical B	25	12.6	5	5	———
(Total)	100	50.4	20	17	3% under

data, interpretation of results initiates reaction from the planning body and from nursing and hospital administration. Explanation of findings ultimately gives future direction to the next major cycle of strategic planning for nursing.

References and notes

1. George A. Steiner, *Strategic Planning* (New York: The Free Press, 1979), p. 44.
2. Henrik L. Blum, *Planning for Health* (New York: Human Sciences Press, 1974), p. 43.
3. Herbert H. Hyman, *Health Planning: A Systematic Approach* (Germantown, Md.: Aspen Systems Corp., 1976), p. 72.
4. Daniel Katz and Robert L. Kahn, *The Social Psychology of Organizations* (New York: John Wiley and Sons, 1966), p. 272.
5. The five principles are adapted from the combined works of George A. Steiner, Henrik L. Blum, Daniel Katz, Robert L. Kahn, James G. March and Herbert A. Simon.
6. Henrik L. Blum, 1974, p. 43.
7. Peter Drucker, *Management: Tasks, Responsibilities, Policies* (New York: Harper & Row, 1974), p. 125.
8. George A. Steiner, *Strategic Planning*, 1979, p. 15.
9. National Commission on Nursing, *Initial Report and Preliminary Recommendations* (Chicago: The American Hospital Association, September 1981), p. 14.
10. Herbert A. Simon, *Administrative Behavior* (New York: The Free Press, 1979), p. 57.
11. George A. Steiner, 1979, p. 42.
12. Joseph A. Litterer, *The Analysis of Organizations* (New York: John Wiley and Sons, 1973), p. 643.
13. George A. Steiner, 1979, pp. 57-59.
14. Herbert A. Simon, 1979, pp. 228-234.
15. Peter Drucker, 1974, p. 121.
16. Samuel Levey and N. Paul Loomba, *Health Care Administration* (Philadelphia: J.B. Lippincott, 1973), pp. 269-275.
17. George A. Steiner, *Top Management Planning* (London: The Free Press, 1969), pp. 1–18.
18. Daniel Katz and Robert A. Kahn, 1966, pp. 271-273.
19. James G. March and Herbert A. Simon, *Organizations* (New York: John Wiley and Sons, 1958), pp. 199-210.
20. The five benefits are adapted from the combined works of George A. Steiner, Henrik L. Blum, Daniel Katz, Robert L. Kahn, James G. March and Herbert A. Simon.
21. Fremont E. Kast and James E. Rosenzweig, "Hospital Administration and Systems Concepts," *Hospital Administration* 11:17-33, Fall 1966.
22. Ludwig von Bertalanffy, "General System Theory—A Critical Review," in Joseph A. Litterer, ed., *Organizations: Systems, Control and*

Adaptation (New York: John Wiley and Sons, 1969), pp. 7–30.

23. Theodore H. Poister, *Public Program Analysis* (Baltimore: University Park Press, 1978), p. 40.

24. Henrik L. Blum, 1974, p. 22.

25. Amitai Etzioni, *Modern Organizations* (Englewood Cliffs, N.J.: Prentice-Hall, 1964), pp. 5–20.

26. George A. Steiner, 1979, p. 125.

27. Stephen P. Shao, *Statistics for Business and Economics* (Columbus, Ohio: Charles E. Merrill, 1976).

28. Steven Makridakis and S.C. Wheelright, *Forecasting: Methods and Applications* (New York: John Wiley and Sons, 1978).

29. George A. Steiner, 1969, p. 202.

30. Henrik L. Blum, 1974, p. 165.

31. George A. Steiner, 1979, pp. 245–267.

32. Joseph A. Litterer, *The Analysis of Organizations,* 1973, pp. 79–91.

33. Samuel Levey and N. Paul Loomba, 1973, pp. 205–228.

34. André L. Delbecq and Andrew H. Van de Ven, "A Group Process Model for Problem Identification and Program Planning," in Warren G. Bennis et al, eds., *The Planning of Change* (New York: Holt, Rinehart, and Winston, 1976), pp. 283–296.

35. Andrew H. Van de Ven, *Group Decision Making and Effectiveness: An Experimental Study* (Kent, Ohio: Kent State University, 1974).

36. André L. Delbecq, Andrew H. Van de Ven, and David H. Gustafson, *Group Techniques for Program Planning* (Glenview Ill: Scott, Foresman, 1975), pp. 16–28.

37. V.H. Vroom, L.D. Grant, and T.J. Cotton, "The Consequences of Social Interaction in Group Problem Solving," *Journal of Applied Psychology* 53(4):338–341, August 1969.

38. Frequently a chosen objective can be reached in several ways. Cost effectiveness analysis is a technique which might be employed in selecting that method operation which would minimize overall costs. This technique, which can be used to solve many institutional problems, is not beyond the capabilities of nurse planners who have a working knowledge of college algebra. Those interested in basic cost effectiveness methodology might consult H.H. Hendricks and G.M. Taylor, *Systematic Analysis: A Primer on Benefit-Cost Analysis and Program Evaluation* (Pacific Palisades, Calif.: Goodyear Publishing, 1972).

39. Theodore H. Poister, 1978, p. 16.

40. Theodore H. Poister, 1978, pp. 6–9.

CHAPTER 32

Accountability and Nursing Diagnosis

by Judith J. Warren

A taxonomy of nursing diagnoses improves communication within the domain of nursing practice. The author contends that use of this tool throughout the health care delivery system could lead to improved management of nursing care. Improvements could be made in identification of staffing requirements, justification of third party payments, development of quality assurance programs, establishment of standard terminology between nurses, and generation of an extensive and valid research data base. Nursing administrators should consider using accepted nursing diagnoses as one of the tools available to improve nursing care and to document nursing accountability.

The administration of a nursing department requires the ability to define nursing. This has become even more true during the past ten years due to both increased participation of third party payments for health care and the increased emphasis on the need to justify each profession's role in the delivery of health care. In addition, nurses are held legally accountable for their practice by those who contract for their services. In 1980, in response to this demand, the American Nurses' Association issued a statement on public accountability: *A Social Policy Statement*[1]. Nursing is the only profession to issue such a statement. This statement defines nursing as the diagnosis and treatment of human responses to actual or potential health problems[1, 2]. One of the ways nurses can document their accountability in practice is with the nursing diagnosis.

Nursing diagnosis, the end result of the assessment phase of the nursing process, defines and communicates to others the specific problems a patient is experiencing which require nursing care[3]. The nurse, therefore, is documenting his/her ability and accountability in nursing practice and is providing a clear articulation of the domain of nursing practice[4, 5]. Shoemaker defines a nursing diagnosis as

a clinical judgment about an individual/family/community which is derived through a deliberate systematic process of data collection and analysis. It provides the basis for pres-

criptions or definitive therapy for which the nurse is accountable. It is expressed concisely and includes the etiology of the condition when known[6].

Moritz agrees with the above definitions, but modifies them in order to exclude any medical diagnoses which nurses may make.

Nursing diagnoses are responses to actual or potential health problems which nurses by virtue of their education and experience are able, licensed, and legally responsible and accountable to treat[7].

The movement toward the use of a taxonomy of nursing diagnoses had been driven by this need to demonstrate and/or document accountability. A taxonomy provides a clear labeling of patient conditions treated by nursing intervention, and provides the scientific base for nursing science. The driving forces behind the development of this taxonomy are standardized communication between nurses, quality assurance programs, third party payments for nursing care, computerization of nursing records, peer review, a unified definition of nursing practice, and theory generation.

Standardized communications between nurses

Communication among nurses has long been hampered by the use of multi-languages. By this it is meant that one group talks about nursing problems, one about patient problems, another about health-related goals, and so on. Some nurses work with negentropy in four dimensional fields, while others work with self-care deficits. Some nurses work with patients who have myocardial infarctions, and others work with patients who have alterations in cardiac output. The problems involved in trying to review the literature pertaining to a topic of interest can be overwhelming—just identifying different labels is a time-consuming task. If we have trouble labeling what it is we do or our "phenomena of concern," is it any wonder that our clients, beginning to lose trust in us, demand accountability measures from us? The development of a common terminology or a diagnostic taxonomy is the goal of the National Group for Classification of Nursing Diagnosis (Exhibit 1). The consensus is

Judith J. Warren, R.N., M.S., is Assistant Professor of Nursing, and Coordinator, Graduate Medical-Surgical Nursing Program, University of Hawaii. She is also a doctoral student in Educational Psychology at the University of Hawaii.

EXHIBIT 1
LIST OF NURSING DIAGNOSES ACCEPTED BY
THE FIFTH NATIONAL CONFERENCE*

Airway Clearance, Ineffective
Activity Intolerance
Anxiety
Bowel Elimination, Alteration in: Constipation
Bowel Elimination, Alteration in: Diarrhea
Bowel Elimination, Alteration in: Incontinence
Breathing Patterns, Ineffective
Cardiac Output, Alterations in: Decreased
Comfort, Alterations in: Pain
Communication, Impaired Verbal
Coping, Ineffective Individual
Coping, Ineffective Family: Compromised
Coping, Ineffective Family: Disabling
Coping, Family: Potential for Growth
Diversional Activity, Deficit
Family Processes, Alteration in
Fear
Fluid Volume Deficit, Actual
Fluid Volume Deficit, Potential
Fluid Volume, Alteration in: Exess
Gas Exchange, Impaired
Grieving, Anticipatory
Grieving, Dysfunctional
Health Maintenance Alteration
Home Maintenance Management, Impaired
Injury, Potential for
Knowledge Deficit (specify)
Mobility, Impaired Physical
Non-compliance (specify)
Nutrition, Alterations in: Less Than Body
    Requirements
Nutrition, Alterations in: More Than Body Requirements
Nutrition, Alterations in: Potential For More Than Body
    Requirements
Oral Mucus Membrane, Alteration in
Parenting, Alterations in: Actual
Parenting, Alterations in: Potential
Powerlessness
Rape-Trauma Syndrome
Self-Care Deficit (specify)
Self-concept, Disturbance in
Sensory Perceptual Alterations
Sexual Dysfunction
Skin Integrity, Impairment of: Actual
Skin Integrity, Impairment of: Potential
Sleep Pattern Disturbance
Social Isolation
Spiritual Distress (Distress of the Human Spirit)
Thought Processes, Alterations in
Tissue Perfusion, Alteration in
Urinary Elimination, Alteration in Patterns
Violence, Potential for

Diagnoses Accepted for Clinical Testing, Fifth National Conference
on Classification of Nursing Diagnosis, St. Louis Mo., April 14-17,
1982.

or patterns, diagnostic labels should refer to that response. As you can imagine, if nurses communicated clinical information according to such a label, professional communications, literature reviews, and measures of accountability could be greatly enhanced. This does not mean that conceptual models of nursing would be discarded. On the contrary, the models describe the interaction or the relationship between the nurse and her patient. The models are crucial structures which allow nurses to label and explore what occurs in a nurse-patient relationship. Nursing diagnoses allow nurses to label and explore what occurs in the patient's response to a health problem. When the vocabulary or labels used in communication become clear, evaluation is facilitated and measures of accountability are more easily articulated.

Quality assurance programs

According to Gordon

Nursing diagnoses describe the independent domain of nursing practice. Thus nurses assume accountability for health problems described by these diagnostic labels. It follows logically that nursing diagnoses should be used to define client populations for care review and that diagnoses provide the ideal tool for writing nursing-specific process and outcome standards, identifying care delivery problems, and planning remedial actions[8].

This should be the basis for quality assurance programs in nursing. Currently, medical diagnoses are used to identify patient populations in these programs. When nurses assume accountability for patient care grouped under medical labels, it implies that they are accountable for care not under their control. Fortunately, most standards derived from this format are actually unlabeled nursing diagnoses. Again, if we assume that nursing has a unique domain of practice, independent from medicine, and wishes to be held accountable for that practice, shouldn't quality assurance programs and documentation of accountability be couched in a nursing vocabulary and diagnostic taxonomy, not medicine's?

Nursing diagnoses facilitate the writing of process and outcome standards which are clearly within the domain of nursing. The etiology and defining characteristics of the nursing diagnosis guide the nurse in defining the time needed to reach a standard and in identifying outcome standards. Theory, research, and expert opinion concerning nursing diagnoses provide the guidance in writing process standards. A nurse with knowledge of nursing diagnoses and nursing process will be ready to meet job responsibilities in the area of quality assurance[9].

Third-party payments for nursing care

Most health consumers do not have direct access to nursing

that, regardless of the specific nursing conceptual framework, nurses diagnose and treat human responses to health problems. Since humans respond in basically human ways

care unless they are able to pay for it directly. Third-party payers currently do not allow payments for nursing care. Before nursing care can be of any benefit, a patient must convince a physician that nursing care is needed so that the physician may order it (while collecting his fee for this service). Consequently, many functional health problems (the domain of nursing) go untreated until disease is present. One example would be a body image alteration after surgery which must progress to a severe depression before treatment is authorized. To assist with the work of gaining third-party reimbursement, the focus should be on the actual and potential health problems (nursing diagnoses) nurses diagnose and treat, rather than on the tasks nurses do.

The second part of this issue is reimbursement for nursing care in the hospital—fee for service. Currently, hospitals receive reimbursement for the number of days a patient stays. Medical diagnoses have provided the framework for this reimbursement system via diagnoses-related groups (DRGs). Thompson suggests that this format could be used for nursing reimbursement by using nursing diagnoses[10]. Currently, a research project, in New Jersey, is exploring this concept[11]. This idea can be taken a step further into developing patient classification systems based on nursing diagnoses. These are better predictors of time required for patient care than are medical diagnoses. This type of patient classification system can be used to establish more effective nurse staffing patterns since these patterns are determined by patient care predictors (nursing diagnoses). Knowing the demands of patient care and the needs of nurses to give that care, structural standards in quality assurance programs can be developed to facilitate quality nursing care[12]. The diagnostic label or the standardized communication is central to the organization of this interrelated system: reimbursement patient classification system, nurse staffing patterns, and quality structural standards. This coordinated effort to establish financial worth (income generating ability) and practice domain within the health care system just may push nursing into its long-sought-after professional status. Naming a thing gives power and control to the user.

Computerization of nursing records

Currently, patient information and information retrieval are based on medical diagnoses. It is difficult to retrieve information concerning a particular nursing intervention or patient response to nursing care. The use of nursing diagnoses facilitates the development of a large computerized nursing data base. A computer program could be developed to retrieve this information according to indexed nursing diagnoses[13]. For example, a nurse researcher would be able to survey a large number of patient records for responses to therapy indicative of ineffective coping patterns. Or, an audit committee could analyze the records for relationships between health care delivery problems and

certain diagnoses. It is evident that accountability measures need to be direct and independent of other health professionals. Romano, et al state

> Because practice is correlated with what nurses document, the development of computerized nursing data bases not only helps to clarify what nurses should document but also helps to define a philosophy of accountable nursing practice[14].

Precision in identifying those nursing functions required for computerization could be obtained through the use of nursing diagnosis.

Peer Review

Peer review is another issue in accountability. How do nurses derive the standards for peer review? Are there process, outcome and structural standards as in quality assurance programs? One such standard could be the ability to make nursing diagnoses. Nurses would have to document and substantiate the diagnosis and identify appropriate nursing interventions and the expected patient outcomes. They would be held accountable for nursing actions based on nursing diagnosis[15]. This would shift the focus from medical handmaiden tasks to a problem-solving nursing practice. Given the patient data base, peers could determine whether or not a nurse was demonstrating competent practice. It would also facilitate in identifying areas for growth and development—achieving more complex levels of practice. This is an exciting concept: can staff consistently and accurately diagnose and treat an alteration in cardiac output or a potential for violence? Follow that question with—what can staff development do to assist their mastery of these diagnoses?

Unified definition of nursing practice

What is nursing? Nursing has been defined vaguely by nurses, by legislators who pass laws regulating practice, by administrators of agencies giving nursing care, by educators designing curricula, and by physicians. Nursing should be an identifiable and measurable discipline defined by nursing research. In the past decade nursing conceptual models have attempted to describe nursing. They have provided a way to think about the nurse and the patient.

> Nursing models serve as a framework for the development of nursing knowledge and thus underpin accountability of the profession through its practice, education, and research [16].

However, a model must generate tools and hypotheses which can be analyzed empirically through research. Most conceptual models represent an initial attempt at this function of development of nursing knowledge and theory. In 1980 the Congress for Nursing Practice of the American

Nurses' Association defined ten actual or potential health problem areas which are the essence of nursing practice[17]. This statement identifies nursing practice by using an inductive approach, not the deductive approach of conceptual models. Also in 1980, the National Group for the Classification of Nursing Diagnosis defined nine patterns of human responses and forty-two diagnoses, again using an inductive approach towards defining the nursing practice domain [18]. In both groups, the components identified were remarkably similar. Both of these are steps in defining in measurable terms the domain of nursing practice.

Theory generation

The effort to identify and classify nursing diagnoses is theory development. Identifying diagnoses is factor-isolating theory building. Classifying diagnoses and defining relationships among them is factor-relating theory building. This particular "theory" (nursing diagnosis development model) has four characteristics that make it amenable to the nursing profession. First, it uses an operational method of reasoning to arrive at content. Second, generation of diagnoses is performed by all nurses, not a select few. Third, it treats man holistically. Fourth, this effort toward a nursing theory leads to constructs and concepts which are well defined and researchable[19]. A proposed paradigm for the evolution of nursing science, then, is this model of theory building—the identification and classification of nursing diagnoses. Kuhn defines a paradigm as an achievement sufficiently unprecedented to attract a group away from competing modes of activity, and sufficiently open-ended to leave problems for the new group to resolve[20]. With this new paradigm, researchers adopt new instruments and look in new places. They even see different things with the old instruments in the old places. It is a scientific revolution. In this respect the new paradigm has so shifted their perceptual field that it could be said they are in a different world. Kuhn likens this to a Gestalt switch[21]. Where before there were many interpretations of the data (conceptual models or nursing tasks), there is now only one that stands out—the nursing diagnosis generated theory of nursing. As Gordon says

> For many years it has been difficult to define the scope of nursing practice. Nursing diagnosis may make it possible to arrive at a clearer definition of nursing's domain of responsibility. Once the domain is defined, research and the development of practice theory can be focused on the health problems that are relevant to nursing[22].

Thus, nursing is at an exciting point in its development. The identification and classification of nursing diagnoses provides nursing with power and authority by naming what nurses do. Nursing administrators will be able to identify needs, document resources, and provide accountable nurs-

ing care. Thus, they will be able to negotiate and maintain nursing's place in the ever changing health care field.

References

1. American Nurses' Association. *A Social Policy Statement.* Kansas City: ANA 1980.
2. Kathryn Barnard: "Social Policy Statement: Implications for Nursing Diagnosis." Fifth Conference for Classification of Nursing Diagnosis, St. Louis, Mo., April 14, 1982.
3. Judith J. Warren: "Problems in Using Nursing Diagnoses: A Descriptive Study of Graduate Nursing Students." Fifth Conference for Classification of Nursing Diagnosis, St. Louis, Mo., April 14, 1982.
4. Marjory Gordon, "Nursing Diagnoses and the Diagnostic Process," *American Journal of Nursing* 76(8): 1298–1300, August, 1976.
5. B. Dossey and Cathy Guzzetta, "Nursing Diagnosis," *Nursing 81* 11(6): 34–38, June, 1981.
6. Joyce Shoemaker: "A Research Study on the Definition of Nursing Diagnosis." Fifth Conference for Classification of Nursing Diagnosis, St. Louis, Mo., April 15, 1982.
7. Derry Moritz, "Nursing Diagnoses in Relation to the Nursing in Relation to the Nursing Process." In MiJa Kim and Derry Moritz (eds.), *Classification of Nursing Diagnosis: Proceedings of the Third and Fourth National Conferences* (New York: McGraw-Hill Book Co., 1982), pp. 53–57.
8. Marjory Gordon, *Nursing Diagnosis: Process and Application* (New York: McGraw-Hill Book Co., 1982), p. 276.
9. Audra McLane, "Nursing Diagnoses in the Master's Practicum." In MiJa Kim and Derry Moritz (eds.), *Classification of Nursing Diagnosis: Proceedings of the Third and Fourth National Conference* (New York: McGraw-Hill Book Co., 1982), pp. 95–105.
10. J.D. Thompson, "Prediction of Nurse Resource Use in Treatment of Diagnosis-Related Groups." In H.H. Werley and M.R. Grier (eds.), *Information Systems* (New York: Springer, 1981), pp. 60–81.
11. Rosalind Toth: "Fee for Service, Reimbursement Mechanism Based on Nursing Diagnosis." Fifth National Conference for the Classification of Nursing Diagnosis, St. Louis, Mo., April 15, 1982.
12. Marjory Gordon, *Nursing Diagnosis: Process and Application,* p. 287.
13. S.J. Spott, "Nursing Information Systems." In MiJa Kim and Derry Moritz (eds.), *Classification of Nursing Diagnosis: Proceedings of the Third and Fourth National Conferences* (New York: McGraw-Hill Book Co., 1982), pp. 76–84.
14. C. Romano, A.A. McCormick and L.D. McNeely, "Nursing Documentation: A Model for a Computerized Data Base, *Advances in Nursing Science* 4(2): 43–56, January, 1982.
15. MiJa Kim, "Issues Related to Research on the Classification of Nursing Diagnosis." In MiJa Kim and Derry Moritz (eds.), *Classification of Nursing Diagnosis: Proceedings of the Third and Fourth National Conferences* (New York: McGraw-Hill Book Co., 1982), pp. 124–137.
16. K.S. Chance, "Nursing Models: A Requisite for Professional Accountability," *Advances in Nursing Sciences* 4(2): 57–65, January, 1982.
17. American Nurses' Association. *A Social Policy Statement,* p. 10.
18. MiJa Kim and Derry Moritz (eds.), *Classification on Nursing Diagnosis: Proceedings of the Third and Fourth National Conferences* (New York: McGraw-Hill Book Co., 1982), pp. 244–245.
19. Phyllis Kritek, "The Generation and Classification of Nursing Diagnosis: Toward a Theory of Nursing." In MiJa Kim and Derry Moritz (eds.), *Classification of Nursing Diagnosis: Proceedings of the Third and Fourth National Conferences* (New York: McGraw-Hill Book Co., 1982), pp. 18–29.
20. Thomas Kuhn, *The Structure of Scientific Revolutions* (Chicago: The University of Chicago Press, 1970), p. 10.
21. Thomas Kuhn, *The Structure of Scientific Revolutions,* p. 111.
22. Marjory Gordon, *Nursing Diagnosis: Process and Application,* p. 292.

CHAPTER 33

Professionalism and Collective Bargaining: A New Reality for Nurses and Management

by Joan Quinn McClelland

The author reviews the literature on labor relations in hospitals, analyzing the opinions and actions of administrators as well as staff. She links collective organization among nurses with a new attitude toward nurses' professionalism, and concludes that health care organizations must accept the "new reality" of collective bargaining. The author further suggests that managers and staff adopt cooperative rather than adversarial roles in order to foster quality patient care and to meet future challenges.

In 1974, the Health Care Amendments of the National Labor Relations Act gave employees of non-profit health care organizations the right to bargain collectively. Since then, nurses have made frequent attempts to unionize. The majority of nurses are employed by hospitals; consequently, hospital nurses have been the focal point of this movement. But the impact of unionization has been felt in other health care organizations as well. Nurses' attempts to unionize have met with varying degrees of resistance and success, but almost always they have been characterized by the kind of conflict between management and workers which has plagued other unionized industries.

The controversy

Some nurses have argued that the concept of collective bargaining is contrary to the nature of professionalism. Others have countered that it is not necessary or even desirable for professional health-care workers and managers to emulate old patterns; instead, they see unionization as

an opportunity to develop a new model of labor relations which will benefit not only employees and management, but health care delivery as a whole.

These issues are especially relevant today. In times of fiscal constraints, managers are expected to examine goals and priorities, and find the best ways to utilize human and material resources. In many health care organizations, considerable energy is diverted into ongoing conflicts between management and staff nurses. This sort of wastefulness deserves as much attention as lagging productivity. The goal of both managers and staff nurses is to provide services to meet the needs of patients; neither management nor employee interests ought to take precedence over patients' needs.

Much of the management literature on labor relations in health care organizations implicitly assumes that collective bargaining by professional nurses is undesirable. Other articles suggest that the long-standing association of labor unions with blue-collar workers in industrial settings is outmoded. These analysts argue that the concept of collective bargaining by professionals is the new reality in service-based organizations.

Views from the literature

According to author Rachel Rotkovitch collective bargaining fosters discord in nursing departments by causing adversarial relationships to develop between nursing administration and staff. She argues further that collective bargaining undermines the nursing administrator's role as a leader in promoting group cohesiveness and commitment to the common goal of quality patient care[1].

In an article describing his successful resistance to unionization in his organization, William Latta writes that management must fight union power with an expertly orchestrated counterattack[2].

Joan Quinn McClelland, R.N., B.S.N., is a Public Health Nurse for the Washtenaw County Health Department and the Huron Valley Visiting Nurses Association in southeastern Michigan. She is a candidate for an M.P.H. degree in public health nursing from the University of Minnesota's School of Public Health.

Laurie Prothro makes the following statement:

As it becomes more apparent that no hospital is safe from this latest army of union organizers, hospitals and their associations are beginning to avail themselves of some of the educational and psychological weapons that do exist to combat unionization[3].

Other authors wish to combat unionization efforts by developing a concept of "preventive labor relations," with an emphasis on better organizational communication and labor relations training for supervisors[4, 5]. Coney and Barmish explain how managers can use industrial relations theory to mitigate "the disequilibrium fomented by national and local union rhetoric"[6]. They advise organizations to hire an industrial relations expert to implement programs which will reduce the risk of "outside interference;" such an expert can also effectively manage relations with a union, should one be elected by the institution's employees[7].

Elliot and Kaiser discuss the implications of case law regarding union organizing. Health care organizations may adopt certain kinds of rules for regulating union organizing activities in the workplace, but the timing of these actions is crucial. According to labor relations law, rules cannot be initiated once a union drive has begun; furthermore, once a bargaining unit is voted in, a hospital's personnel practices can be changed or eliminated only through collective bargaining[8, 9].

Several groups have systematically investigated the reasons why nurses pursue the collective bargaining option. A Kansas City employee and labor relations consulting firm studied the attitudes of hospital employees and professional nurses to determine why they join unions, and to discover how union organizers garner their support. The study was intended to define management strategies to "eliminate the need for outside representation of professional nurses[10]. Instead they concluded:

A myth widely subscribed to by hospital management is that big powerful unions organize professional nurses. In fact, unions do not organize professional nurses, professional nurses organize themselves. They do this because administrators and nursing supervisors fail to recognize and address nurses' individual and collective needs[11].

Many investigators feel that while economic concerns and working conditions may at one time have been the principal motivators for collective action, the primary issue now is control of nursing practice. Parlette, O'Reilly and Bloom, an interdisciplinary team from the Schools of Public Health and Business Administration at the University of California at Berkeley, found that nurses who engage in collective bargaining believe it is the only solution to a management-employee power struggle. They conclude that nurses decide to unionize because of their ". . . inability to communicate with management and their perception of authoritarian behavior on the part of management"[12].

In addition, nurses do *not* consider collective bargaining

to be incompatible with professionalism. Professionals have traditionally relied on collective action to achieve professional goals, through the lobbying efforts of their professional organizations. Virginia Cleland suggests that collective bargaining provides an opportunity for the nursing profession to exercise control over nursing practice by providing a mechanism to redistribute power within the health-care organization. "The power bestowed upon the nursing profession should derive not from hospital administrators' benevolence but rather from a public's view of the value of the services provided by practitioners"[13].

Professions are characterized by a long period of specialized education which prepares individuals to provide a service to society. Because of their expertise and by virtue of the value society places on the service they provide, professionals are granted a measure of autonomy in the work setting. Traditionally nursing has been organized along bureaucratic rather than professional lines; the profession has placed a high value on obedience and following the directions of others, rather than on independent judgment and decision making[14]. But such notions have become outmoded as health care delivery has become more complex and technical. Nurses are now called upon to assume responsibility for complicated decisions and to use their professional expertise in new and sophisticated ways.

Nevertheless, the outmoded assumptions and bureaucratic structures remain in place. Ada Jacox is critical of nursing departments that fail to acknowledge that nurses are professionals. In her view, the authority for professional practice must rest with the profession collectively. "The idea that a single administrator can or should be solely responsible for the quality of service given by a group of professionals is misguided and anti-professional"[15]. She suggests that collective bargaining through the professional organization may be a means for nurses to implement the concept of collective professional responsibility.

In an article entitled "The Constructive Orchestration of Chaos," James Affleck describes the needs of a "new worker, . . . educated well beyond the narrow limits of professional specialties and the scope of specific job assignments"[16]. He feels that managers must "grasp the essential quality of the collective will of the people. . . which ultimately determines where and how the organization will actually move regardless of orders issued from the top"[17].

Conclusion

Management and nurses are mutually dependent on one another. Their relationship is characterized by symbiosis, not domination and submission. The struggle for power and perrogative is a quagmire in which neither nursing nor management can win and the patient will most certainly lose. We must recognize that health care organizations and health care professionals must play complementary roles rather than competing roles in order to respond constructively to society's rapidly evolving health care needs and expectations.

References

1. Rachel Rotkovitch, "Do Labor Union Activities Decrease Professionalism?," *Supervisor Nurse* 11(9): 16, September 1980.
2. William A. Latta, "What You Should Do When a Union Knocks on Your Door," *Medical Group Management* 27(6):19, November–December 1980.
3. Laurie Prothro, "Hospital Unions: Which Way for the West?," *Hospital Forum* 23(2):10, March 1980.
4. Laurie Prothro, "Hospital Unions," p. 8
5. Frank K. Whitney, "Communication During a Strike Threat," *Hospital Forum* 23(2): 5, March 1980.
6. Aims C. Coney and Ascher S. Barmish, "What to Do When Organized Labor Comes Calling," *Hospitals* 53(24):85, December 16, 1979.
7. Coney and Barmish, "What to Do When Organized Labor Comes Calling," p. 85.
8. Coney and Barmish, "What to Do When Organized Labor Comes Calling," p. 90.
9. Clifton L. Elliot and Gina Kaiser, "Patients, Not Unions, First Concern of Hospitals," *Hospitals* 53(21):78, November 1, 1979.
10. Bruce K. Stickler and James C. Velghe, "Why Nurses Join Unions," *Hospital Forum* 23(2):14, March 1980.
11. Stickler and Velghe, "Why Nurses Join Unions," p. 14.
12. Nicholas G. Parlette, Charles A. O'Reilly, and Joan R. Bloom, "The Nurse and the Union," *Hospital Forum* 23(6):16, September–October 1980.
13. Virginia S. Cleland, "Taft-Hartley Amended: Implications for Nursing—The Professional Model," *The Journal of Nursing Administration* 11(7):17, July 1981.
14. Ada Jacox, "Collective Action: The Basis for Professionalism," *Supervisor Nurse* 11(9):22, September 1980.
15. Ada Jacox, "Collective Action," p. 23.
16. James G. Affleck, "The Constructive Orchestration of Chaos," *The Journal of Nursing Administration* 10(3):17, March 1980.
17. James G. Afleck, "The Constructive Orchestration of Chaos," p. 18.

CHAPTER 34

Networking: A Managerial Strategy for Research Development in a Service Setting

by Valerie Hunt, June L. Stark, Frances Fisher,
Kathryn Hegedus, Loretta Joy, and Karyl Woldum

An innovative managerial strategy—networking—used to establish and promote a nursing research program within three teaching hospitals in Boston is outlined in this article. Networking provides an opportunity for research and program development experts to share resources to meet common needs and goals. One of the advantages of a research network is that it can provide educational offerings that will stimulate all levels of professional nursing staff independent of their research background. Results of a survey the network conducted to determine a citywide profile of nursing research needs are presented.

Nursing administration within a service setting must articulate the value of research to clinical practice by creating a climate conducive to research. This is done by incorporating research goals into departmental philosophies, beliefs, and by-laws, by including research objectives in position descriptions, and by raising the level of research awareness and skill through nursing research committee activities and program offerings. The incorporation of research skills into all levels of practice has been mandated by the American Nurses' Association:

> Nurses prepared in all programs have an active role in the process of developing scientific knowledge and incorporating that knowledge into practice. No one group of nurses is

expected to assume responsibility for the total process of developing knowledge and ensuring its impact on the practice of nursing[1].

Within three Boston teaching hospitals different models to implement and promote nursing research were in operation. At the Beth Israel Hospital, the Brigham and Women's Hospital, and New England Medical Center research activities were defined, positions designated, studies being conducted, and educational offerings provided. All three hospitals had institutional review boards and nursing research committees in various stages of development and operation. Strengths and weaknesses within each program had been identified. Each hospital possessed its own special talents and resources. However, recognizing each other's uniqueness, there was still the need to share and expand beyond each hospital's existing program. The climate at all three hospitals was conducive for professional nurses to learn from one another's expertise in order to accomplish the following goals:

- Bond for professional growth
- Reinforce and refine nursing research knowledge
- Clarify research standards of practice
- Share developed tools, techniques, and strategies
- Provide a creative outlet

Staging of the network

The level of receptivity at the three hospitals was high and only a catalyst was needed to launch the first stage of the network. The concept of networking between nurse professionals as well as the formation of educational consortia to share information and solve problems has been described in the literature[2]. Many articles define networking as sharing of resources or collaborative sponsorship of programs, both of which definitions are correct. But a network is also a high-level group process, a creative thinking group. Establishing a network, as the Nursing Research Network of Boston experienced it, occurs in five stages (see Exhibit 1).

Valerie Hunt, R.N., M.S., was formerly Assistant Director, Staff Education, Brigham and Women's Hospital and is presently Director, Nursing Education, St. Elizabeth's Hospital of Boston.

June L. Stark, R.N., B.S.N., is Critical Care Instructor, New England Medical Center, Boston.

Frances Fisher, R.N., M.S., was formerly Head Nurse, Clinical Research Unit, Beth Israel Hospital and is presently Clinical Director of Surgical Nursing, St. Elizabeth's Hospital of Boston.

Kathryn Hegedus, R.N., D.N.Sc., is Director of Nursing Research/Quality Assurance, Beth Israel Hospital, Boston.

Loretta Joy, R.N., M.S.N., is Coordinator of Quality Assurance, Brigham and Women's Hospital, Boston.

Karyl Woldum, R.N., M.S., is Associate Chairman of Ambulatory Nursing, New England Medical Center, Boston.

1. Idea initiation

The first stage occurs even before the group first convenes, when interest reaches a level conducive to the formation of a network. The idea initiator, the person who first gathers the group together, has a need to seek and share resources outside of his or her institution. The initiator also must have the notion that a group approach or network of experts can accomplish a task more successfully than an individual effort. Prospective members are receptive to the idea initiator and see the value in sharing ideas and resources.

Participants involved at this stage are the charter members of the group. They include the idea initiator and one or two other members who find themselves engaged in frequent brainstorming sessions before the first network meeting to generate ideas and do some initial planning. The energy level among the charter members is very high.

2. Role clarification

The idea initiator begins the formal networking by contacting prospective members of the group to set the date for the first meeting. The group's purpose at first is often a goal-directed activity such as cosponsoring a program. In the initial meetings members seek to explain their roles and function within their professional setting and establish territoriality. The idea initiator generally emerges as the group leader and facilitator of group process.

During this stage members strive to protect their title and have strong institutional affiliation. While they are involved in the group, they do not necessarily *believe* in the idea of the group. Group dynamics are multilevel and the atmosphere intense. Individuals identify with the institutions that employ them; rather than saying, "I believe" or "I feel," they begin statements with the words, "At the X Hospital we do. . . ."

3. Negotiation

In the negotiation phase members assess territorial gains, expertise, and goals of other members and bargain on issues to reach common ground. They balance the values of their respective institutions. Common goals are established. The group decides what work is to be done and formulates a plan.

Testing behaviors continue as group members begin to move away from institutional identities and establish their individual professional identities. Often members begin to seek each other out outside of the network meeting for discussions and to establish stronger relationships. Follow-

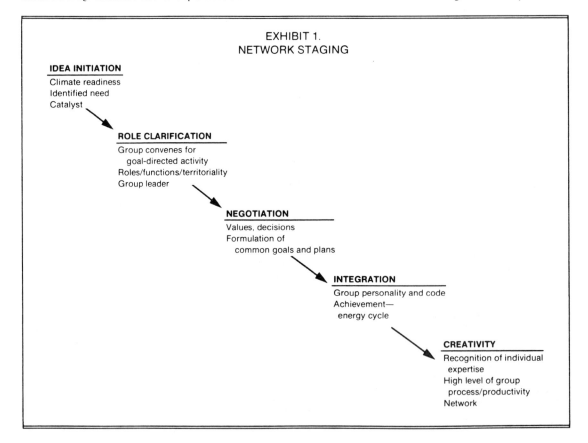

EXHIBIT 1.
NETWORK STAGING

IDEA INITIATION
Climate readiness
Identified need
Catalyst

ROLE CLARIFICATION
Group convenes for
  goal-directed activity
Roles/functions/territoriality
Group leader

NEGOTIATION
Values, decisions
Formulation of
  common goals and plans

INTEGRATION
Group personality and code
Achievement—
  energy cycle

CREATIVITY
Recognition of individual
  expertise
High level of group
  process/productivity
Network

ing our meetings some group members would stay and informally carry over discussions on practice issues that had arisen during the meeting. Issues such as autonomy and scope of practice were discussed.

4. Integration

Eventually a group personality or code emerges. The group has negotiated for territory and resolved values conflicts to become a cohesive unit. The group is productive and goals are accomplished. Getting work done, especially if results are successful, energizes the group. This is the *achievement-energy* cycle.

Group attention and activity is still focused on the accomplishment of identified goals such as program development. But now members take more risks and share ideas more. Our group began sharing the tools we used to review research proposals. The group also expressed the need to formalize the organizational structure by electing a chairperson and formulating a one-year plan. Thus the group members showed that they believed in the *idea* of the group.

5. Creativity

During the final phase of establishing a network members of the group extend beyond the group as a functioning unit to display creative talents. Group members are very comfortable with territorial issues and seek out the unique contributions and expertise of individual members. The level of group process and productivity is high. The group has finally become a network.

This is a time when individuals acknowledge their own areas of expertise as well as those of other members. For example, we began volunteering to present sections in the workshops or seeking out our own members to serve as speakers. Also, outside of the network meeting time group members contacted one another to share ideas and projects that were not necessarily related to research.

Reflecting on how the stages just described worked for our network, the idea initiation phase began with the need to clarify nursing research roles within our respective agencies, to develop a cohesive system for the conduct and evaluation of nursing research studies, and to share resources, strategies, and concerns with other nursing research experts and program specialists. Role clarification not only served as a means of integrating the group but helped us all understand how research responsibilities were incorporated into different nursing positions in a service setting. Negotiation and integration occurred as the group worked together on developing and presenting a nursing research workshop. And finally creativity was realized as we began conducting our own nursing research and publishing our results.

Composition of the network

Nurses belonging to the research network represented a variety of backgrounds and positions. The heterogeneous complexity of our own group reflects the state of research in the profession itself. Since no one group has assumed the charge for research development we found that members of the network all functioned in different jobs. Yet we shared research responsibilities. Unlike other consortia who most often are groups of nurses functioning in the same position,

---

"The group has negotiated for territory and resolved values conflicts to become a cohesive unit."

---

we were homogeneous only in that research functions were incorporated into respective job descriptions. Clinical, administrative, education, and nursing research specialists were all part of the group. Therefore we were able to offer education programs as well as conduct research projects, generate revenue, and provide the professional stimulation and creative expertise necessary for research role clarification. The roles and functions of the individual members and how they interfaced with the network are outlined in Exhibit 2.

Managerial strategy of networking

As the group assembled, each institution valued the concept that research is an integral part of professional practice. Members of the network each came with their own set of institutional values and goals. These ideas were discussed and translated into group goals attainable by utilizing the network. The goals were then broken into sets of tasks to be accomplished by the network or others recruited for that purpose. The common goals of three institutions were to be met through the combined efforts of the network. The network can be viewed as a managerial strategy, since management entails getting work done through the work of others.

For the first ten months the network functioned as a task force, with the nurse representative who first convened the group acting as the coordinator. As the group became an integrated unit and highly productive the members felt the need to become a network and formalize the organizational structure and functions. Thus in the first several meetings of the eleventh month, the group delineated organizational structure (Exhibit 3) so that the network became its own organizational entity: "a body of persons relating through some structured system for a specific purpose"[4]. United for the specific purpose of support for nursing research, the network functioned independently. The coordinator was elected chairperson and maintained the same role functions. She continued to coordinate and direct the individual group tasks and recorded the group's progress in minutes. The group also identified a list of network functions that interfaced smoothly with the functions of the institutional research committees. The three teaching institutions represented in the network each has a different nurse practice system, organizational structure, and research program. General discussions were held during the first several meetings to clarify how each institution would retain its managerial rights regarding decision making and finances.

The decision that each member of each institution would retain the authority and responsibility for decisions affecting their institutions only was an important one. This meant that the group could not decide policy affecting all three institutions. The interest and expertise in nursing research would be shared while individual institutional autonomy was maintained.

Finances were divided equally without benefit of a joint account. Sigma Theta Tau (Theta Chapter, Boston University) agreed to sponsor the first workshop. Mailing costs, duplicating costs, and other expenses incurred were shared. From educational programs offered a profit of $600.00 was realized and divided equally among the sponsoring body and the three hospitals. The logo of each institution was to appear on all fliers or posters so that each institution would have fair representation and equal publicity.

Each member of the network was able to share skills and knowledge without a direct commitment to the two other institutions. The commitment was to effect the goals of the network. The responsibility to influence an individual institution was the sole responsibility of the members of that institution. Without direct risk, sharing and problem solving was done in a nonthreatening atmosphere, with each member taking the information or idea needed.

The managerial functions of the group included problem solving, assembling resources, decision making, motivating, organizing, directing, supporting, and reappraising[3]. Within these functions there was agreement on issues of territory, individual professional autonomy, and maintenance of each institution's managerial rights. The professional concepts shared were as follows:

- Research is a component of professional practice and the basis of knowledge.
- Information and resources should be shared.
- Collegial relationships foster collaboration.

Professional aspect of networking

The varied membership of the network afforded it a wealth of information and creative thought. Each member offered the group expertise and support. Individuals' autonomy as nurses and professionals was emphasized. The responsibility of nurses to share and support colleagues regardless of institutional identity or professional title was supported.

The professional aspects of the network are highlighted by Batey, who states:

Research represents a collection of tools designed for the discovery of knowledge and evaluation of action. Professions require a continuing replenishment of knowledge in order

---

EXHIBIT 2.
COMPOSITION OF NURSING RESEARCH NETWORK

Position	Areas of Specialization	How Research Fits into Role; Research Responsibilities	How Network Is Utilized
Head nurse	Administration Nursing research	Head nurse of research unit Member, nursing research committee Member, IRB committee	Sponsors educational offerings for nursing department
Asst. director	Administration Staff development	Chairperson, nursing research committee Consultation for nursing staff research	Provides forum for sharing of institutional tools or techniques Sponsors educational offerings for nursing department
Director	Administration Nursing research Quality assurance	Designated nurse researcher Member, nursing research committee Member, IRB committee	Sponsors educational offerings for nursing department
Instructor	Staff development	Chairperson, nursing committee Consultation for nursing staff research	Assists with development of nursing research committee Sponsors educational offerings for nursing department
Nurse leader	Administration Nursing research	Member, nursing research committee Consultation for nursing staff research	Assists with development of nursing research committee Sponsors educational offerings for nursing department
Coordinator	Quality assurance	Member, nursing research committee	Sponsors educational offerings for nursing department

that their practice may be of maximum service to the actual and potential consumers of their services. For this to become a reality and not just an ideal, attention must be given to the conduct, dissemination, and utilization of research in the initial and continuing preparation of practitioners and the environment when nursing is practiced[5].

The network provided an environment of support and encouragement for this to happen. The educational programs held would encourage and direct professionals into research. The effective problem solving, and future research projects would provide the nursing community at large with better methods and information in the practice of nursing. Newer and more scientific approaches would affect patient care outcomes positively.

Research profile

The network evolved out of an administrative climate that favored research occurring at the level of clinical practice. This fostered the commitment within the network group to the conduct of its own research. Network members decided that every possible opportunity to survey participants attending the educational presentations would be utilized. The surveys were to obtain information on the level of research preparation and learning needs of nurses within our region and their past experiences and attitudes or values toward nursing research. An exposure to this kind of data would assist the network to maintain a contemporary approach to the development of continuing education pro-

grams and to sponsor programs that would continue to meet the rapidly changing needs of the participants as their involvement in research increased.

During the first eight-hour program a sixteen-item questionnaire was distributed to the 110 participants; a total of 100 questionnaires was returned. The demographics revealed an interesting variety of professional positions reflective of the many and varied levels of nurses involved in the conduct of nursing research. There were 49 nurses in clinical positions, of whom 35 were staff nurses, 12 were clinical specialists, and 2 were nurse practitioners. Among the 33 nurses representing administration were 13 head nurses, 8 assistant head nurses, 6 nurse coordinators or supervisors, 5 directors, and 1 assistant director. A total of 3 research nurses attended. Eleven participants were in academia or service education—8 instructors, 2 professors, and 1 unit teacher. The 4 nurse specialists were 2 quality assurance coordinators and 2 nurse consultants.

As for educational preparation, 78 percent of the audience had a BS or higher degree and 35 percent an MS or PhD. A correlation of level of educational preparation to number of research projects conducted revealed that as educational preparation increased so did the number of projects conducted. While all of the MS- and PhD-prepared participants reported having completed one or more research projects, 30 percent of the BS participants reported none, 50 percent of the AD participants reported none, and 62 percent of the diploma participants reported none. From the MS-prepared participants 38 percent

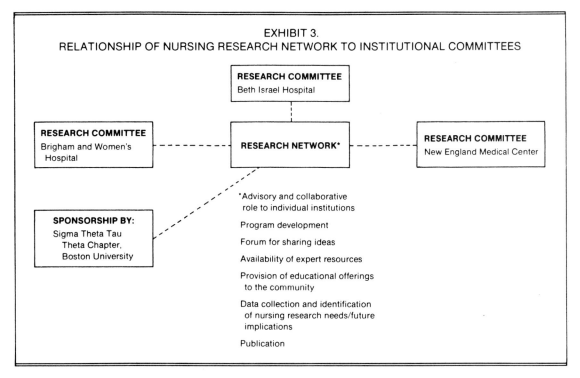

EXHIBIT 3.
RELATIONSHIP OF NURSING RESEARCH NETWORK TO INSTITUTIONAL COMMITTEES

RESEARCH COMMITTEE
Beth Israel Hospital

RESEARCH COMMITTEE
Brigham and Women's
Hospital

RESEARCH NETWORK*

RESEARCH COMMITTEE
New England Medical Center

SPONSORSHIP BY:
Sigma Theta Tau
Theta Chapter,
Boston University

*Advisory and collaborative
role to individual institutions

Program development

Forum for sharing ideas

Availability of expert resources

Provision of educational offerings
to the community

Data collection and identification
of nursing research needs/future
implications

Publication

reported completing four or more research projects and 100 percent of the PhD participants reported the same. A combined total of only 28 percent of the BS, AD, and diploma graduates stated they had completed four or more projects. To determine attitudes and values regarding the nursing research process the audience was asked to respond to some value statements. When asked whether research should be conducted only by nurses at the MS level, 91 percent disagreed. The audience was divided when trying to decide if participating in a physician's study was a form of nursing research (44 percent agreed, 37 percent disagreed and 19 percent were undecided). A total of 71 percent disagreed with the statement "Nursing research is beyond my everyday nursing activities."

Summary

Numerous articles continue to describe the methodology for implementing research in a variety of settings, yet not one approach has been accepted as ideal for encouraging and developing nurse researchers. The diversity of knowledge, motivation, and performance is reflective of the state of research in the nursing profession today and presents a special challenge for anyone trying to foster the development of a nursing research program in a hospital setting. The Nursing Research Network of Boston believes that one successful managerial strategy for research development is networking.

References

1. Carolyn A. Williams, et al. *Guidelines for the Investigative Functions of Nurses* (Kansas City: American Nurses' Association, 1982), p. 2.
2. Adrienne B. Code, "Consortium: A New Direction for Staff Development," *Journal of Continuing Education in Nursing* 7(2):18–22, 1976.
   Terri Koenig and Christy Dachelet, "Meeting the Challange of Inservice Education in Rural Minnesota Hospitals," *Journal of Continuing Education in Nursing* 11(5):20–24, 1980.
3. Barbara Stevens, *The Nurse as Executive* (2nd Edition) (Rockville, MD: Aspen Systems Publication, 1983), p. 29.
4. Barbara Stevens, 1983, p. 35.
5. Marjorie Batey, "Nursing Research: Conflict of Congruence with Nursing Service Goals," in *Conflict Management: Fight, Negotiate,* a National League for Nursing Publication from Forum for Nursing Service Administrators, Western Regional Assembly of Constituents for League of Nursing, Seattle, WA, October 1975, p. 12.

CHAPTER 35

Negotiating Cooperative Agreements Between Health Organizations

by Anita Werner O'Toole and Richard O'Toole

Comprehensive care and continuity of care are often dependent upon cooperation and coordination between organizations. Nursing administrators who understand the process through which cooperative agreements between health care organizations are negotiated can plan, direct, and monitor the process. This article covers four major aspects of the negotiations process and their implications for nursing administrators.

Nursing administrators and practitioners realize that the solutions to health care problems cannot be found in a single organization. Comprehensive care and continuity of care require cooperation among hospitals and agencies. However, we all know of many cases where care was not provided because of interorganizational problems of cooperation and coordination. All too often the system fails, not for lack of skilled and dedicated professionals, adequate technology or sufficient funding, but because of inadequate cooperation or coordination. Thus, nursing administrators must understand the negotiations process through which agreements can be reached in order to produce change in the health care system.

We find Strauss' analysis of negotiation useful in making sense out of the complicated, often incomprehensible, maze of interactions which occur when hospital and agency representatives attempt to coordinate programs[1]. We hope that nursing administrators will find this analysis not only useful in negotiating cooperative programs between their organization and other agencies in the health care system, but also in reaching agreements with other administrators in their own organization.

Strauss identified four essential aspects to consider when analyzing the negotiations process:

1. Who are the negotiators? The number of negotiators, their relative experience in negotiations, whom they represent, and their theories of negotiation.
2. The nature of their respective stakes in the negotiation.
3. The number and complexity of the issue negotiated.
4. The visibility of the transactions to others; that is, their overt and covert characters.

In this article we apply Strauss' framework to the problems faced by nursing administrators. We also draw upon our research observations and interviews, our personal experiences as negotiators, and relevant research literature[2,3,4].

First, we consider issues related to the selection of negotiators. Those who hope to initiate a cooperative or coordinated health care program often are able to form a team of negotiators and to select its members. What are the advantages of a team? Who should be selected? Why? Is is also possible to have some input concerning the negotiators who will represent the other agency(s)? Second, we discuss the stakes of those valuables which can be gained, lost, or shared by the participants and their respective organizations. In particular, we show how self-esteem becomes a stake in the negotiations. Third, we draw upon our research data to analyze a tendency for the number of issues and their complexity to increase during the course of the negotiations. What factors contribute to the escalation of issues? How can this escalation be anticipated and alleviated? Finally, we discuss the visibility of the negotiations. What are the advantages of covert over overt negotiations at different stages of the process?

Anita Werner O'Toole, R.N., Ph.D., is Professor of Nursing at Kent State University, Kent, Ohio.

Richard O'Toole, Ph.D, is Professor of Sociology at Kent State University, Kent, Ohio.

The authors express their appreciation to Susan L. Jones, R.N., Ph.D. and Ellen Rudy, R.N., Ph.D. for their critique of an earlier version of this article.

Selection of negotiators

While some relatively simple cooperative programs can be negotiated by two individuals, each representing one of the involved organizations, additional persons are often required because of their knowledge, resources, or organizational or community positions. This necessity results from the complexity of the health care system and the framework of issues that often must be negotiated to secure change. Our research shows that a team of negotiators is beneficial in planning and orchestrating the many activities which are necessary to secure cooperative agreements.

In planning for cooperation or coordination of agency effort toward health care goals, the administrator must analyze the situation so that the issues which will emerge can be anticipated. At the same time, the make-up of the team and the characteristics of individual team members also must be considered. What are the major problems that must be solved? What agreements will be necessary in order to plan and implement the new program? Who should be involved at each stage of the negotiation process? Who has the authority, knowledge, and ability to secure resources, the commitment to the new program, and the negotiation experience that will be required by the team? Of those who meet these criteria, which individuals will work well together as a team for what may be an extended period of time in often trying conditions?

Some strategies which suggest answers to these questions are provided in one of the cases we researched. In this situation, negotiations led to the formation of a rehabilitation complex comprised of eleven member agencies[5]. The successful outcome of the negotiations, according to our analysis, was due in part to: (1) the characteristics of the individuals who made up the negotiation team that initiated the coordination plan, (2) the members' commitment to the plan, (3) team members' positions in community power and resource networks, (4) their understanding of the negotiation process, and (5) the negotiations' initiators selecting as representatives people they personally knew in the other agencies for the early stages of the negotiations process.

The plan for the rehabilitation complex was initiated and the negotiations conducted by a team comprised of one agency's chief administrator and two influential members of its board of trustees. Each person has considerable negotiation experience and, equally important, each was dedicated to the success of the project and willing to spend considerable time in developing the rehabilitation complex. They worked well together as a team. Relationships were based upon respect, mutual trust, and a division of labor which took into consideration expertise, roles in the agency, personal contacts and connections with other individuals and organizations. They selected as co-negotiators their counterpart trustees and administrators in other agencies, often on the basis of previous relationships. In some cases co-negotiators were board members of two or more agencies

involved in the negotiations and, thus, were able to influence the process from various sides. Trustees who hold similar positions in other agencies are refered to as interorganizational leaders by Perrucci and Pilisuk[6]. As interorganizational leaders, trustees could use their positions in community power and resource networks to secure needed information, to influence decision making, and to provide resources to barter in the negotiations.

Initially, the team did not attempt to implement an extensive coordination effort, as is often the model in formal planning. Instead, based on their experience, the negotiators sought limited goals to serve as a foundation for higher level goals. Using what Strauss called *multiple and linked negotiations*, the negotiators first contacted agencies they believed would be easier to recruit and then, on the basis of these alliances, approached the more difficult organizations[7]. They did not attempt to develop a rigid plan for the rehabilitation complex or the procedures for attaining it. At critical junctures plans were revised, new and unforeseen developments capitalized upon, and new goals were developed to meet the needs and desires of other agency representatives.

The stakes

The innovative administrator with a plan for the coordination of health care is aware of the benefits that can be gained in terms of improved patient care, development of role potential for nurses, and cost savings. In order to sell the plan to various groups and prepare for negotiating necessary agreements, the administrator will analyze the benefits (stakes) for these groups, and study the costs of interorganizational coordination efforts as they are perceived by the individuals, professions, organizations, and community interest groups that may become involved. Who will represent whom and what are the potential stakes in the negotiations deserves a good deal of administrator attention.

Fear of loss of autonomy is a major stake for individuals, professions and organizations. Lack of full autonomy in decision making with regard to goals, service programs, and clients may be seen as a loss. Yet, some compromise often is required in one or more of these decision-making areas. The team which negotiated the formation of the rehabilitation complex used what we called a "cost-reward-involvement formula" as a strategy in dealing with this problem. On the basis of their knowledge of the other agencies, the team offered rewards for coordination, specified financial costs of participation and stipulated contingencies for membership. According to the formula, the greater the agency's involvement in the coordination plan, the greater its costs. Therefore, the agency had to be offered greater rewards for participation. The group pointed to such rewards as savings through shared use of facilities, equipment, and services for staff and clients. In particular, goals which an organization could not achieve alone were offered as rewards for cooperation[8]. The negotiations were restricted to fiscal issues and, thus, each agency's financial costs were clearly outlined. Also, they developed a "peer type" coordinating organization in which each agency was a voting member and therefore, reduced fears for autonomy[9].

Organizations are not, however, the only units to which the cost-reward involvement formula applies. Individuals also experience personal gains and losses both during the negotiations and as a result of coordination between organization. Thus, analysis of the stakes that are involved must include such factors as impact on individual prestige, satisfaction of personality needs, and individual career interests.

Early phases of the process often involve negotiating identities and roles for participants, although such issues are not confined only to beginning stages. We have observed several cases of failure of severe difficulty in reaching or maintaining coordination agreements due to lack of resolution of what we came to call "the identity problem". If not resolved, these problems become magnified. This is because other issues and stakes acquire values, in part, according to identities and role relationships among participants. For example, an administrator who believes that he or she is the senior and most qualified person present will expect to be so identified and to have his or her ideas reacted to accordingly. A problem develops when the administrator's counterpart across the table may feel the same way. It may be difficult to recognize this attitude in oneself or to tell one's peer or superior that he or she has this problem, but it may be necessary for successful negotiations. Male negotiators may expect deference from their female counterparts. Directors of programs, or representatives of professions or organizations that have been competitive in the past may see coordination proposals as a test of their ability to gain the upper hand and to capture rewards for their organization and themselves. Issues then take on personal self-esteem stakes. Due, perhaps, to basic personality differences or needs, we have observed negotiators continually clash over what appear to be relatively minor issues. Identity issues then become the "hidden agenda" for meetings. In a situation involving interdisciplinary research negotiations, we saw minor issues become highly controversial because of the personal conflict that developed between a psychologist and a physician. Other participants were expected to be either "on *my* side or *his* side" of every issue.

Career interests of negotiators and the persons they represent have to be taken into account. Coordination can be the capstone of a career or bring on fear of career destruction. For example, in merger situations staff of each organization may worry about role and and career autonomy. We also have found that some individuals interpret interorganizational negotiations as an extra and unnecessary burden added to their current administrative tasks and, therefore, resist participation. Having seen attempts to coordinate services come and go, they may passively attend meetings and wait for this plan to fade away. Administra-

tors must, therefore, provide themselves and subordinates with sufficient time to deal with the negotiations process. Also, effort invested in negotiations to coordinate programs must be rewarded.

One way to analyze personal and interpersonal influences on negotiations is to ask "*Who* is negotiating which *issues*, with *whom*, on *whose* behalf, at which *time*, with what *success*? What kind of identity problems are hindering the negotiations? How can they be resolved?" Such issues should be taken into account in selecting a negotiation team. The administrator often can select co-negotiators at least in the initial stages of the process. Awareness of the "identity problem" when selecting the negotiation team and approaching co-negotiators who will represent the other agency helps restrict the number of issues. Another way to limit personal and interpersonal influences is to limit the number of negotiators.

Trust, an important interpersonal ingredient in negotiations, often is based on previous relationships among negotiators or on developing informal relationships. Interpersonal factors are so important in interorganizational relations that we have seen negotiations put on hold until a person left one of the organizations. This seems a rather high price to pay for health care goals that could be attained through cooperative effort. If identity problems can be handled, the negotiations have a better chance of success.

As we discuss later, it may be necessary for covert meetings to be held between individuals to help solve the identity problem. Not as many personal stakes are involved in covert when compared to overt meetings because the audience is limited and often there is no formal record of the interactions.

The issues

The number of issues and their complexity is one of the major sources of concern in the administrator's analysis of proposed interorganizational agreements. We have observed a tendency for both the number of issues and their complexity to escalate in the negotiations process. In several cases costs have been added to the negotiations from additional issues which were not related, or only peripherally related, to the actual problems currently being discussed. Our research shows that strategies can be used to restrict both the number and complexity of issues. First, the scope of the problems that will be negotiated must be discussed. Second, the problems to be encountered when different levels and offices in each of the participating organizations become involved in the negotiations must be considered.

The scope of problems discussed may escalate for a variety of reasons, but it is particularly noticeable when negotiations involve different professions, different specialties within the same profession, different schools of thought, or when the participants are representatives of organizations with different goals such as nursng educators and nursing service administrators. Also, each profession has a number of unresolved issues and continuing disputes over philosophy, theory, practice, rights, or territory. Negotiators often believe that these should be untangled and resolved as a part of, or a necessary precursor to, an agreement. Such discussions may increase participation costs, in addition to confirming the participants worst fears concerning one another. Each person's time costs are increased without the rewards of progress. Real issues of coordination appear lost in a quagmire of unresolved problems. Thus, the interorganizational situation may appear hopeless. In the negotiations to establish the rehabilitation complex, the negotiation team avoided an escalation of problems by limiting discussion to financial and physical plant concerns while they recruited other agencies to join the complex. The financial and physical plant issues were more easily identified and, therefore, more easily negotiated. Initially, no attempt was made to coordinate programs or share staff. That would come later.

In another situation we observed negotiations for cooperative educational programs and interdisciplinary research. Based on that experience we think negotiators should not stick their heads in the sand regarding tough issues. However, they need to decide which problems require resolution and when to agree to disagree on an issue. Then they can proceed to negotiate the specific program agreements. At times it is difficult to decide which issues require debate and resolution and which do not. Some unresolved issues provide an undercurrent of frustration and conflict which may block the program from reaching its goals. Some problems are easier to resolve once the rewards of successful cooperation have been achieved. Participants would not feel that continued negotiations denote failure. Often, more negotiations are necessary to meet new contingencies and to renegotiate past agreements. And, as Strauss points out, we must expect negotiations to lead to further negotiations[10].

Further complexity develops as the negotiators begin to identify all the different offices in each of the organizations which may be involved in the negotiations process. To accomplish an interorganizational agreement, different levels and offices within an organization must negotiate agreements with their counterparts in one or more of the other organizations. In anticipation of these meetings, or as they begin a number of new issues may be perceived as relevant by individuals, professions, and administrators from each organization.

It is imperative that professionals who will actually implement the new program, as well as their immediate supervisors, should be involved early in the negotiations so that their ideas and needs will be reflected in the plan. We observed one case in which top level administrators negotiated a cooperative referral program without involving their respective staffs. The program never functioned well and, after a few months, it ceased to exist.

Negotiations between two universities concerning cooperative graduate programs illustrates the need to contract at different levels of each organization. The following offices and administrative units became involved: directors of graduate programs, deans of nursing, faculty groups, graduate deans, vice presidents for academic affairs and for financial affairs, directors of admissions, registrars, presidents, and boards of trustees. A number of persons and organizations outside the universities further affected the negotiations process: accrediting agencies, professional organizations, funding agencies, and agencies providing placements for clinical practice, agencies employing program graduates and, of course, potential students.

As issues go up and down the administrative line, organizational problems are raised which change the issue and the stakes. In some departments, administrators will use the new program to bring up past problems or to piggyback their own proposals for change. An administrator initiating an interorganizational program may feel that he or she has opened Pandora's box, and may wonder if it is all really worth it. However, if the process of negotiating interorganizational coordination is to be successful and health care goals realized, the process must be planned, orchestrated, and monitored.

Organizational charts would have us believe that interactions involving interorganizational relations would take place in a rational style. We have yet to observe, however, a case where a coordination plan was developed, agreed upon, and then implemented according to bureaucratic procedures. To achieve coordination, negotiations must be managed carefully. The administrator preparing for complex negotiations must be able to budget the time such complex series of negotiations require. Some responsibilities may need to be assigned to subordinates or to others on the negotiation team. Selection of the negotiation team members should certainly take into account the potential problems within the administrative hierarchy of the organization. Additionally, interactions and negotiations between individuals within one organization or between representatives of other agencies may work best when they are informal or covert. Others, will have to be overt.

Visibility—overt and covert negotiations

While some individuals may have a positive or a negative interpretation of the words overt and covert, we use these terms to refer only to the amount of visibility given to the negotiation process. Many negotiations involved in constructing a coordinated program will be covert in nature, although they may not be kept invisible by design. Much of the covert aspects of negotiations may be informal. For example, when two administrators meet at a nursing conference they may discuss informally the possibility of a cooperative program between their organizations. They may map out some of the major ingredients of the joint program, and later meet to discuss problems once the negotiations are underway. Their previous friendship allows for trust and an easy give and take of ideas, suggested compromises, and strategy discussions. By restricting negotiators, they restrict issues.

In the negotiations to form the rehabilitation complex, informal covert meetings were conducted with selected representatives of other organizations. Through a network of informal relationships the team secured limited agreements with representatives of other organizations. On the basis of those agreements, the team informally approached members of agencies where the negotiations would be more difficult. Team members also served as mediators between agencies that did not want to confront one another directly or did not want to make their disagreements known in a public forum. In open meetings agreements were announced, without revealing the disagreement and bargaining which had taken place. Significant agreements were reached in covert negotiations. Overt negotiations conducted in formal meetings served mostly expressive and public relations functions. A "peer type" coordinating organization was established as the structure for overt negotiations. However, most issues already had been argreed upon in covert informal meetings. Mott points out that while "peer type" coordinating organizations reduce member agencies' fears for autonomy, they lack hierarchial means to accomplish goals[9]. In this case power maneuvers were employed in covert negotiations, thus, permitting continuation of peer relationships in the formal meetings.

In each case we observed, informal covert negotiations were equivalent to the functions performed by informal groups in formal organizations. Administrators are well aware of the vital role that informal groups and relationships play in the functioning of an organization. This knowledge must also be used as individual representatives of organizations interact to negotiate interorganizational agreements.

Implications for nursing administrators

Nursing administrators need to become part of networks which provide power, influence, information, funds, and social contacts. These resources are vital in the negotiations process to secure interorganizational agreements. Network linkage to all sectors of the community is important: business, politics, religion, education, voluntary groups, as well as, health care associations. Special attention should be given to developing contacts with planning boards, funding sources, and various governmental bodies. It is no accident that special interest groups, professions, and corporations attempt to place their members in key power positions where they can act as gatekeepers or innovators of change. Nursing administrators need to become community interorganizational leaders, and thus acquire the resources useful in the negotiations process. Traditionally, women have

been excluded from such networks, but those who hope to use their resources must somehow gain access to them. This access will require group effort, working through local, state and national nursing organizations.

Summary

Our analysis demonstrates the significance of careful planning, orchestration, and monitoring of the negotiations to attain cooperation and coordination between organizations. Similarly, our research shows that flexibility and compromise are key elements in the negotiations process. In particular, the following strategies deserve consideration.

1. *Use a carefully selected negotiations team.* The team should be small enough to act quickly as a unit, but large enough to include members with the necessary knowledge, resources, authority, and contacts to do the job. Members should also be selected on the basis of their ability to work well both with team members from their own organization and those representing other parties in the transactions.

2. *Analyze the stakes.* A cost-reward-involvement formula can be applied to maximize rewards while minimizing costs to all concerned.

3. *Restrict the number of issues and their complexity.* It is possible to "agree to disagree" on some issues and still cooperate in a joint venture. It may also be necessary to demonstrate the effectiveness of cooperation in achieving limited goals before more complex joint efforts can be proposed. Also, plan for a series of *multiple and linked negotiations* between offices and their counterparts in the other organizations. While we advise following usual channels of communication, we caution administrators to expect and plan for exceptions to official administrative protocol.

4. *Consider using covert as well as overt negotiations.* An administrator should understand how the visibility of the negotiations affects the outcome of the process. Informal covert meetings are often the first step in the process of determining the plausibility of joint effort.

Finally, we believe that negotiations should be viewed as a process not a procedure. There is probably no regular series of steps which can ensure success. However, understanding the negotiations process places the nursing administrator in a better position to negotiate cooperative programs to improve the health care.

References

1. Anselm Strauss, *Negotiations: Varieties, Contexts, Processes and Social Order* (San Fransisco: Josey-Bass Publishers, 1978) p. 238.
2. Richard O'Toole and Anita W. O'Toole, "Negotiating Interorganizational Relations," *Sociological Quarterly* 22(1):29–41, 1981.
3. Richard O'Toole and Anita W. O'Toole, "The Myth of Comprehensive Care," *U.S.A. Today* 108(2410):55–57, 1979.
4. Richard O'Toole et al., *The Cleveland Rehabilitation Complex: A Study of Interagency Coordination* (Cleveland: Vocational Guidance and Rehabilitation Services, 1972).

5. O'Toole et al., 1972.
6. Robert Perrucci and Marc Pilisuk, "Leaders and Ruling Elites: The Interorganizational Bases of Community Power," *American Sociological Review* 35(6):1040–1057, 1970.
7. Strauss, 1978.
8. Sherif et al., *Intergroup Conflict and Cooperation: The Robbers Cave Experiment* (Norman, Oklahoma: University of Oklahoma, Institute of Group Relations, 1964) p. 191.
9. Basil Mott, Coordination and Inter-organizational Relations in Health. In Paul White and George Vlasak (Eds.), *Inter-Organizational Research in Health* (Washington D.C.: National Center for Health Services Research and Development, 1970) pp. 55–69.
10. Strauss, 1978, p. 124.

INDEX